A Clinician's Guide to Sleep Disorders

A Clinician's Guide to Sleep Disorders

Editor: Destiny Lockhart

AMERICAN
MEDICAL PUBLISHERS
www.americanmedicalpublishers.com

AMERICAN
MEDICAL PUBLISHERS
www.americanmedicalpublishers.com

Cataloging-in-Publication Data

A clinician's guide to sleep disorders / edited by Destiny Lockhart.
p. cm.
Includes bibliographical references and index.
ISBN 978-1-63927-087-3
1. Sleep disorders. 2. Nervous system--Diseases. 3. Sleep disorders--Guidebooks.
I. Lockhart, Destiny.
RC547 .C55 2022
616.849 8--dc23

American Medical Publishers,
41 Flatbush Avenue,
1st Floor, New York,
NY 11217, USA

ISBN 978-1-63927-087-3 (Hardback)

Contents

Preface

Sleep disorders influence or disturb the sleep pattern of a person. They are broadly categorized into 3 groups, namely, dyssomnia, circadian rhythm sleep disorders and parasomnias. The most common type of sleep disorder is insomnia, which falls under the category of dyssomnia. A person suffering from this disorder has difficulty in falling asleep or getting adequate amount of sleep. A sleep disorder that causes a frequent need to get up and urinate at night is referred to as nocturia. There are various other sleep disorders such as periodic limb movement disorder, night terror and narcolepsy. They can be caused due to various reasons such as traumatic childhood experiences, heredity and traumatic brain injury. Various treatments and therapies are provided to the person suffering from sleep disorders including music therapy, allergy treatment and melatonin. Music therapy is used to improve sleep quality in both acute and chronic sleep disorders. This book contains some path-breaking studies in the field of sleep disorders. It presents researches and studies performed by experts across the globe. The book will provide comprehensive knowledge to the readers.

This book is a comprehensive compilation of works of different researchers from varied parts of the world. It includes valuable experiences of the researchers with the sole objective of providing the readers (learners) with a proper knowledge of the concerned field. This book will be beneficial in evoking inspiration and enhancing the knowledge of the interested readers.

In the end, I would like to extend my heartiest thanks to the authors who worked with great determination on their chapters. I also appreciate the publisher's support in the course of the book. I would also like to deeply acknowledge my family who stood by me as a source of inspiration during the project.

Editor

Accelerated Diagnosis and Treatment of Sleep Apnea in Hospitalized Patients: Practice Improvement Method for Ensuring Follow up

Rose A Franco* **and Dheeraj Dhotre**

Department of Medicine – Division of Pulmonary, Medical College of Wisconsin, Milwaukee, Wisconsin, USA

***Corresponding author:** Rose A Franco, 9200 W. Wisconsin Avenue, Suite E5200, Milwaukee, Wisconsin, 53226, USA, E-mail: rfranco@mcw.edu

Abstract

Background: Sleep Apnea Syndrome is common and underdiagnosed in the hospitalized patient population. Protocols for evaluation of sleep apnea in the inpatient setting are not standardized.

Study question: Does requiring a sleep and breathing consultation when requesting a type 3 portable monitor to evaluate for sleep apnea syndrome in the inpatient setting lead to better follow up and continuous positive airway pressure device (CPAP) use than open access to this testing.

Methods: Retrospective chart review of patients who underwent a type 3 portable sleep study between 2008 to 2010 from a tertiary care, academic medical center. Midway through the period of review the process of ordering was changed to include mandatory pulmonary consultation. 105 patient records were analyzed for outcomes including diagnosis and ongoing care for sleep disordered breathing.

Results: The number of studies adequate for interpretation was not impacted by addition of a mandatory consult (87% vs. 92%), nor was the number of positive studies with an AHI >5 (80% vs. 73%). Follow up after undergoing a diagnostic type 3 study was significantly higher in the post intervention group (51% vs. 76%, P=0.04). Medical follow up as outpatient and CPAP initiation for those with a positive study was also significantly higher with the consultation requirement (55% vs. 84%, P=0.024).

Conclusion: In the hospitalized setting, a type 3 portable monitor for evaluation of sleep apnea when paired with a consultation from a sleep/pulmonary specialist can significant improve the likelihood outpatient follow up and improved likelihood of ongoing adherence for those who are initiated on CPAP. Large controlled multicenter studies are needed to determine if a protocol for identifying at risk hospitalized patients coupling type 3 testing with an experienced consultant in the evaluation of sleep disordered breathing translates to improved value based care.

Keywords: Type 3 portal monitor; Continuous positive airway pressure; CPAP adherence; Sleep apnea

Introduction

Undiagnosed sleep apnea is common in hospitalized patients. The National Hospital Discharge Survey from 2004 registered that only 5.8% of inpatients diagnosed with sleep apnea were provided with CPAP therapy during hospitalization [1].

As far back as 1998, sleep researchers detected an increase in healthcare utilization in cardiac patients who had untreated OSA [2]. Sleep disordered breathing in general remains a significant co-morbidity that factors into readmissions. In a recent observation cohort study Central Sleep Apnea (CSA) was an independent risk factor for 6 months' cardiac readmissions and the effect size exceeded that of all known predictors of heart failure readmissions. In this same study, severe OSA was also an independent predictor of readmissions with an adjusted rate ratio of 1.49 (P=0.04) [3].

Two 2008 population-based studies, one from the United States, [4] and one from Australia, [5] also showed increased all-cause mortality in subjects with moderate-to severe OSA. The adjusted hazard ratios in both studies ranged from 3.0-6.2 for subjects with moderate-to-severe disease compared with no disease.

Cost to Benefit analyses support that the treatment of sleep apnea reduces the total cost of care through better control of comorbidities resulting in decreased health care utilization including readmissions and improvement in co-morbid conditions such as obstructive lung disease and congestive heart failure [6].

Current guidelines recommend overnight polysomnography in a monitored setting (type 1 PSG) for the diagnosis of OSA [4,7-9]. Home-based diagnosis and therapy for OSA with limited monitoring channels designed to detect sleep apnea primarily has provide an alternative to the type 1 PSG and improves access for patient care. In carefully selected patients (generally those with a high pretest probability of disease and without comorbidities), a home-based approach using the type 3 portable monitor (minimum requirement:one oximetry channel, one airflow channel, one effort belt channel) had similar clinical outcomes to those patients studied in the laboratory [10,11].

According to current American academy of Sleep Medicine (AASM) clinical guidelines, type 3 portable monitoring (PM) is not appropriate for OSA diagnosis when dealing with inpatients who have significant comorbid conditions that may degrade the accuracy of PM, including but not limited to, moderate to severe pulmonary disease, neuromuscular disease, or CHF. However, they go on to state the PM may be indicated for OSA diagnosis if a Type 1 PSG cannot be done due to immobility, age, or critical illness [12].

Many patients cared for in the inpatient setting have co-morbid sleep apnea. A significant proportion is undiagnosed at the time of the hospital stay. For those with a substantial co-morbid condition such as heart failure or obstructive lung disease where the co-existing untreated sleep apnea increases the likelihood of morbidity and mortality, rapid diagnosis and initiation of therapy is appealing. Factors such as decompensated heart failure, narcotics, sepsis and delirium states that result in poor sleep/little sleep need to be weighed again the risks of discharging a patient with underlying sleep disordered breathing that ultimately contributes to costs of care and may result in readmission for the same or related condition before an outpatient evaluation of the sleep disordered breathing can be completed. Inpatient evaluation of sleep disordered breathing at this time is limited to non-validated methods as the type 1 PSG is in general not widely accessible for inpatient testing. While the type 3 PM can be an effective diagnostic tool patient factors that can result in over diagnosis and under diagnosis of sleep disordered breathing need to also be considered in the inpatient setting. The appropriateness of testing and the timing of the testing require knowledge of these factors and experienced clinicians are a necessary component of any inpatient screening program.

Inpatient diagnosis of obstructive sleep apnea (OSA) may improve our ability to expedite the initiation of continuous positive airway pressure (CPAP) treatment for the more frail patients with sleep disordered breathing when a laboratory based PSG is not practical.

Prior to June 30, 2009 our academic practice offered inpatient testing using the type 3 portable monitor to evaluate for sleep apnea at the treating physician's request. Physicians were given general guidelines that the patient should be as close to discharge as possible to allow for any acute medical issues to have the least impact on the test results and that the patient could not be on more than 4 liters of oxygen as that had led to less reliable airflow signal. Results were reported to the requesting physician and documented in the patient chart. Coordinating any follow up and initiation of PAP therapy was the responsibility of the discharging physician. In reviewing standards for care across the practice, it was noted by primary care physicians that many of these patients who had undergone inpatient testing were not aware of the test results nor were they given specific instructions regarding the results or need for follow up. This raised concerns that the open access model did not provide patients with adequate communication on results or guarantee outpatient treatment or follow up. As a result we added a mandatory pulmonary consult to the the request for the inpatient type 3 portable monitor testing in hopes that it would improve patient follow up upon discharge. In this quality improvement process, we evaluated retrospectively whether the outcomes for outpatient follow up and adherence improved when testing was directed by experienced clinicians.

Methods

This was a practice quality improvement project. Retrospective chart review was done for those patients undergoing type 3 portable sleep studies from 2008 to 2010 in our tertiary care, academic medical center. Beginning July 1, 2009 a mandatory pulmonary consultation was added to the requirements for sleep testing for hospitalized patients. The patient outcomes were evaluated comparing those before and after this added requirement.

Inclusion criteria as follows: 1) age ≥ 18 years, 2) inpatient generated request for portable monitoring for evaluation of sleep apnea, 3) Type 3 PM testing completed during the time period of July 2008 to December 2010. The outcomes assessed were the proportion of ordered studies usable for analysis of sleep apnea, (AHI>5), proportion of patients tested that had follow up after discharge, and proportion that had ongoing PAP therapy after discharge.

A Type 3 PM device (Somnostar Orbit) with 4 channels including nasal flow, chest and abdominal movement belts and oximetry channels was used for all the patients [13]. A minimum of 4 hour of recording was required for a usable test. The studies were scored a trained respiratory therapist and reviewed and edited by a board certified sleep specialist. The scoring following the American Academy of Sleep Medicine 2007 scoring requirements. Criteria for failed testing were less than 4 hours recording time or lost signal channels preventing interpretation. Failed testing did not eliminate the subject from analysis for endpoints. Subgroup analysis for obstructive versus central apnea was not done due to the nature of the type 3 monitor's design and intended purpose specific to screening for obstructive sleep apnea only. The criteria for initiating PAP therapy was at the discretion of the physician who ordered the type 3 portable monitor test and included consideration for co-morbid cardiovascular disease, hypersomnia or sleep dysfunction in the context of an AHI of at least 5 or more events per hour.

At the time of the quality assessment, patients were interviewed when possible via telephone at the time of the chart review to report on their status of medical follow up after discharge regarding the suspected sleep apnea. They were also asked if they were currently using PAP therapy. Medical follow up for the sleep apnea was defined as the presence of an adherence download in the medical record, a Type 1 PSG completed as an outpatient after the inpatient evaluation, or an outpatient follow up visit for which the sleep apnea as a problem addressed during the visit. The outpatient chart audit for follow up documentation included specialists (either sleep or pulmonary) and the primary care physician. Data was analyzed using STATA software for Windows OS. Analysis was carried out using Fishers Exact test. The P-value of <0.05 were considered as statistically significant.

Results

A total 105 patients underwent testing during the period of chart review. Fifty six patients underwent inpatient PM testing prior to the requirement of pulmonary consultation and 49 underwent evaluation after the intervention (Table 1).

	Follow up with positive(POS) study	PAP Follow up with usable study (POS+NEG)	Follow overall All tested
PRE intervention	17/ 31	18/35	21/56
POST intervention	21/25	25/33	28/49
Fishers exact test	P=0.02	P=0.04	P=0.05

Table 1: Quality Initiative Outcomes. Follow up on results and PAP therapy initiation was significantly higher across all groups after the addition of the mandatory consultation (intervention) associated with

ordering an inpatient type 3 PM to assess for sleep disordered breathing. A positive study (POS) was defined as at least 4 hours of study with an AHI >5. Those with AHI <5 were considered negative (NEG). Some tests were failure (unusable due to lead failure). Follow up was significantly improved in all categories after addition of the pulmonary consultation.

The number of usable studies was similiar comparing groups(pre intervention 87% vs. post intervention 92% usable, P=ns), as was the number of positive studies with an AHI >5 (pre intervention 80% vs. post intervention 73%, P=ns). The average recording time was 9.1 hours for those undergoing testing prior to the intervention of a mandatory consultation intervention and 7.75 hours for those after the intervention.

Documented outpatient medical follow up for the sleep apnea was significantly higher in the post intervention group (Pre intervention 51% vs. post intervention 75%, P=0.04). For those with a positive study, PAP initiation and ongoing use was significantly higher with the consultation requirement (pre intervention 55% vs. post intervention 84%, P=0.02).

Phone contact was not possible in 26 of the 56 (46%) pre-intervention patients with 13 of them having died prior to the start of the study. Phone contact was not possible in 20 of the 49 (40%) post intervention (P=ns) with 3 dead prior to the study. For those with whom we were able to discuss their current status, their reports of use of cpap were added to the medical follow up statistics when they were not being followed at our institution (Figure 1).

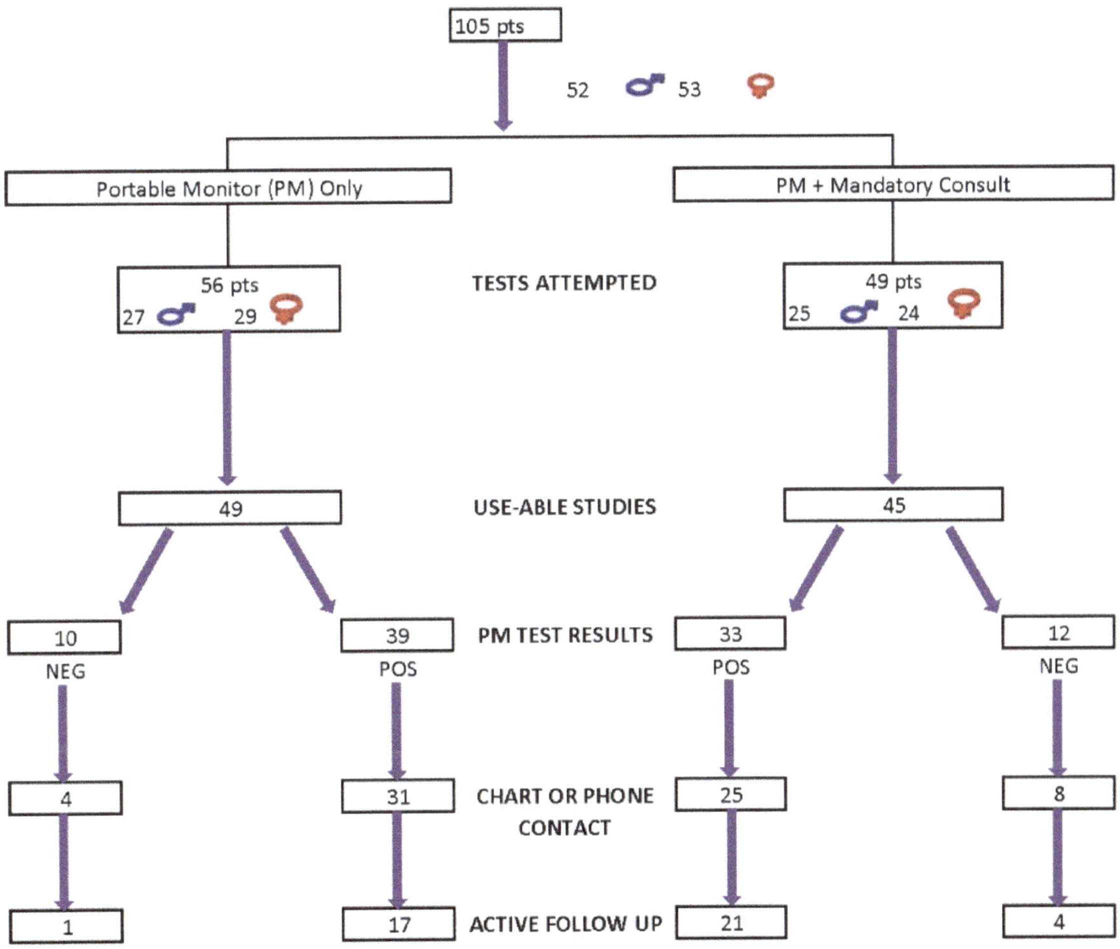

Figure 1: Study Design. PM=Portable Monitor Level 3. A total of 105 charts were surveyed. 56 patients underwent testing as requested by the hospital physician. After institution of a mandatory consult 49 patients underwent testing. Several studies were not usable in both arms (not significantly different between groups). Those with positive tests (39 pre intervention and 33 post intervention) and well as negative tests (10 vs. 12) who were contacted and /or the charts reviewed confirming communication of results.

Discussion

As a practice improvement project, the addition of a mandatory pulmonary consultation linked to the Type 3 PM testing did lead to significant improvement in outpatient follow up and ongoing PAP therapy for all those seen in consultation based on the documentation in the patients' medical records. The reason why adding the consultative requirement to the inpatient testing request improved the outpatient follow up and PAP adherence may in part be the result of ownership in communication and active management on the part of the consultants during and beyond the inpatient setting. Engaging in discussion with the patient throughout the process on the impact of sleep apnea on health reinforced through repeat bedside visits and outpatient office follow up visits may have decreased drop outs.

As a retrospective review, there were several weaknesses inherit in our study. The cohorts were fixed based on the time they underwent testing. The cohort without a mandated consultation was tested at an earlier time period. A prospective controlled study was not possible and same time comparison analysis could not be done due to insufficient numbers tested during the time prior the implementation of manadatory consultation for all requested inpatient studies. Public awareness of sleep apnea and treatment has steadily increased over time, so there is possibility of improved adherence in the group with the mandated consultation as a result of having been tested in an environment of better awareness of the value of treatment that the pre-intervention cohort.

Conclusion

Untreated sleep apnea is a common condition in hospitalized patients. Untreated sleep disordered breathing is considered a risk factor for readmission when coupled with co-morbid diseases. As more and more focus is brought on improving quality of care through reducing readmission rates, addressing sleep disordered breathing for hospitalized patients will become a necessary component of the inpatient practice of medicine. We have demonstrated that the Type 3 portable monitor coupled with involvement at the outset by the pulmonologist can result in improved likelihood for ongoing treatment for some patients. Consistent application of diagnostic and treatment protocols for the hospitalized patients will be necessary to realize the full savings in healthcare utilization costs associated with addressing sleep disordered breathing in the hospital setting.

A larger prospective controlled study of accelerated diagnostic and treatment clinical pathways for the hospitalized patient will be needed to explore the potential of subsequent health care savings associated with treatment of sleep disordered breathing.

References

1. Spurr KF, Graven MA, Gilbert RW (2008) Prevalence of unspecified sleep apnea and the use of continuous positive airway pressure in hospitalized patients, 2004 National Hospital Discharge Survey. Sleep Breath 12: 229-234.
2. Peker Y, Hedner J, Norum J, Kraiczi H, Carlson J (2002) Increased incidence of cardiovascular disease in middle-aged men with obstructive sleep apnea: a 7-year follow-up. Am J Respir Crit Care Med 166: 159-165.
3. Khayat R, Abraham W, Patt B, Brinkman V, Wannemacher J, et al. (2012) Central sleep apnea is a predictor of cardiac readmission in hospitalized patients with systolic heart failure. J Card Fail 18: 534-540.
4. Young T, Finn L, Peppard PE, Szklo-Coxe M, Austin D, et al. (2008) Sleep disordered breathing and mortality: eighteen-year follow-up of the Wisconsin sleep cohort. Sleep 31: 1071-1078.
5. Rich J, Raviv A, Raviv N, Brietzke SE (2012) All-cause mortality and obstructive sleep apnea severity revisited. Otolaryngol Head Neck Surg 147: 583-587.
6. Peker Y, Hedner J, Johansson A, Bende M (1997) Reduced hospitalization with cardiovascular and pulmonary disease in obstructive sleep apnea patients on nasal CPAP treatment. Sleep 20: 645-653.
7. Hiestand DM, Britz P, Goldman M, Phillips B (2006) Prevalence of symptoms and risk of sleep apnea in the US population: Results from the national sleep foundation sleep in America 2005 poll. Chest 130: 780-786.
8. Flemons WW (2004) Measuring quality of life in patients with sleep apnoea: whose life is it anyway? Thorax 59: 457-458.
9. Fleetham J, Ayas N, Bradley D, Ferguson K, Fitzpatrick M, et al. (2006) Canadian Thoracic Society guidelines: diagnosis and treatment of sleep disordered breathing in adults. Can Respir J 13: 387-392.
10. Berry RB, Hill G, Thompson L, McLaurin V (2008) Portable monitoring and autotitration versus polysomnography for the diagnosis and treatment of sleep apnea. Sleep 31: 1423-1431.
11. Kuna ST, Gurubhagavatula I, Maislin G, Hin S, Hartwig KC, et al. (2011) Noninferiority of functional outcome in ambulatory management of obstructive sleep apnea. Am J Respir Crit Care Med 183: 1238-1244.
12. Mulgrew AT, Fox N, Ayas NT, Ryan CF (2007) Diagnosis and initial management of obstructive sleep apnea without polysomnography: a randomized validation study. Ann Intern Med 146: 157-166.
13. Littner MR (2005) Portable monitoring in the diagnosis of the obstructive sleep apnea syndrome. Semin Respir Crit Care Med 26: 56-67.

2

A Retrospective Examination of Sleep Disturbance across the Course of Bipolar Disorder

Jennifer C Kanady[1], **Adriane M Soehnera**[2] **and Allison G Harvey**[1*]

[1]*Department of Psychology, University of California, Berkeley, Berkeley, CA, USA*

[2]*Department of Psychiatry, University of Pittsburgh, School of Medicine, Pittsburgh, PA, USA*

[*]**Corresponding author:** Allison G. Harvey, Ph.D., 3210 Tolman Hall #1650, Berkeley, CA, 94720-1650, USA, E-mail: aharvey@berkeley.edu

Abstract

Background: Sleep disturbance is a prevalent and clinically significant feature of bipolar disorder. However, there are aspects of sleep and bipolar disorder that have been minimally characterized. This study aims to fill several gaps in the literature by examining the prevalence, coexistence, and persistence of sleep disturbance retrospectively across a five-year period in bipolar disorder.

Methods: Fifty-one people with bipolar disorder I and comorbid insomnia who were currently inter-episode completed the NIMH Retrospective Life-Charting Methodology (the life chart). The life chart was used to document the prevalence, coexistence, and persistence of insomnia, hypersomnia, delayed sleep phase, reduced sleep need, and irregular sleep patterns across the course of five years.

Results: Across the five year period, manic months were primarily characterized by reduced sleep need (62.8%) and insomnia (38.1%), depressive months by hypersomnia (56.0%) and insomnia (51.9%), mixed months by all five types of sleep disturbance, and inter-episode months by insomnia (67.4%). There was coexistence in the types of sleep disturbance experienced. Further, each type of sleep disturbance demonstrated persistence across the five years, with persistence rates being the highest for insomnia (49.0–58.8%).

Conclusions: Sleep disturbance is a prevalent and complex feature across mood episodes and inter-episode periods of bipolar disorder. Further, there is variation in the types of sleep disturbance experienced.

Keywords Bipolar disorder; Sleep disturbance; Prevalence; Coexistence; Persistence

Introduction

Bipolar disorder is a severe disorder characterized by mood episodes; namely, periods of elevated or irritable mood, referred to as mania, periods of depression, and mixed manic and depressed states [1]. Bipolar disorder is further characterized by periods identified as neither depressive nor manic, a phase referred to as the inter-episode period [2-4]. Although there have been important advances in psychological and pharmacological treatments for bipolar disorder, it remains a severe and chronic psychiatric illness with a lifetime prevalence of approximately 1.0% [5] and is one of the 10 most disabling conditions worldwide [6]. Further, bipolar disorder is associated with significant impairment across numerous functional and health domains and this impairment often persists during the inter-episode period [2,3,7-9]. Sleep is one important domain that is often impaired in bipolar disorder and is the focus of the current study.

Sleep disturbance is a common feature of bipolar disorder. Within the Diagnostic and Statistical Manual of Mental Disorders (DSM-5), sleep disturbance is listed as a diagnostic criterion of mania, depression, and mixed episodes [1]. Moreover, sleep disturbance persists during the inter-episode period and as many as 70% of people with bipolar disorder report clinically significant sleep disturbance during inter-episode states [10]. Different types of sleep disturbance characterize bipolar disorder. Insomnia, for example, is highly prevalent [11] with as many as 100% of people with bipolar disorder report experiencing insomnia while depressed [12] and 55% reporting insomnia during the inter-episode period [10]. Episodes of depression are also characterized by hypersomnia [13] and 25% of people endorse symptoms of hypersomnia during the inter-episode period [14]. A reduced need for sleep is often exhibited during mania [15] and mixed episodes are characterized by decreases in total sleep time [16]. Furthermore, people with bipolar disorder are more likely to report circadian dysfunction, such as a delayed sleep phase preference, when compared to healthy individuals, [17,18] and irregular sleep patterns are commonly reported [19-21].

Notably, these different types of sleep disturbance can coexist and sleep disturbance is often persistent. For example, two studies have examined the coexistence of sleep disturbance in the context of depression and found that 10% of children with Major Depressive Disorder [22,23] and 8-11% of older adults in a depressive episode [23] experience insomnia and hypersomnia simultaneously. Moreover, in general population studies, 6% of adults [24] and 8% of young adults [25] also reported comorbid insomnia and hypersomnia. The coexistence of other types of sleep disturbance has yet to be examined. Sleep disturbance is also persistent. Longitudinal studies in healthy, aging, and depressed samples have shown insomnia persistence rates ranging from 40-74% [25-29]. Insomnia relapse rates are high and 25% of individuals who remit report at least one relapse over a 3-year period [30]. Furthermore, individuals with symptoms of insomnia, who do not meet diagnostic criteria for insomnia, are more likely to relapse and report worsening of insomnia over time [30]. Few studies have examined the persistence of other types of sleep disturbance. However, one study found that the lifetime prevalence of hypersomnia alone is 8.2% and the lifetime prevalence of hypersomnia in conjunction with insomnia is 8% [25].

Taken together, it is clear that sleep disturbance is a prevalent and variable feature of bipolar disorder and sleep disturbance may coexist and be persistent. However, a number of unanswered questions remain. For instance, no studies have examined the course or variability of sleep disturbance across several mood episodes and inter-episode periods of bipolar disorder. Previous studies examining sleep disturbance in bipolar disorder have typically focused on a single mood episode or a single period of time. Moreover, previous research has typically focused on just one type of disturbance and therefore, the potential coexistence of different types of sleep disturbance during a single period of time has yet to be determined. A second gap is that the persistence of sleep disturbance across the course of bipolar disorder has yet to be established. Sleep disturbance is a common feature of both mood episodes and the inter-episode period. However, it is unclear if, and how, sleep disturbance endures or changes from year to year.

The goal of the present study was to contribute to the process of closing these important gaps in the literature by examining the course of sleep disturbance across bipolar disorder. The first aim was to retrospectively examine the prevalence and coexistence of insomnia, hypersomnia, delayed sleep phase, reduced sleep need, and irregular sleep patterns across mood episodes and inter-episode periods over the last five years. Based on previous research, we hypothesized that sleep disturbance would be a prevalent feature across this five-year period and that the different types of sleep disturbance would coexist. The second aim was to retrospectively examine the persistence of each type of sleep disturbance across the same five-year period. Based on previous research, we hypothesized that sleep disturbance would be a persistent feature across this same five-year period. Information about the course of the different types of sleep disturbance in bipolar disorder is important for a number of reasons. First, it will pave the way to improving our understanding of this prominent but understudied feature of mood episodes and inter-episode periods. Second, sleep disturbance is a prominent correlate of mood disruption [31-37] and better understanding the course of sleep disturbance across bipolar disorder may aid in the prevention of relapse. Finally, understanding the course of sleep disturbance will help guide the development of more focused interventions.

Methods

Participants

The aims of the present study were addressed in the context of an NIMH-funded trial examining the effectiveness of treating insomnia during inter-episode bipolar disorder with cognitive behavior therapy for insomnia [CBT-I; e.g., 38]. Hence, all participants met criteria for bipolar I disorder and current insomnia and were inter-episode at the time of assessment.

Fifty-one people who met DSM-IV-TR criteria [15] for bipolar I disorder were included in the study. Bipolar diagnoses were assessed using the Structured Clinical Interview for Axis I Disorders [SCID; 39]. Ethnicity and race of the participants reflected the diversity of Alameda County (63% Caucasian, 11.1% African American, 9.3% Asian, 9.3% more than one ethnicity, 3.7% declined to answer, 1.9% American Indian/Alaska Native, 1.9% other). Participants were inter-episode (i.e., not currently manic or depressed) at the time of the assessment. An inter-episode period was defined by a score of 24 or less on the Inventory of Depressive Symptomatology, Clinician Rating [IDS-C; 40] and a score of 12 or less on the Young Mania Rating Scale, [YMRS; 41] which are standard measures and cutoffs in the bipolar literature. Participants were required to be on a stable medication regimen for at least four weeks prior to enrollment in the study and under the care of a treating physician or nurse practitioner who manages their bipolar disorder. All participants were at least 18 years old and reported English fluency, which was necessary as all aspects of the protocol were in English.

Participants also met criteria for current insomnia. Insomnia was defined as a subjective report of difficulty falling asleep (>30 minutes), difficulty maintaining sleep (wake after sleep onset >30 minutes), and/or waking up too early (early morning awakening >30 minutes), with associated daytime complaints, at least three times a week for at least one month. Further, these sleep difficulties had to occur despite adequate opportunity to sleep. These criteria reflect a combination of Research Diagnostic Criteria, [42] International Classification of Sleep Disorders [ICSD-2; 43] and DSM-IV-TR standards [15]. The Duke Structured Interview for Sleep Disorders [DSISD; 44], a valid and reliable semi-structured interview, was used to establish all insomnia diagnoses.

Exclusion criteria for the study included the following: an alcohol and/or substance abuse or dependence diagnosis within the past three months based on DSM-IV-TR criteria [15]; a current post-traumatic stress disorder diagnosis based on DSM-IV-TR criteria [15]; an active or progressive neurodegenerative disease or physical illness; evidence of sleep apnea, restless legs syndrome, or periodic limb movements during sleep; employment as an overnight shift worker in the last three months; current suicidal risk, specifically endorsements of active suicidal intent and/or a specific suicide plan; attempted suicide within the past 6 months; current homicidal risk; and pregnancy and/or breast-feeding mothers.

Procedure

All procedures described were approved by the Committee for Protection of Human Subjects at the University of California, Berkeley and represent the pre-treatment stage of the larger NIMH-funded trial. Participants were recruited through Internet advertisements and flyers distributed to psychiatric clinics in the community. Participants were first screened over the phone to determine if they were preliminarily eligible. Once determined eligible over the phone, they were invited for a detailed in-person assessment. After written informed consent was obtained, the SCID and DSISD diagnostic interviews were administered, demographic data were recorded, and a current inter-episode state was established. The life chart was administered during the in-person assessment.

The NIMH retrospective life-charting methodology

The National Institute of Mental Health Retrospective Life-Charting Methodology [the life chart; 45] was used to retrospectively examine the prevalence, coexistence, and persistence of sleep disturbance across a five-year period of bipolar disorder. The life chart is a validated, standard, and often utilized measure for recording retrospective features of bipolar disorder including the number, duration, and severity of mood episodes, inter-episode periods, and medication use [19,46-50] Using the life chart, we focused on the last five years because of the evidence of accurate retrospective recollection of details about life events over as much as a 5-year period [49] and the evidence that interview formats that include easy to recall anchor points are able to elicit life event information over periods ranging from 1-16 years [50].

The life chart does not include an assessment of sleep. Hence, for the present study, the life chart was carefully modified to include comorbid sleep disturbance; namely: insomnia, hypersomnia, reduced sleep need, delayed sleep phase, and irregular sleep patterns. For the purpose of the life chart, definitions of each type of sleep disturbance were based on DSM-IV-TR and ICSD-2 criteria [15,43]. Insomnia was defined as difficulty falling asleep, staying asleep, and/or waking up too early. Hypersomnia was characterized as persistent and excessive daytime sleepiness and abnormally prolonged sleep periods. Reduced sleep need was described as sleeping very little, but feeling energized despite the inadequate amount of sleep. Delayed sleep phase was defined as a circadian rhythm disorder in which the major sleep episode is two or more hours later relative to the desired bedtime, which causes difficulty waking at the desired time. Finally, irregular sleep patterns were classified as inconsistent and fragmented sleep and an erratic sleep-wake routine. In order to qualify as sleep disturbance, each type of sleep disturbance, with the exception of reduced sleep need, had to be associated with daytime complaints and/or distress.

The life chart was completed collaboratively with the participant and trained psychology doctoral students. Information about mood and sleep were collected using month-to-month units across the course of a five-year period. Previous studies have used the life chart to examine the total number of weeks ill in the past year [46]. However, since this study examined the past five years, we decided to use a less specific and easier to recall unit–months. To aid in life chart administration and participant recollection, the participant was provided with definitions and examples of mild, moderate, and severe mood episodes; definitions of the different types of sleep disturbance; and a list of life events that aided in recollection (e.g., high school graduation, loss of a job). Furthermore, participants were asked to consult diaries, medical records, doctors, friends, and family members to further ensure recollection and accuracy. Notably, a substantial proportion of participants arrived to their appointments with relevant records and associated notes.

Analysis plan

To examine the prevalence and coexistence of sleep disturbance across bipolar disorder, the life chart data were collapsed into several variables: (a) the total number of manic, depressive, mixed and inter-episode months across the five-year period; and (b) the total number of manic, depressive, mixed and inter-episode months with comorbid insomnia, hypersomnia, reduced sleep need, delayed sleep phase and irregular sleep patterns across the same five year period. Percentages of manic, depressive, mixed, and inter-episode months characterized by each type of sleep disturbance were then calculated.

To examine the persistence of sleep disturbance across bipolar disorder, persistence was conceptualized in two ways. First, we examined the persistence of insomnia, hypersomnia, delayed sleep phase, reduced sleep need, and irregular sleep patterns across each year of the five-year period: Year 1, Year 2, Year 3, Year 4, and Year 5. Within each year, we calculated the percentage of the year that was characterized by each type of sleep disturbance. We then categorized the percentage of sleep disturbance into tertile ranges. For each year, and each type of sleep disturbance within each year, we established tertile membership. We then categorized the change in—or endurance of—sleep disturbance by examining tertile transitions from Year 1 to Year 2, Year 2 to Year 3, Year 3 to Year 4, and Year 4 to Year 5. The change in sleep disturbance was then categorized by one of the following: Developed, Persisted, Worsened, Improved, or Remitted [51]. Developed was defined as transitioning from no sleep disturbance to having sleep disturbance the following year. Persisted was defined as remaining in the same tertile categorization from one year to the next. Worsened was defined as an increase in tertile categorization from one year to the next. Improved was defined as decreasing in tertile categorization from one year to the next. Remitted was defined as transitioning from having a sleep disturbance to not having sleep disturbance the following year.

We were also interested in examining the persistence of sleep disturbance across mood episodes and inter-episode periods. To address this aim, we separately calculated the percentage of total mood months (i.e., depressed, manic, mixed) and total inter-episode months across the five year period that were characterized by each type of sleep disturbance. Paired sample t-tests were used to examine the difference between percentage of mood months and percentage of inter-episode months characterized by each type of sleep disturbance. We operationalized a non-significant t-value as indicative of considerable sleep disturbance persistence across mood episodes and inter-episode periods.

Results

Participant characteristics

The demographic and clinical characteristics for the 51 participants are presented in Table 1. The average age of onset for sleep disturbance was significantly earlier than the average age of onset for mood disturbance in this sample, $t(50)=2.35$, $p=0.01$.

Gender (% female)	60.8% female
Employment Full-time (% of participants) Part-time (% of participants) Unemployed (% of participants)	17.90% 28.6 % 53.60%
Age (Years)	Mean ± SD 36.5 ± 11.1
Education (Years)	15.5 ± 3.7
Age at Onset Bipolar Disorder (Years)	21.2 ± 9.0
Age at Onset Sleep Disturbance (Years)	18.3 ± 9.7
Number of Manic Episodes Across the Five Year Period	1.5 ± 1.5
Duration of Manic Episodes Across the Five Year Period (Months)	2.5 ± 2.2
Number of Depressed Episodes Across the Five Year Period	1.9 ± 2.1
Duration of Depressed Episodes Across the Five Year Period (Months)	4.2 ± 3.5

Number of Mixed Episodes Across the Five Year Period	0.5 ± 1.3
Duration of Mixed Episodes Across the Five Year Period (Months)	3.0 ± 1.3
Number of Mood-Related Hospitalizations Across the Five Year Period	0.5 ± 0.8

Table 1: Demographic and Clinical Characteristics of People with Bipolar Disorder.

Percentages were calculated to examine the prevalence and coexistence of insomnia, hypersomnia, delayed sleep phase, reduced sleep need, and irregular sleep patterns across mood episodes and inter-episode periods of bipolar disorder. The prevalence of each type of sleep disturbance is presented in Figure 1.

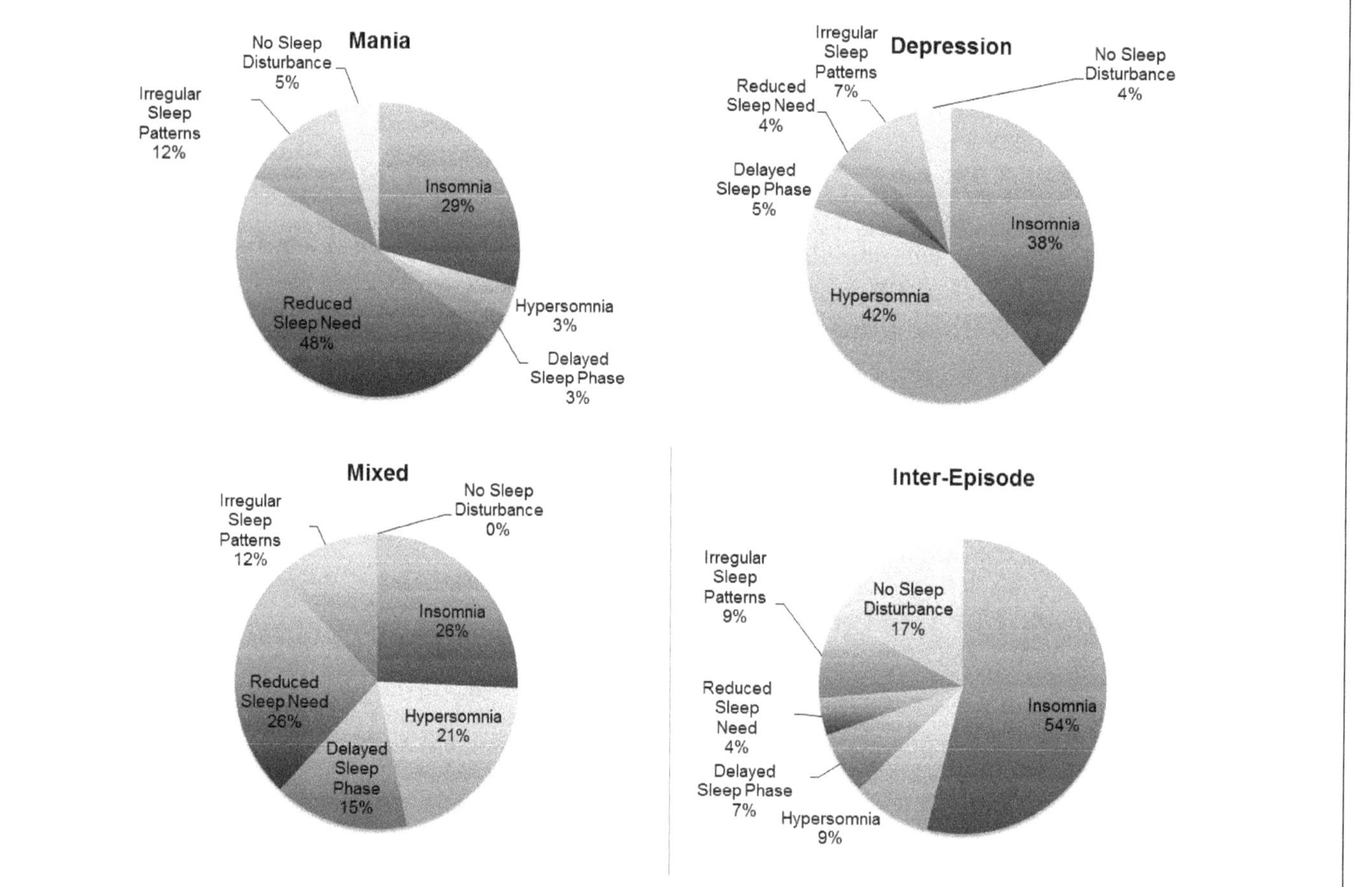

Figure 1: The Prevalence of Sleep Disturbance in Mood Episodes and the Inter-episode Period of Bipolar Disorder. (The percentages represent the percentage of months within each mood or inter-episode state characterized by each type of sleep disturbance).

Across the course of five-years, manic months were largely characterized by reduced sleep need and insomnia. Hypersomnia and insomnia were highly prevalent during depressive months and all five types of sleep disturbance were present during mixed months. No mixed months were characterized by a lack of sleep disturbance and across manic and depressive months, having a lack of sleep disturbance was infrequent. Moving on to inter-episode months, over half of the inter-episode months were characterized by insomnia and less than a quarter was characterized by no sleep disturbance. Overall, delayed sleep phase and irregular sleep patterns were the least common features of each type of mood episode and the inter-episode period.

The coexistence of sleep disturbance is depicted in Table 2. Across mood episodes and inter-episode periods of bipolar disorder, there was coexistence in the types of sleep disturbance experienced. During manic months, the most frequently reported coexistence was for insomnia and reduced sleep need, followed by coexistence of insomnia and irregular sleep patterns. However, the percentage of months characterized by these two types of coexistence was low with percentages of 9.2% and 6.3%, respectively. Insomnia and hypersomnia coexisted in 7.9% of depressive months and 14.4% of mixed months were characterized by both hypersomnia and reduced sleep need. Lastly, inter-episode months were most prominently characterized by coexistence of insomnia and delayed sleep phase, although this percentage is small at 5.9%. The coexistence of more than two types of sleep disturbance was rare, with the exception of during mixed episode months. Mixed episode months were characterized by coexistences of: (a) insomnia, hypersomnia, and delayed sleep phase, (b) insomnia, delayed sleep phase, and reduced sleep need, and (c) insomnia, reduced sleep need, and irregular sleep patterns. The prevalence of these coexistences ranged from 6.9–8.3 %.

Sleep Disturbance	Mania	Depression	Mixed	Inter-Episode
	Mean % ± SD	Mean % ± SD	Mean % ± SD	Mean % ± SD
Insomnia Alone	16.5 ± 33.8	29.7 ± 42.0	16.7 ± 38.9	55.4 ± 43.8
Hypersomnia Alone	1.6 ± 7.2	39.2 ± 43.6	10.0 ± 28.9	6.0 ± 22.4
DELAY Alone	--	--	8.3 ± 28.9	0.5 ± 2.7
REDUC Alone	47.3 ± 44.9	0.9 ± 2.9	12.8 ± 29.5	1.0 ± 3.6
IIRREG Alone	0.8 ± 3.3	0.9 ± 3.9	12.8 ± 29.5	2.8 ± 11.9
Insomnia & Hypersomnia	--	7.9 ± 25.4	1.4 ± 4.8	0.5 ± 2.9
Insomnia & DELAY	2.8 ± 16.7	4.0 ± 14.6	--	5.9 ± 21.5
Insomnia & REDUC	9.2 ± 28.3	0.2 ± 0.9	--	0.3 ± 1.8
Insomnia & IRREG	6.3 ± 23.5	2.9 ± 16.9	--	3.2 ± 13.1
Hypersomnia & DSP	--	--	--	--
Hypersomnia & REDUC	0.4 ± 2.4	0.5 ± 2.3	14.4 ± 30.5	--
Hypersomnia & IRREG	--	1.3 ± 7.3	--	--
DELAY & REDUC	--	--	--	--
DELAY & IRREG	1.4 ± 8.3	0.1 ± 0.7	--	0.1 ± 0.9
REDUC & IRREG	3.5 ± 14.7	0.3 ± 1.7	--	--
Insomnia, Hypersomnia, & DELAY	--	2.8 ± 14.0	8.3 ± 28.9	0.1 ± 0.6
Insomnia, Hypersomnia, & REDUC	--	--	--	--
Insomnia, Hypersomnia, & IRREG	1.4 ± 6.3	1.4 ± 6.0	--	--
Insomnia, DELAY, & REDUCb	--	0.2 ± 1.4	8.3 ± 28.9	--
Insomnia, DELAY, & IRREG	--	--	--	2.1 ± 14.6
Insomnia, REDUC, and IRREG	1.7 ± 7.1	--	6.9 ± 24.1	--
Hypersomnia, DELAY, & REDUC	--	--	--	--
Hypersomnia, DELAY, & IRREG	--	--	--	--
Hypersomnia, REDUC, & IRREG	0.5 ± 3.0	--	--	0.4 ± 2.9
REDUC, DELAY, & IRREG	--	--	--	--
Insomnia, Hypersomnia, DELAY, & IRREG	--	--	--	--
Insomnia, Hypersomnia, DELAY, & REDUC	--	--	--	--
Insomnia, Hypersomnia, REDUC, & IRREG	0.3 ± 1.5	2.9 ± 16.9	--	--
Insomnia, DELAY, REDUC, & IRREG	--	--	--	--
Hypersomnia, DELAY, REDUC, & IRREG	--	--	--	--

Insomnia, Hypersomnia, DELAY, REDUC & IRREG	--	--	--	--

Table 2: The Prevalence and Coexistence of Sleep Disturbance across Mood Episodes and Inter-episode Periods of Bipolar Disorder. (The percentages represent the percentage of months within each mood or inter-episode period characterized by each type of sleep disturbance. DELAY = Delayed Sleep Phase; REDUC = Reduced Sleep Need; IRREG = Irregular Sleep Patterns).

Persistence was operationalized in two ways. First, we were interested in determining whether each type of sleep disturbance developed, persisted, worsened, improved, or remitted from year to year. The results are presented in Table 3.

Sleep Disturbance	Year 1 - Year 2	Year 2 - Year 3	Year 3 - Year 4	Year 4 - Year 5
	% of participants	% of participants	% of participants	% of participants
Insomnia				
Developed	9.8	5.9	9.8	11.8
Persisted	56.9	49	58.8	58.8
Worsened	5.9	3.9	9.8	13.7
Improved	3.9	11.8	3.9	3.9
Remitted	11.8	3.9	5.9	5.9
Hypersomnia				
Developed	5.9	11.8	11.8	19.6
Persisted	9.8	11.8	15.7	7.8
Worsened	3.9	3.9	2	5.9
Improved	2	2	3.9	9.8
Remitted	3.9	3.9	7.8	9.8
Delayed Sleep Phase				
Developed	5.9	3.9	5.9	3.9
Persisted	7.8	5.9	3.9	7.8
Worsened	0	0	2	2
Improved	0	0	0	0
Remitted	0	7.8	3.9	2
Reduced Sleep Need				
Developed	9.8	9.8	11.8	15.7
Persisted	7.8	5.9	7.8	5.9
Worsened	0	3.9	0	3.9
Improved	0	3.9	0	3.9
Remitted	15.7	3.9	15.7	5.9
Irregular Sleep Patterns				
Developed	7.8	2	2	13.7
Persisted	11.8	13.7	9.8	5.9

Worsened	2	0	2	3.9
Improved	0	2	2	3.9
Remitted	2	5.9	3.9	2

Table 3: The Persistence of Sleep Disturbance Across a Five-Year Period in Bipolar Disorder. (The percentages represent the percentage of participants within each year that experienced either a developing, persisting, worsening, improving, or remitting of each type of sleep disturbance).

Insomnia developed in 5.8–11.8% of participants across the five years. Persistence rates for insomnia were high, ranging from 49–59%, and 3.9–13.7% of participants reported that their insomnia worsened from year to year. Finally, improvement and remission rates for insomnia were low, ranging from 3.9–11.7%. Hypersomnia developed in 5.9–19.6% of participants and persisted in 7.8–15.7% of participants. Few participants reported that their hypersomnia worsened, with percentages ranging from 2.0–5.9%. A slightly larger percentage of participants reported that their hypersomnia improved or remitted from year to year (2.0–9.8%). Delayed sleep phase was reported by a small percentage of participants. The majority of participants that reported having delayed sleep phase syndrome reported that their delayed sleep phase developed and persisted from year to year (3.9–7.8%). However, some improvement was noted as well, with 7.8% of participants reporting remission from year 2 to year 3. Reduced sleep need was primarily characterized by "developing," "persisting," or "remitting" from year to year. Few participants reported that their reduced sleep need worsened (3.9%) and improved (3.9%) from one year to the next. Finally, irregular sleep patterns primarily developed (1.9–13.7%) or persisted (5.9–13.7%) across the five-year period. Irregular sleep patterns also demonstrated some improvement and 5.8% of the participants reported remission from year 2 to year 3.

Second, we examined the persistence of sleep disturbance across mood episodes and inter-episode periods by conducting paired sample t-tests for each type of sleep disturbance. Non-significant t-values were conceptualized as indicative of considerable sleep disturbance persistence across mood episodes and inter-episode states. The results are presented in Figure 2.

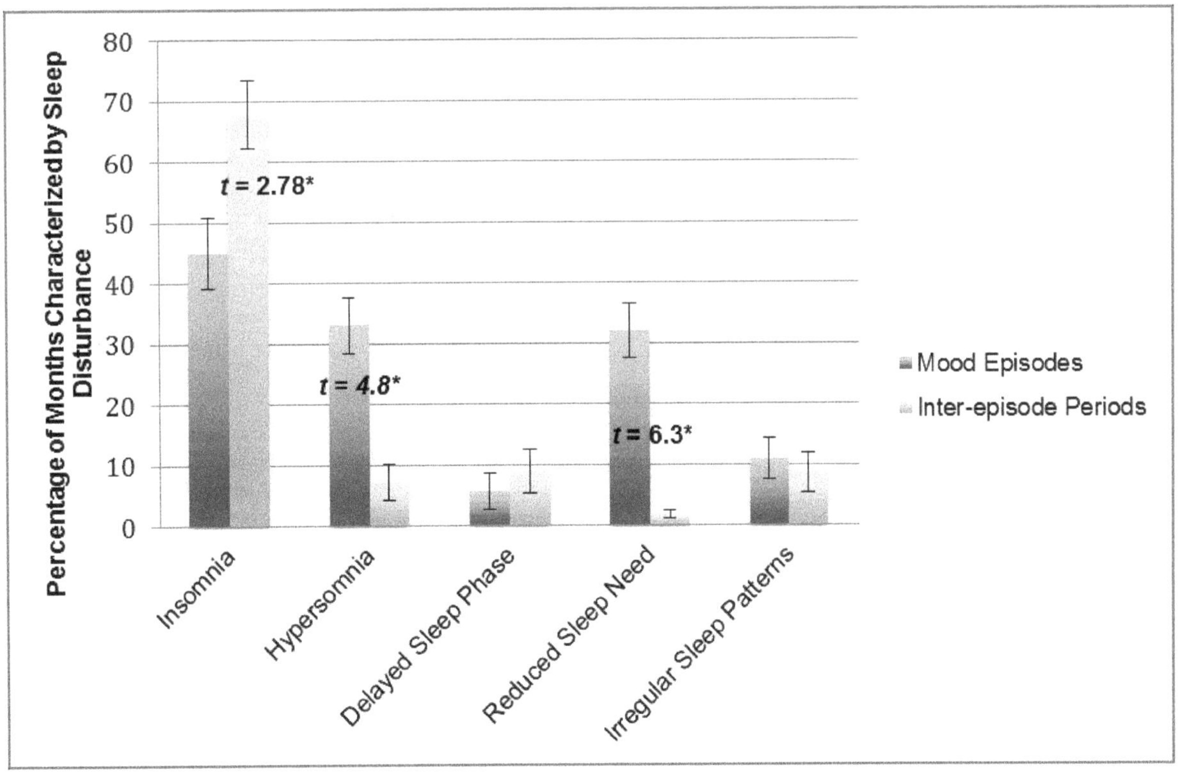

Figure 2: The Persistence of Sleep Disturbance: Mood Episodes vs. Inter-episode Periods. (The percentage of months within mood episodes and inter-episode periods characterized by each type of sleep disturbance are depicted in this bar graph. t-values represent the difference between mood episode and inter-episode percentage means. *p<0.01).

There were significant t-values for hypersomnia and reduced sleep need, with participants reporting significantly greater hypersomnia and reduced sleep need during mood episodes compared to the inter-episode period. There was also a significant t-value for insomnia;

however the percentage of insomnia during the inter-episode period was greater than the percentage of insomnia during mood episodes. T-values for both delayed sleep phase and irregular sleep patterns were not significant, pointing to the possibility that these types of sleep disturbance persist across mood episodes and inter-episode periods.

Discussion

The present study was designed to extend knowledge about sleep and bipolar disorder by addressing the prevalence, coexistence, and persistence of sleep disturbance across a five-year period. At the outset, we wish to emphasize two important limitations. First, this study was part of a larger NIMH-funded study. Hence, all participants met diagnostic criteria for current insomnia. Given their current symptoms, we cannot rule out the possibility that participants may have exhibited biased recall of their previous sleep disturbance [e.g., 52]. Future research is needed to test whether these results are generalizable to people with bipolar disorder without current insomnia. The second limitation is that we used the NIMH Retrospective Life-Charting Methodology. Although ample recollection aids were provided, the accuracy of participant recollection cannot be verified. However, previous research demonstrates that retrospectively collecting details about life events over as much as a 5-year period is reliable [49] and that interview formats that include easy-to-recall anchor points are able to elicit life event information over periods ranging from 1-16 years [50]. Moreover, although we utilized a retrospective design, many of our results are consistent with previous cross-sectional and prospective reports that did not rely on long periods of recall [e.g., 10,16,22,53]. Nonetheless, longitudinal studies are needed. Given the limitations of this study, these results should be interpreted with caution. Nonetheless, to the best of our knowledge, this is the first study to examine the course of sleep disturbance across bipolar disorder.

Not surprisingly, results of this study demonstrated that sleep disturbance is a prevalent feature across bipolar disorder. Consistent with previous research, we found that 62.8% of manic months were characterized by reduced sleep need [16,54,55]. Interestingly, insomnia occurred in 38.1% of manic months. Whereas some studies have reported sleep continuity problems during mania, [55,56,57] to the best of our knowledge, the present study is the first to suggest that distress or impairment is associated with these sleep problems. Recall that sleep discontinuity and distress or impairment are required for a diagnosis of insomnia [15,43]. Depressive months were largely characterized by hypersomnia and insomnia, which is consistent with prior work [11,58]. Sleep during mixed episodes has been less-extensively characterized with only one study reporting that mixed episodes were associated with decreases in total sleep time [16]. Building on this study, the present results suggest that the percentage of mixed months characterized by insomnia, hypersomnia, delayed sleep phase, reduced sleep need, and irregular sleep patterns were roughly similar, with insomnia and reduced sleep need being at the upper end of the range at approximately 42%, and irregular sleep patterns being at the lower end of the range at 19.7%. Moreover, in contrast to manic, depressed, and inter-episode months, months spent in mixed states were characterized by sleep disturbance 100% of the time. Lastly, across the course of the disorder and consistent with the literature, [10,53] over two thirds of inter-episode months were characterized by insomnia.

Importantly, there was coexistence in the types of sleep disturbance experienced across manic, depressed, mixed, and inter-episode months. Approximately 10% of manic months were characterized by both reduced sleep need and insomnia. This is a novel finding. These data suggest that in addition to experiencing reduced sleep need during mania, a subset of people also experience problems initiating and/or maintaining sleep and have associated daytime complaints. Depressed months were predominantly characterized by a coexistence of insomnia and hypersomnia (7.9%), a finding that is consistent with the depression literature [22]. The most notable coexistence during mixed months was the comorbidity of hypersomnia and reduced sleep need (14.4%). A possible explanation for this finding is that perhaps within the same month, people are experiencing a decrease in the amount of sleep they are receiving (i.e., reduced sleep need) and try to compensate for this sleep loss by spending an excessive amount of time in bed [59]. Further, mixed episode months were characterized by having more than two types of sleep disturbance within a single month. These findings coupled with the fact that mixed months were characterized by sleep disturbance 100% of the time, demonstrate that sleep disturbance is a prevalent and complicated feature of mixed states. Coexistence of sleep disturbance during inter-episode months was rare. The highest coexistence was insomnia and delayed sleep phase, reported in 5.9% of inter-episode months.

There was considerable variation in the pattern of sleep disturbance across the five-year period. Notably, insomnia was the most persistent with rates ranging from 49.0–58.8%. Consistent with prior work, [26] these percentages demonstrate that insomnia is a persistent disorder with comparatively low rates of improvement and remittance (3.9–11.8%). Remarkably, even though this was an insomnia sample, a notable percentage of participants reported experiencing hypersomnia, reduced sleep need, delayed sleep phase, and irregular sleep patterns across the five-year period. The pattern of endurance and/or change varied depending on the type of sleep disturbance. However, for every type of sleep disturbance, a greater percentage of participants reported that their sleep disturbance developed or persisted compared to improved or remitted from one year to the next.

An examination of persistence across mood episodes and inter-episode periods revealed that hypersomnia and reduced sleep need are not persistent and are more commonly reported during mood episodes. This suggests that hypersomnia and reduced sleep need may be more mood state-dependent. On the other hand, there wasn't a significant difference between delayed sleep phase and irregular sleep patterns across mood episodes and inter-episode periods, pointing to the possibility that these two types of sleep disturbance are more persistent, regardless of mood-state. Interestingly, insomnia was reported more frequently during the inter-episode period than during mood episodes. This may be a product of our sample and this finding requires replication. The assumption that non-significance is indicative of persistence requires validation.

A particularly noteworthy finding was that the average age of onset for sleep disturbance was significantly earlier than the average age of onset for mood disturbance. There is a parallel finding that is quite robust in unipolar depression. Multiple longitudinal studies have reported that sleep disturbance often precedes episodes of depression and may be a risk factor for first and recurrent episodes of depression [25,60-62]. The current findings extend these results to bipolar disorder and suggest that sleep disturbance may be an early marker for bipolar disorder and an ideal target for early intervention. Using electroencephalogram [63,64], self-report measures, and clinical interviewing, it is possible that we can identify sleep disturbance early and intervene to improve to improve quality of life.

In sum, these findings demonstrate that sleep disturbance is a prevalent and complex feature across mood episodes and inter-episode periods of bipolar disorder. Some particularly noteworthy results include the findings that mixed episodes are characterized by sleep disturbance 100% of the time, 10% of manic months are characterized by both reduced sleep need and insomnia, and sleep disturbance tended to develop or persist over time and across mood–to–inter-episode states. These results have important implications. Due to the unequivocal relationship between sleep disturbance and mood disruption in bipolar disorder [31-37], it is possible that by further understanding the nature of sleep disturbance across the course of bipolar disorder, we can better prevent relapse into a mood episode and improve quality of life. In light of these results, it is recommended that current treatments for sleep disturbance, that encompass the complexities uncovered, should be adapted for use in bipolar disorder [58,65].

Acknowledgement

The authors thank Dr. Polina Eidelman for her contributions to the study protocol, Jason Lee for his contributions to data collection, and Kerrie Hein for her continued support throughout the study. This project was supported by a National Institute of Mental Health Grant No. R34MH080958 award to AGH.

References

1. American Psychiatric Association (2013) Diagnostic and Statistical Manual of Mental Disorders (5th edn), American Psychiatric Association, Washington, DC.
2. Judd LL, Akiskal HS, Schettler PJ, Coryell W, Endicott J, et al. (2003) A prospective investigation of the natural history of the long-term weekly symptomatic status of bipolar II disorder. Arch Gen Psychiatry 60: 261-269.
3. MacQueen GM, Marriott M, Begin H, Robb J, Joffe RT, et al. (2003) Subsyndromal symptoms assessed in longitudinal, prospective follow-up of a cohort of patients with bipolar disorder. Bipolar Disord 5: 349-355.
4. Robb JC, Cooke RG, Devins GM, Young LT, Joffe RT (1997) Quality of life and lifestyle disruption in euthymic bipolar disorder. J Psychiatr Res 31: 509-517.
5. Merikangas KR, Jin R, He JP, Kessler RC, Lee S, et al. (2011) Prevalence and correlates of bipolar spectrum disorder in the world mental health survey initiative. Arch Gen Psychiatry 68: 241-251.
6. World Health Organization (2001) World Health Report 2001. Mental Health: New Understanding, New Hope. Geneva, Switzerland: World Health Organization.
7. Huxley N, Baldessarini RJ (2007) Disability and its treatment in bipolar disorder patients. Bipolar Disord 9: 183-196.
8. Martínez-Arán A, Vieta E, Reinares M, Colom F, Torrent C, et al. (2004) Cognitive function across manic or hypomanic, depressed, and euthymic states in bipolar disorder. Am J Psychiatry 161: 262-270.
9. Sanchez-Moreno J, Martinez-Aran A, Tabarés-Seisdedos R, Torrent C, Vieta E, et al. (2009) Functioning and disability in bipolar disorder: an extensive review. Psychother Psychosom 78: 285-297.
10. Harvey AG, Schmidt DA, Scarnà A, Semler CN, Goodwin GM (2005) Sleep-related functioning in euthymic patients with bipolar disorder, patients with insomnia, and subjects without sleep problems. Am J Psychiatry 162: 50-57.
11. Harvey AG1 (2008) Sleep and circadian rhythms in bipolar disorder: seeking synchrony, harmony, and regulation. Am J Psychiatry 165: 820-829.
12. Winokur G, Clayton PJ, Reich T (1969) Manic Depressed Illness. St Louis, CV Mosby.
13. Detre T, Himmelhoch J, Swartzburg M, Anderson CM, Byck R, et al. (1972) Hypersomnia and manic-depressive disease. Am J Psychiatry 128: 1303-1305.
14. Kaplan KA, Gruber J, Eidelman P, Talbot LS, Harvey AG (2011) Hypersomnia in inter-episode bipolar disorder: does it have prognostic significance? J Affect Disord 132: 438-444.
15. American Psychiatric Association (2000) Diagnostic and Statistical Manual of Mental Disorders (text revised 4th edn) American Psychiatric Association, Washington, DC.
16. Cassidy F, Murry E, Forest K, Carroll BJ (1998) Signs and symptoms of mania in pure and mixed episodes. J Affect Disord 50: 187-201.
17. Giglio LM, Magalhães PV, Andersen ML, Walz JC, Jakobson L, et al. (2010) Circadian preference in bipolar disorder. Sleep Breath 14: 153-155.
18. Staton D1 (2008) The impairment of pediatric bipolar sleep: hypotheses regarding a core defect and phenotype-specific sleep disturbances. J Affect Disord 108: 199-206.
19. Eidelman P, Talbot LS, Gruber J, Harvey AG (2010) Sleep, illness course, and concurrent symptoms in inter-episode bipolar disorder. J Behav Ther Exp Psychiatry 41: 145-149.
20. Jones SH, Hare DJ, Evershed K (2005) Actigraphic assessment of circadian activity and sleep patterns in bipolar disorder. Bipolar Disord 7: 176-186.
21. Millar A, Espie CA, Scott J (2004) The sleep of remitted bipolar outpatients: a controlled naturalistic study using actigraphy. J Affect Disord 80: 145-153.
22. Liu X, Buysse DJ, Gentzler AL, Kiss E, Mayer L, et al. (2007) Insomnia and hypersomnia associated with depressive phenomenology and comorbidity in childhood depression. Sleep 30: 83-90.
23. Roberts RE, Shema SJ, Kaplan GA, Strawbridge WJ (2000) Sleep complaints and depression in an aging cohort: A prospective perspective. Am J Psychiatry 157: 81-88.
24. Ohayon MM1 (2012) Determining the level of sleepiness in the American population and its correlates. J Psychiatr Res 46: 422-427.
25. Breslau N, Roth T, Rosenthal L, Andreski P (1996) Sleep disturbance and psychiatric disorders: a longitudinal epidemiological study of young adults. Biol Psychiatry 39: 411-418.
26. Buysse DJ, Angst J, Gamma A, Ajdacic V, Eich D, et al. (2008) Prevalence, course, and comorbidity of insomnia and depression in young adults. Sleep 31: 473-480.
27. Foley DJ, Monjan A, Simonsick EM, Wallace RB, Blazer DG (1999) Incidence and remission of insomnia among elderly adults: an epidemiologic study of 6,800 persons over three years. Sleep 22 Suppl 2: S366-372.
28. Janson C, Lindberg E, Gislason T, Elmasry A, Boman G (2001) Insomnia in men-a 10-year prospective population based study. Sleep 24: 425-430.
29. Morphy H, Dunn KM, Lewis M, Boardman HF, Croft PR (2007) Epidemiology of insomnia: a longitudinal study in a UK population. Sleep 30: 274-280.
30. Morin CM, Bélanger L, LeBlanc M, Ivers H, Savard J, et al. (2009) The natural history of insomnia: a population-based 3-year longitudinal study. Arch Intern Med 169: 447-453.
31. Jackson A, Cavanagh J, Scott J (2003) A systematic review of manic and depressive prodromes. J Affect Disord 74: 209-217.
32. Colombo C, Benedetti F, Barbini B, Campori E, Smeraldi E (1999) Rate of switch from depression into mania after therapeutic sleep deprivation in bipolar depression. Psychiatry Res 86: 267-270.
33. Leibenluft E, Albert PS, Rosenthal NE, Wehr TA (1996) Relationship between sleep and mood in patients with rapid-cycling bipolar disorder. Psychiatry Res 63: 161-168.
34. Wehr TA, Sack DA, Rosenthal NE (1987) Sleep reduction as a final common pathway in the genesis of mania. Am J Psychiatry 144: 201-204.
35. Barbini B, Bertelli S, Colombo C, Smeraldi E (1996) Sleep loss, a possible factor in augmenting manic episode. Psychiatry Res 65: 121-125.

36. Gruber J, Harvey AG, Wang PW, Brooks JO 3rd, Thase ME, et al. (2009) Sleep functioning in relation to mood, function, and quality of life at entry to the Systematic Treatment Enhancement Program for Bipolar Disorder (STEP-BD). J Affect Disord 114: 41-49.
37. Krüger S, Seminowicz D, Goldapple K, Kennedy SH, Mayberg HS (2003) State and trait influences on mood regulation in bipolar disorder: blood flow differences with an acute mood challenge. Biol Psychiatry 54: 1274-1283.
38. Edinger JD, Wohlgemuth WK, Radtke RA, Marsh GR, Quillian RE (2001) Cognitive behavioral therapy for treatment of chronic primary insomnia: a randomized controlled trial. JAMA 285: 1856-1864.
39. First MB, Spitzer MB, Gibbon M, Williams JB (1995) Structured Clinical Interview for DSM-IV Axis I Disorders-Patient Edition (SCID-I/P, Version 2.0). New York, Biomedics Research Department, New York State Psychiatric Institute.
40. Rush AJ, Gullion CM, Basco MR, Jarrett RB, Trivedi MH (1996) The Inventory of Depressive Symptomatology (IDS): psychometric properties. Psychol Med 26: 477-486.
41. Young RC, Biggs JT, Ziegler VE, Meyer DA (1978) A rating scale for mania: reliability, validity and sensitivity. Br J Psychiatry 133: 429-435.
42. Edinger JD, Bonnet MH, Bootzin RR, Doghramji K, Dorsey CM, et al. (2004) Derivation of research diagnostic criteria for insomnia: report of an American Academy of Sleep Medicine Work Group. Sleep 27: 1567-1596.
43. American Academy of Sleep Medicine (2005) International Classification of Sleep Disorders, (2nd edn). American Academy of Sleep Medicine, Washington, DC.
44. Edinger JD, Wyatt JK, Olsen MK, Stechuchak KM, Carney CE, et al. (2009) Reliability and validity of the Duke Structured Interview of Sleep Disorders for insomnia screening. Sleep Supplemental 32: A810.
45. Leverich GS, Post RM (1993) The NIMH life chart manual for recurrent affective illness: The LCMS-S (Self Version). NIMH Mongraph, Biological Psychiatry Branch.
46. Denicoff KD, Ali SO, Mirsky AF, Smith-Jackson EE, Leverich GS, et al. (1999) Relationship between prior course of illness and neuropsychological functioning in patients with bipolar disorder. J Affect Disord 56: 67-73.
47. Denicoff KD, Smith-Jackson EE, Disney ER, Ali SO, Leverich GS, et al. (1997) Comparative prophylactic efficacy of lithium, carbamazepine, and the combination in bipolar disorder. J Clin Psychiatry 58: 470-478.
48. Roy-Byrne P, Post RM, Uhde TW, Porcu T, Davis D (1985) The longitudinal course of recurrent affective illness: life chart data from research patients at the NIMH. Acta Psychiatr Scand Suppl 317: 1-34.
49. Brown EW, Harris T (1982) Fall-off in the reporting of life events. Soc Psychiatry 17: 23-28.
50. Roy-Byrne P, Geraci M, Uhde TW (1987) Life events obtained via interview: the effect of time of recall on data obtained in controls and patients with panic disorder. J Affect Disord 12: 57-62.
51. Bonuck KA, Chervin RD, Cole TJ, Emond A, Henderson J, et al. (2011) Prevalence and persistence of sleep disordered breathing symptoms in young children: a 6-year population-based cohort study. Sleep 34: 875-884.
52. Bradley BP, Mogg K, Williams R (1995) Implicit and explicit memory for emotion-congruent information in clinical depression and anxiety. Behav Res Ther 33: 755-770.
53. Brill S, Penagaluri P, Roberts RJ, Gao Y, El-Mallakh RS (2011) Sleep disturbances in euthymic bipolar patients. Ann Clin Psychiatry 23: 113-116.
54. Clayton PJ, Pitts FN Jr (1965) Affect disorder. IV. Mania. Compr Psychiatry 6: 313-322.
55. Hudson JI, Lipinski JF, Frankenburg FR, Grochocinski VJ, Kupfer DJ (1988) Electroencephalographic sleep in mania. Arch Gen Psychiatry 45: 267-273.
56. Linkowski P, Mendlewicz J (1993) Sleep electroencephalogram and rhythm disturbances in mood disorders. Curr Opin Psychiatr 6: 35-37.
57. Winokur G, Tanna VL (1969) Possible role of X-linked dominant factor in manic depressive disease. Dis Nerv Syst 30: 89-94.
58. Plante DT, Winkelman JW (2008) Sleep disturbance in bipolar disorder: therapeutic implications. Am J Psychiatry 165: 830-843.
59. Kaplan KA, Harvey AG (2009) Hypersomnia across mood disorders: a review and synthesis. Sleep Med Rev 13: 275-285.
60. Ford DE, Kamerow DB (1989) Epidemiologic study of sleep disturbances and psychiatric disorders. An opportunity for prevention? JAMA 262: 1479-1484.
61. Perlis ML, Smith LJ, Lyness JM, Matteson SR, Pigeon WR, et al. (2006) Insomnia as a risk factor for onset of depression in the elderly. Behav Sleep Med 4: 104-113.
62. Weissman MM, Greenwald S, Niño-Murcia G, Dement WC (1997) The morbidity of insomnia uncomplicated by psychiatric disorders. Gen Hosp Psychiatry 19: 245-250.
63. Yaghouby F, Modur P, Sunderam S (2014) Naive scoring of human sleep based on a hidden Markov model of the electroencephalogram. Conf Proc IEEE Eng Med Biol Soc 2014: 5028-5031.
64. Yaghouby F, Sunderam S2 (2015) Quasi-supervised scoring of human sleep in polysomnograms using augmented input variables. Comput Biol Med 59: 54-63.
65. Harvey AG (2011) Sleep and circadian functioning: critical mechanisms in the mood disorders? Annu Rev Clin Psychol 7: 297-319.

3

Association between Subjective Sleep Quality, Hypertension, Depression and Body Mass Index in a Nigerian Family Practice Setting

Shittu RO[1]*, Issa BA[2], Olanrewaju GT[2], Odeigah LO[3], Sule AG[4], Sanni MA[5], Aderibigbe SA[6], Uthman MB[6] and Nyamngee AA[7]

[1]*Department of Family Medicine, Kwara State Specialist Hospital, Nigeria*
[2]*Department of Behavioral Sciences, University of Ilorin Teaching Hospital, Nigeria*
[3]*Department of Family Medicine, University of Ilorin Teaching Hospital, Nigeria*
[4]*Department of Family Medicine, Ahmadubello University, Teaching Hospital, Nigeria*
[5]*Department of Hematology, Kwara State Specialist Hospital, Nigeria*
[6]*Department of Epidemiology and Community Health, University of Ilorin Teaching Hospital, Nigeria*
[7]*Department of Medical microbiology and parasitology, College of Health, Sciences, University of Ilorin, Nigeria*

Abstract

Objectives: Poor subjective sleep quality in primary care has not been widely studied in Nigeria; hence this study was aimed to evaluate the subjective sleep quality and to find the association with blood pressure, depression and body mass index.

Methodology: Pittsburg Sleep Quality Index (PSQI) questionnaire was administered. Good sleep quality was defined as PSQI less than 5. The level of depression was assessed using the Patient Health Questionnaires (PHQ–9).

Results: The sample consisted of 400 subjects in the age group 18-70years. The overall mean age did 48.0 + 13.2 years, with the age group 41-50years constitute 29.5% of the studied subjects. Whilst 240 (60%) had normal blood pressure, 29(7.5%) had stage 1 and 43 (10.8%) had stage 2 hypertension. One hundred and thirty eight (34.5%) had normal weight, while 108 (27.0%) were obese. Overall sleep quality was very good, fairly good, fairly bad, and very bad in, 30.8%, 33.2%, 19.5%, and 16.5% of the respondents respectively. The prevalence of poor sleep quality was 44.0%. There was strong statistical association between poor sleep quality, blood pressure (p-value 0.002), depression (p-value 0.000) and body mass index (p-value 0.05).

Conclusion: A substantial proportion of the subjects had poor sleep quality associated with high blood pressure, increased body mass index and depression.

Keywords: Sleep quality; Hypertension; Depression; Body mass index

Introduction

Sleep is a vital reparative, restorative and physiological phenomenon, and impaired sleep has significant negative impact on health [1]. The quality of sleep is a measure of both the quantitative and qualitative component of sleep. The quantitative component involves the duration of sleep whereas the qualitative components is a subjective measure of the depth and feeling of restfulness upon awakening [2]. Sleep quality is an important clinical entity for two major reasons. In the first instance, complaints about sleep quality are common; epidemiological surveys indicate that 15-35% of the adult population complain of frequent sleep quality disturbance, such as difficulty falling asleep or difficulty maintaining sleep [3]. In addition, poor sleep quality can be an important symptom of many sleep and medical disorders. One frequently measured component of sleep quality, sleep duration, may even have a direct association with mortality [4]. According to the National Sleep Foundation adults should get between 7 and 9 hours of sleep each night [5].

Sleep quality complaints are particularly relevant to physicians. Factors relating to anxiety and stress are one of the most important concomitants of sleep complaints in the general population [6]. Sleep quality represents a complex phenomenon that is difficult to define and measure objectively. It varies with sex and age. Females have higher risk of poor sleep quality [7]. Increased age is also associated with indices of poor sleep quality [8]. Bansil et al. reported that combinations of sleep disorders short sleep duration and quality of sleep were associated with increased risk in the prevalence of hypertension [9]. In another study, subjective sleep duration was negative related to depressive state [10].

The largest and longest study on adult sleep habits and weight was the Nurses' Health Study, which followed 68,000 middle-age American women for 16 years [11]. Compared to women who slept seven hours a night, women who slept five hours or less were 15 percent more likely to become obese over the course of the study. Abdulsalam et al. [12] found no significant correlation between age, weight, height, BMI and sex of students.

Subjective Sleep quality had been associated with hypertension, depressive symptoms and higher body mass index (BMI) with paucity of data in Nigeria, hence the need for this study.

Methodology

This study was conducted at the General Outpatients Clinic

***Corresponding author:** Shittu RO, Department of Family Medicine, Kwara State Specialist Hospital, Nigeria, E-mail: oorelopehospital@gmail.com

(GOPD) of Kwara State Specialist Hospital, Ilorin, and north Central Nigeria. The target populations were the newly registered patients attending the clinic.

The sample size was estimated using the Fisher's Formula [13], $n = \frac{Z^2 p(1-p)}{e^2} = \frac{(1.96)^2 0.325(1-0.325)}{(0.05)^2} = 337.1$ using 32.5% from a previous study [14], as the best estimate of poor sleep quality among medical students at a Nigerian University, a minimum sample size of 337.1 was calculated, but 400 was used to increase the reliability of the study.

A systematic random sampling method was used in recruiting respondents for this study, from the period of study from October 30 to November 30, 2013. Already identified depressed subjects who were on treatment and those who refused to give consent were excluded from the study. Pretesting was carried out at the Kwara State Civil Service Hospital, using 40 respondents (10% of the sample size). Ethical approval was obtained from the Ethical Review Committee of the Kwara State Ministry of Health before the commencement of the study.

The Pittsburgh Sleep Quality Index (PSQI) was used for the subjective assessment of sleep quality [2]. The PSQI is a questionnaire consisting of 19 items which are coded on a 4-point scale (0-3) to obtain seven sub-categories, including sleep duration, sleep efficiency, sleep satisfaction, and medication use. The sum of all sub scores represents the total sleep quality score, ranging between 0-21, with higher scores representing lower sleep quality. The individuals were categorized as follows: good sleep quality (less than 5) and poor sleep quality (greater than or equal to 5). Psychometric properties have demonstrated good reliability internal consistency 0.89; test retest reliability 0.85) and good construct validity for the English language version [15].

The Patients Health Questionnaire (PHQ-9) [16] is a brief, 9 - item, patients self-report depression assessment tool that was derived from the interview-based PRIME-MD [17]. It was specifically developed for use, in primary care. It is the only tool that was specifically developed for use as a patient self-administered depression diagnostic tool, rather than as a severity or screening tool. It is the only short self-report tool that can reasonably be used both for diagnosis of DSM-4 major depression as well as for tracking of severity of major depression over time [18]. Psychometric evaluation of the PHQ-9 revealed a sensitivity ranging from 62%-92% and a specificity between 74%-88% [16-18]. All subjects screened positively for depression using Patients Health Questionnaire - 2 (PHQ-2), which was the first two questions of PHQ-9, triggered full diagnostic interviews by the behavioral scientists. Respondents who scored one and more were assessed clinically for depression. Scoring and level of depression was assessed viz: (1-4) minimal depression, (5-9) mild depression, (10-14) moderate depression, (15-19) moderately severe depression, and (20-27) severe depression. Some direct depression care, such as care support, coordination, case management, and treatment was embarked on.

Height and weight were measured according to standardized procedures. Body Mass Index (BMI) was calculated as weight in Kg divided by height in m^2 (kg/m^2). The international classification of BMI was used. The principal cut-off points were as follows: moderate thinness (16.00-16.99), mild thinness (17.00-18.49), normal (18.50-24.99), pre-obese (25.00-29.99), obese class I (30.00-34.99), obese class II (35.00-39.99), obese class III (>40.00).

An Accosson Mercury sphygmomanometer was used to measure the resting blood pressure of the subjects in a sitting position. Classification of hypertension was made according to the seventh report of the Joint National Committee on Prevention, Detection, Evaluation and Treatment of high blood pressure (JNC 7) [19] recommends the following classification of blood pressure for adults aged ≥ 18 years

Normal: Systolic: <120 mm Hg Diastolic: <80 mm Hg

Pre-hypertension: Systolic: <120-139 mm Hg Diastolic: <80-89 mm Hg

Stage 1 hypertension: Systolic: <140-159 mm Hg Diastolic: <90-99 mm Hg

Stage 2 hypertension: Systolic: ≥ 160 Hg Diastolic: ≥ 100 mm Hg

Completed questionnaire and measurements were entered into a computer data base. The data were analyzed using the epidemiological information (Epi-info) 2005 software package of Center for Disease Control and Prevention (CDC).Stepwise multiple regression analysis was conducted and poor sleep quality was significantly correlated with hypertension, depression and body mass index, the level of significance and values less than 0.05 were regarded as statistically significant.

Results

Table 1 displays the socio-demographic characteristics of the respondents. 400 newly registered patients were recruited. Subject with the age group 41-50 constituted 29.5% of the respondents with an overall mean age of 48.0 + 13.2. Female outnumbered males. The respondents were predominantly Yoruba, 384 (96.0%) and Muslims, 354 (88.5%). Majority, 238 (59.5%) had no formal education; they were mostly traders, 156 (39.0%). Thirty (7.5%) agreed to alcohol intake. Thirty six (9.0%) formerly engaged in smoking, while 8 (2.0%) were currently smoking Table 2 shows the association between socio-demographic factors and PSQ 1 scores. Marital status (p-value .020) and ethnicity (p-value .053) were significant.

Table 3 shows that the overall sleep quality was very good, fairly good, fairly bad, and very bad in 30.8%, 33.2%, 19.5%, and 16.5% of the subjects respectively.

Table 4 shows the association between blood pressure, depression, body mass index and psqi among the subjects, at the family practice clinic.

Figure 1 evaluates the Pittsburgh Sleep Quality Index Score. Two hundred and twenty four (56%) scored ≤ 5 indicating good sleepers, while 176 (44.0%) scored >5 indicated poor sleepers.

Discussion

The prevalence of poor sleep quality among the subjects was 44%. This was consistence with Suen and co-workers [20], in the US, who reported 42% and also similar to the findings of Krishna and colleagues with the prevalence of 42% [21], but higher than the CDC surveillance report of 35.3% [22] and the findings of Bawo and co-workers, at a Nigerian University with 32.5% [14], On the other hand, the result was lower than Seblewngel and colleagues [23], who found that the prevalence of poor sleep quality was 55.8%, Cheng et al. [24], who reported 54.7% and Adewole et al. while studying sleep disorders and sleep quality among adult's patients presenting at the General Outpatients Department in ObafemiAwolowo University Teaching Hospital Complex (OAUTHC) in Nigeria, who reported prevalence of 50% [25].

The apparently high prevalence in this study may be attributed to lower health-related quality of life, low socio-economic status

Variable	Frequency	(%)	Mean	Std. Deviation
Age				
≤ 20	4	1.0	48.0	13.16
21-30	58	14.5		
31-40	64	16.0		
41-50	118	29.5		
51-60	100	25.0		
≥ 61	59	14.0		
Gender				
Male	96	24		
Female	304	76		
Ethnicity				
Hausa	8	2.0		
Yoruba	384	96.0		
Igbo	6	1.5		
Others	2	0.5		
Religion				
Christianity	46	11.5		
Islam	354	88.5		
Marital Status				
Married	250	62.5		
Single	24	6.0		
Divorced	14	3.5		
Separated	26	6.5		
Widow	82	20.5		
Widower	4	1.0		
Educational Level				
Non-formal	238	59.5		
Primary	48	12.0		
Secondary	62	15.5		
Tertiary	52	13.0		
Occupation				
Trader	156	39.0		
Civil Servant	56	14.0		
Self Employed	126	31.0		
Unemployed	50	24.0		
Student	12	76.0		
Alcohol Intake				
Yes	30	7.5		
No	370	92.5		
Smoking Status				
Never	356	89.0		
Former	36	9.0		
Current	8	2.0		

Table 1: Socio-Demographic Characteristics of The Respondents.

and concomitant poor medical conditions, and to snoring which is common among hypertensive subjects in South Western Nigeria [26]. In addition, it could also results from Obstructive sleep apnea (OSA) was high in Nigeria [27]. In this study, the overall sleep quality was very good, fairly good, fairly bad, very bad in 30.8%, 33.2%, 19.5%, and 16.5% of the subjects respectively. This result was higher than that of Vivek et al. [28], in Banasthali University Rajasthan, India, where distribution of sleep quality were excellent 20.4%, good 38.5%, satisfactory 35.8%, poor 4%, very poor, 1.3%.

Seblewengel et al. found out that approximately 25% had very good and 60% fairly good overall sleep quality [23].

Consistent with previous studies [29,30], poor sleep quality was associated with depression [31,32]. Depression was significantly associated with sleep complaints; a finding that was consistent with previous reports [33]. The relationship between depression and sleep disturbances was so strong that it was one of the diagnostic criteria of major depression [34]. High degree of depression and anxiety were found to be the influencing factors of poor sleep among Chinese adolescents [35].

There was a strong statistical association between body mass index and PSQI Score. Obese class 3 was poor sleepers. This was similar to the finding of Pearson et al. [36] who found that obese patient had difficulty with sleep. This result was consistence to the findings of Anne et al. [37]. However Abdul Salam et al. [12] found no significant correlation between age, weight, height and BMI.

Several studies had indicated that insufficient sleep, less than five or six hours were associated with weight gain [38]. The result of this study contrasted with Watson et al. [38] who found no relationship between subjective sleep quality and BMI and to Aylin et al. [30] who found no significant relationship between body measurement and PSQI scores

Variables	PSQI SCORES		Total	p-value
	<=5	>5		
Age Groups				
<=20	3	1	4	.775
21-30	35	23	58	
31-40	33	31	64	
41-50	62	56	118	
51-60	59	41	100	
>=61	32	24	56	
Total	224	176	400	
Sex				
Male	48	48	96	.174
Female	176	128	304	
Total	224	176	400	
Ethnicity Hausa	3	5	8	.053
Yoruba	220	164	384	
Igbo	1	5	6	
Others	0	2	2	
Total	224	176	400	
Religion				
Christianity	22	24	46	.235
Islam	202	152	354	
Total	224	176	400	
Marital Status				
Married	149	101	250	.020
Single	7	17	24	
Divorced	11	3	14	
Separated	11	15	26	
Widow	44	38	82	
Widower	2	2	4	
Total	224	176	400	
Level of Education				
Non-formal	135	103	238	.547
Primary	23	25	48	
Secondary	38	24	62	
Tertiary	28	24	52	
Total	224	176	400	
Occupation				
Trader	94	62	156	.398
Civil Servant	27	29	56	
Self Employed	68	58	126	
Unemployed	30	20	50	
Student	5	7	12	
Total	224	176	400	

Table 2: Association between Socio Demographic Factors and Psqi Scores at the Family Practice Clinic.

Sleep Quality	Frequency	(%)
Very good	123	30.8
Fairly good	133	33.2
Fairly bad	78	19.5
Very bad	66	16.5
Total	400	100

Table 3: Subjective Sleep Quality.

Variables	PSQI SCORES		Total	p-value
	<=5	>5		
Blood Pressure Normal	150	90	240	.002
Pre-HTN	46	42	88	
Stage 1	9	20	29	
Stage 2	19	24	43	
Total	224	176	400	
Depression Minimal Depression	212	129	341	.000
Mild Depression	12	42	54	
Moderate Depression	0	2	2	
Severe Depression	0	3	3	
Total	224	176	400	
Body Mass Index Moderate thinness	0	4	4	.045
Mild thinness	9	11	20	
Normal	84	54	138	
Pre-obese	72	58	130	
Obese class 1	38	34	72	
Obese class 2	15	5	20	
Obese class 3	6	10	16	
Total	224	176	400	

Table 4: Association between Blood Pressure, Depression, Body Mass Index and Psqi among the Subjects, At the Family Practice Clinic.

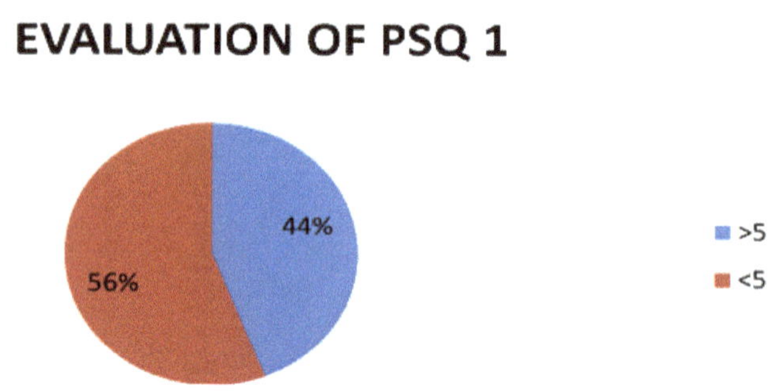

Figure 1: Evaluation of Psq 1.

[39]. Also, Van and Knutson [40] found no association between sleep quality and BMI.

In this study, there was statistical association between high blood pressure and PSQI (p-value = .002). Pooja et al. [9] found out that among people with both sleep disorder and short sleep, the likelihood of hypertension was slightly more than twice that for people with no sleep problems. This relationship may, in part, be the result of biologic mechanisms, suggesting that sleep deprivation may alter cortisol stress hormones and the sympathetic nervous system, resulting in elevated BP. In the sleep Heart Health Study, subjects sleeping ≤5 h/night had a higher frequency of prevalent hypertension [41] The Whitehall II [42] study also found that, women sleeping ≤ 5h/night had a higher risk of hypertension compared with those sleeping 7 h/night.

Conclusion

A large proportion of adults, attending the Kwara State Specialist Hospital, Ilorin Nigeria are poor sleepers with associated hypertension, depression and increased body mass index. Taking into account that poor sleep quality has major negative long term impact on health, prevention programs should be put in place.

References

1. Guilleminault C, Brooks SN (2001) Excessive daytime sleepiness: a challenge for the practicing neurologist. Brain 124: 1482-1491.
2. Buysse DJ, Reynolds CF 3rd, Monk TH, Berman SR, Kupfer DJ (1989) The Pittsburgh Sleep Quality Index: a new instrument for psychiatric practice and research. Psychiatry Res 28: 193-213.
3. Mellinger GD, Balter MB, Uhlenhuth EH (1985) Insomnia and its treatment. Prevalence and correlates. Arch Gen Psychiatry 42: 225-232.
4. Kripke DF, Simons RN, Garfinkel L, Hammond EC (1979) Short and long sleep and sleeping pills. Is increased mortality associated? Arch Gen Psychiatry 36: 103-116.
5. National sleep foundation (2012) How much sleep do we need? And how much sleep are we getting?
6. Karacan I, Thornby JI, Williams RL (1983) Sleep/Wake Disorders: natural History, Epidemiology, and Long-Term Evolution. New York: Raven Press, 37-60.
7. Oluwole OS (2010) Sleep habits in Nigerian undergraduates. Acta Neurol Scand 121: 1-6.
8. Dregan A, Armstrong D (2010) Adolescence sleep disturbances as predictors of adulthood sleep disturbances--a cohort study. J Adolesc Health 46: 482-487.
9. Bansil P, Kuklina EV, Merritt RK, Yoon PW (2011) Association between sleep disorders, sleep duration, quality of sleep and hypertension: results from the National Health and Nutrition Examination Survey, 2005 to 2008. J Chin Hypertens (Greenwich) 13:739-743.
10. Kawada T (2012) Quality of sleep, Sleep duration and depressive state. The Journal of Clinical Hypertension14: 479-82.
11. Patel SR, Malhotra A, White DP, Gottlieb DJ, Hu FB (2006) Association between reduced sleep and weight gain in women. Am J Epidemiol 164: 947-954.
12. Abdulsalam, Salman MT, Gupta S, Trivedi M, Farooqi M (2013) Poor quality of sleep and its relationship with depression in first year medical students. Advances in life science and technology 12: 17-21.
13. Araoye MO (2003) Data Collection in: Research methodology with statistics for health and social sciences. Nathadex Publishers130-159.
14. James BO, Omoaregba JO, Igberase OO (2011) Prevalence and correlates of poor sleep quality among medical students at a Nigerian university. Annals of Nigerian Medicine 5:1-4.
15. Shochat T, Tzischinsky O, Oksenberg A, Peled R (2007) Validation of the Pittsburgh Sleep Quality Index Hebrew translation (PSQI-H) in a sleep clinic sample. Isr Med Assoc J 9: 853-856.
16. Kroenke K, Spitzer RL, Williams JB (2003) The Patient Health Questionnaire-2: validity of a two-item depression screener. Med Care 41: 1284-1292.
17. Spitzer RL, Williams JB, Kroenke K, Linzer M, deGruy FV 3rd, et al. (1994) Utility of a new procedure for diagnosing mental disorders in primary care. The PRIME-MD 1000 study. JAMA272: 1749-1756.
18. Kroenke K, Spitzer RL, Williams JB (2001) The PHQ-9: validity of a brief depression severity measure. J Gen Intern Med 16: 606-613.
19. Chobanian AV, Bakris, GL, Black HR, Cushman WC, Green LA, et al. (2003) The Seventh Report of the Joint National Committee on Prevention, Detection, Evaluation and Treatment of High Blood Pressure: the JNC 7 report. JAMA 289: 2560-2572.

20. Suen LK, Hon KL, Tam WW (2008) Association between sleep behavior and sleep-related factors among university students in Hong Kong. ChronobiolInt 25:760-775.

21. Pushpa K, Shwetha S (2008) Sleep quality and correlates of sleep among medical students. The Indian Journal of Sleep Medicine. 3: 58-61.

22. CDC (2014) Youth Risk Behaviour Surveillance (YRBSS).

23. Lemma S, Gelaye B, Berhane Y, Worku A, Williams MA (2012) Sleep quality and its psychological correlates among university students in Ethiopia: a cross-sectional study.BMC Psychiatry 12: 237.

24. Cheng SH, Shih CC, Lee IH, Hou YW, Chen KC, et al. (2012) A study on the sleep quality of incoming university students. Psychiatry Res 197: 270-274.

25. Adewole TO, KuteyiBA,Ezeoma I, Bello I (2013) Sleep disorders and sleep quality among adults patients presenting at a General Outpatient Department in Ile Ife, Nigeria- A preliminary report. European Respiratory Society. 12: 50-54.

26. Alebiosu OC, Ogunsemi OO, Familoni OB, Adebayo PB, Ayodele OE (2009) Quality of sleep among hypertensive patients in a semi-urban Nigerian community: a prospective study. Postgrad Med 121: 166-172.

27. Akintunde AA, Okunola OO, Oluyombo R, Oladosu YO, Opadijo OG (2012) Snoring and obstructive sleep apnoea syndrome among hypertensive Nigerians: prevalence and clinical correlates. Pan Afr Med J 11: 75.

28. Jain V, Tomar R, Jha J, Pareek A, Ratan Y, et al. (2013) Sleep quality and sleep associated problems in female pharmacy students. Chronicles of young scientists 4: 138-143.

29. Moo-Estrella J, Pérez-Benítez H, Solís-Rodríguez F, Arankowsky-Sandoval G (2005) Evaluation of depressive symptoms and sleep alterations in college students. Arch Med Res 36: 393-398.

30. Eller T, Aluoja A, Vasar V, Veldi M (2006) Symptoms of anxiety and depression in Estonian medical students with sleep problems. Depress Anxiety 23: 250-256.

31. Breslau N, Roth T, Rosenthal L, Andreski P (1996) Sleep disturbance and psychiatric disorders: a longitudinal epidemiological study of young adults. Biol Psychiatry 39: 411-418.

32. Sahraian A, Javadopur A (2010) Sleep disruption and its correlation to psychological distress among medical students. Med J 11: 12-17.

33. Ford DE, Kamerow DB (1989) Epidemiologic study of sleep disturbances and psychiatric disorders. An opportunity for prevention? JAMA 262: 1479-1484.

34. American Psychiatric Association (1994) Diagnostic and statistical manual of mental disorders, (4thedn), Text Revision (DSM-IV-TR).

35. Xu Z, Su H, Zou Y, Chen J, Wu J, et al. (2012) Sleep quality of Chinese adolescents: distribution and its associated factors. J Paediatr Child Health 48: 138-145.

36. Pearson NJ, Johnson LL, Nahin RL (2006) Insomnia, trouble sleeping, and complementary and alternative medicine: Analysis of the 2002 national health interview survey data. Arch Intern Med 166: 1775-1782.

37. Hayley AC, Williams LJ, Berk M, Kennedy GA, Jacka FN, et al. (2013) The relationship between excessive daytime sleepiness and depression and anxiety disorders in women. Aust NZ J Psychiatry 47: 772-778.

38. Watson NF, Harden P, Buchwald D, Schur E, Goldberg J (2011) Sleep duration modifies the heritability of body mass index. Poster presented at the Annual Meeting of the association Professional Sleep Societies.

39. Aylin A, Esra AK, Duygu O (2012) Pittsburgh sleep quality index score and its relationship between body measurements in late menopause patients.

40. Van Cauter E, Knutson KL (2008) Sleep and the epidemic of obesity in children and adults. Eur J Endocrinol 159 Suppl 1: S59-66.

41. Gottlieb DJ, Redline S, Nieto FJ, Baldwin CM, Newman AB, et al. (2006) Association of usual sleep duration with hypertension: the Sleep Heart Health Study. Sleep 29: 1009-1014.

42. Cappuccio FP, Stranges S, Kandala NB, Miller MA, Taggart FM, et al. (2007) Gender-specific associations of short sleep duration with prevalent and incident hypertension: the Whitehall II Study. Hypertension 50: 693-700.

4

Benefits of Thalassotherapy with Sleep Management on Mood States and Well-being, and Cognitive and Physical Capacities in Healthy Workers

Mounir Chennaoui[1,2*], Danielle Gomez-Merino[1,2], Pascal Van Beers[1,2], Mathias Guillard[1,2], Catherine Drogou[1,2], Didier Lagarde[2] and Clément Bougard[1,2]

[1] *Institut de Recherche Biomédicale des Armées (IRBA), Département Environnements Opérationnels, 91223 Brétigny sur Orge, France*

[2] *Université Paris Descartes, Hôtel Dieu, EA7330 VIFASOM (Vigilance Fatigue et Sommeil), 75004 Paris, France*

[*] **Corresponding author:** Mounir Chennaoui, PhD, Institut de Recherche Biomédicale des Armées (IRBA), Département Environnements Opérationnels, 91223 Brétigny sur Orge, France and Université Paris Descartes, Hôtel Dieu, EA7330 VIFASOM (Vigilance Fatigue et Sommeil), 75004 Paris, France,
E-mail: mounirchennaoui@gmail.com

Abstract

Objective: Thalassotherapy, which combines seawater hydrotherapy and the marine climate, improves mood, fatigue, general well-being, and physical capacities in the working population, but little is known on the interest to add sleep management to cares. We investigated effects of three days of thalassotherapy cares combined with sleep management on psychological and physical capacities using subjective and objective tests in healthy workers.

Methods: Cares were undertaken in the morning after tests (10:15-12:15) and in the afternoon (14:15-16:15). Participants were asked to go to sleep from 22:30 to 07:00. Tests were performed at 09:00 before arriving to the resort (T0), the day after arrival (T1), the days following cares (T2, T3, T4), the day after week-end at home (T5) and after three days working (T6).

Results: Polysomnographic sleep analysis showed that Total Sleep Time was significantly higher (+6%) the second night compared to the first, indicating an immediate positive effect of hydrotherapy cares. Self-reported mood states and health outcomes scores were improved at T2 in comparison with T1 (-67% for total mood disturbances, -17% for anxiety, -71% for fatigue, +23% for general well-being), as was daytime sleepiness (-26%). The number of lapses in the Psychomotor Vigilance Test (as objective marker of sustained attention) was significantly lower (-59%) at T2 compared to T1, whereas a delayed increase of lower limb flexibility was observed at T4 compared to T1 (+38%).

Conclusion: Three days of thalassotherapy combined to sleep management have immediate beneficial effects on self-reported mood states, anxiety, fatigue, well-being and daytime sleepiness, as well as on the objective evaluation of sustained attention, in healthy workers. Beneficial effects on lower limb flexibility are observed after 3 days of cares. Positive effects were still observed after the weekend back home and after 3 days of return to work.

Keywords: Thalassotherapy; Sleep; Psychological state; Sustained attention; Flexibility

Introduction

In western countries, professionally active populations (e.g. health care professions, drivers, soldiers) are prone to sleep loss with daytime sleepiness, fatigue, mood disorder, and cognitive deficits [1,2]. Several approaches are available for improving sleep and general well-being and fatigue, and there has been a growing interest in this last decade for treatments in health thalassotherapy resorts both in healthy subjects with non-specific disorders and in patients with defined health conditions [3]. Thalassotherapy is a therapy that is linked to the sea and is one of the most important of the climatotherapeutic methods. It refers to a combination of different techniques, including hydrotherapy (pool, baths, showers, and saunas), balneotherapy, spas, aquatic exercises, massages supervised by physiotherapists [3]. The duration of the sessions and the temperature of the water may vary between treatments [4,5].

The cares in health resorts can be applied to different groups of people, e.g. healthy subjects, persons with non-specific disorders and patients with defined health conditions [3]. Stays in thalassotherapy resorts are currently proposed with a limited number of cares (healthcare) selected for their specific actions. Thus, it has been evidenced that sea water exercises bring more advantages related to emotional aspects when compared to water pool in women with fibromyalgia [6]. Moreover, the warmth and buoyancy of water reduces pressure on the bones, joints and muscles which may facilitate movement and may block nociception by acting on thermal receptors and mechanoreceptors [7]. Warm water causes peripheral vasodilatation, a reduction in vascular resistance, enhances cardiac output and stroke volume which may dissipate algogenic chemicals and facilitate muscle relaxation [8]. In accordance with these principles, it has been shown that in the case of various pathologies or aging, thalassotherapy can improve flexibility, postural control, and articular amplitude, contribute to tissues detoxification, which may last for several weeks [3].

Relative to the interest of hydrotherapy for sleep, Horne, et al. [9] evidenced, using EEG recording, an increase of sleepiness at bed-time, and increases of N3, N4 and reduction of REM sleep after 90 min of passive body heating in a warm bath (41°C) in young healthy women. The spa resort and balneotherapy use are also beneficial for health-related quality of life, sleep, sickness absence, and fatigue in the working population [10-12] but this has been reported mainly after several weeks of cares. Frequent spa resort users (a large population of 3341 employees) were more likely to have better quality of sleep, and better physical and mental health [10]. Vitorino et al. [13] also already reported, using sleep logs data, an improvement in TST (by at least 1 hour) and quality of life in fibromyalgia patients after three weeks of hydrotherapy care (60 min per day, three times per week). Recently, a 12-day balneotherapy programme was found to improve significantly pain, mood state, sleep and depression (all through questionnaires and VAS scales) in healthy elderly [14]. A 3-week resort-based spa therapy was found to improve quality of sleep, fatigue, distress, reduced motivation, in working individuals with mild burnout (i.e. increased emotional exhaustion) and individuals with a full burnout syndrome (i.e. increased exhaustion plus social detachment and/or performance dissatisfaction) [15]. However, polysomnographic sleep and cognitive capacities have been only weakly studied. Being constantly exposed to professional and family constraints, workers may suffer from insufficient rest and reduced daily sleep time [16]. This chronic sleep debt and repeated sleep/wake cycle disturbances induced behavioral changes (diurnal sleepiness, anxiety, fatigue) and impairments of cognitive and physical capacities (decreases of sustained attention and physical capacity, increase of mistakes, fatigue, pain, etc) [17,18]. Implementing a sleep extension programme was recently shown to improve sleep and sustained attention with beneficial changes in stress hormone expression among professional athletes [19].

The aim of this study was to evaluate the effects of 3 days of thalassotherapy cares combined with sleep management in a thalassotherapy resort (Saint-Malo, North Brittany, France, Les Thermes Marins) on objective and subjective measures of sleep, mood states, well-being, health outcomes and cognitive (sustained attention) and physical capacities in healthy middle-aged workers.

Subjects and Methods

Subjects

After being informed of the procedures, 11 healthy workers (7 men and 4 women; age: 41.1 ± 11.9 years) were volunteer to take part in the experiment. They all signed an informed consent before being included in this study which is conformed to The Code of Ethics of the World Medical Association (Declaration of Helsinki) for experiments involving humans. The study was reviewed and approved by the local Institutional Review Board of the medical committee.

Exclusion criteria were as follows: to not present an extreme chronotype (moderately morning=4, intermediate=3, moderately evening=3) based on the Horne and Östberg questionnaire (1976) [20] nor any sleep troubles (PSQI scores<6) [21], to not suffer from excessive diurnal sleepiness (Epworth scores<11) [22], and to not use nap during the day. Participants were nonsmokers, had no medical treatment, and did not suffer from an articular or functional disease (rheumatoid arthritis, osteoarthritis…).

Protocol Design

After the inclusion visit, participants remained working during 2 weeks. During this period, they wore a wrist activity monitor (Actiwatch7, CamNtech2008®, Cambridge Neurotechnology, Cambridge, Cambridgeshire, UK) and filled out a sleep diary to control sleep/wake activity rhythm. At the end of this period (Thursday), they come to the laboratory to spend one night with electrophysiological recording of nocturnal sleep (Night 0 as a baseline night) followed the day after, between 9:00 to 10:00, by the first testing (T0 as baseline) (detailed further) (corresponding to D-3, 3 days before the transfer to the thalassotherapy resort). Then, participants spend the weekend at home, and on Monday (D1) they moved for thalassotherapy cares (3 days) in Saint-Malo, North Brittany, France (Les Thermes Marins). Participants arrived in the afternoon at the resort and spent the first night (Night 1) without having received any cares. The day after and during 3 days (D2, D3 and D4), they were submitted to the test battery (T1, T2, and T3) (from 9:00 to 10:00) followed by hydrotherapy cares (detailed further) (H1, H2, and H3) from 10:15 to 12:15 and from 14:15 to 16:15. After the fourth night (Night 4) and after completion of the last test session (T4) in the morning, participants returned to their home for the week-end and came back next day to the laboratory (D8) for tests in the morning (T5). Then, after working 3 days (D9 to D11), participants had to complete the last morning tests session (T6) at D12. During the four nights in the resort, the participants were instructed to have sleep opportunity by staying in bed between 22:30 and 07:00 (510 min). From living the thalassotherapy resort to D12, participants wore a wrist activity monitor and filled out a sleep diary (Figure 1).

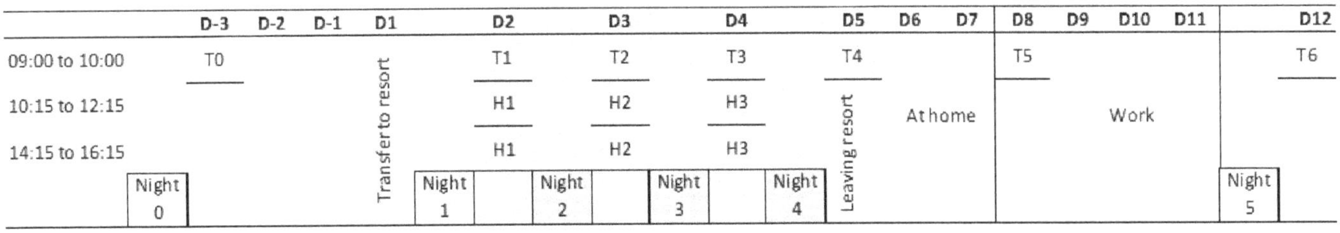

Figure 1: Protocol design. D-3 is the baseline day (3 days before transfer to the thalassotherapy resort); D1 is day of transfer; D2 to D4 are days with cares; D5 day leaving the resort; D6 and D7 are week-end at home; D9 to D11 working days; and D12 the last day with tests. T0 to T6: tests between 09:00 and 10:00; H1 to H3: hydrotherapy cares between 10:15 and 12:15 and between 14:15 and 16:15. The stay in the resort is in gray

During the two weeks of work before beginning the protocol, and during returning at home and working after the thalassotherapy stay, the mean of the total sleep time (according to wrist actigraphy and sleep diaries) of the participants was 347 ± 57 min and 345 ± 67 min.

Hydrotherapy treatments

During the three days of treatments, the participants received 4 different cares each day, determined by the technical staff. Thalassotherapy treatments in the Saint-Malo resort involve hydrotherapy treatments with warm seawater (31°C-34°C). On H1, they had a marine draining (12 min), underwater showerheads, pool with lombar jets (15 min) and modelling under affusions (25 min). On H2, the participants had a jets bath with essential oils (20 min), dynamic affusions (15 min), seaweed body wrap (25 min), aquarelaxing. On H3, they had a marine draining, underwater showerheads (15 min), pool with cervical jets (15 min) and modelling under affusions. In addition, during the half-day of cares, the participants had an unlimited open access to an aquatonic® pool, hammam, sauna and a sea mist room.

Measurements

Nocturnal sleep: Sleep parameters were analyzed by polysomnographic (EEG, EMG, EOG and EKG) recordings [23] using miniaturized multi-channel ambulatory devices (Actiwave®, CamNtech Ltd England) during the baseline night (Night 0), the four nights in the resort (Nights 1, 2, 3, 4), and the night after 3 days of recovery and 3 days of work (Night 5). Bio-electrical signals were digitized at a sampling frequency of 200 Hz with a 16-bit quantization between −500 and 500 μV, within a bandwidth of 0-48 Hz. All the data were stored into computer files using the standard EDF data format.

Daytime sleepiness: The subjective feeling of diurnal sleepiness was measured by the Karolinska Sleepiness Scale (KSS) [24]. The dependent measure was the subject's sleepiness rating. This scale was completed during test sessions at T0, T1, T2, T3, T4, T5, and T6.

Mood states and fatigue assessment: The POMS-f (French version) is a 65-item questionnaire measuring six mood states (Tension, Depression, Anger, Vigor, Fatigue, Confusion) on a 5-point Likert scale, in relation to the context [25]. The Total Mood Disturbance [(Tension+Depression+Anger+Fatigue+Confusion)−Vigor] was calculated. In addition, the raw scores for each item were analyzed to further investigate changes in mood states.

The subjective feeling of fatigue was measured using the Pichot's questionnaire which consisted in 8 items rated from 0 (not at all) to 4 (extremely) [26]. The sum of the different items was retained for analysis.

Anxiety and depression: The Hospital Anxiety and Depression (HAD) questionnaire was used which comprised 14 items, 7 items related to anxiety and 7 related to depression [27]. Each item of the questionnaire is scored from 0 to 3. The summed score for each symptom was retained for analysis.

Visual analog scales: Relaxation, perceived soreness, well-being were evaluated using visual analog scales [6]. Participants had to estimate these 3 dimensions by placing a cursor on a 10 cm line. Each scale was defined with an adjective at each extremity (0 cm=Not at all; 10 cm=extremely). The higher the scores for relaxation and well-being, the better for health. In contrast, the lower the scores for perceived soreness, the better for health.

Sustained attention: The 3-min Psychomotor Vigilance Task (PVT-Brief version) [28] was performed at T0, T1, T2, T3, T4, T5, and T6. The inter-stimulus intervals varied randomly from 1-4 sec. Subjects were instructed to press the response button as soon as each stimulus appeared, in order to keep RT as low as possible, but not to press the button too soon (which yielded a false start warning on the display). An auditory signal was given after a 30-sec period without response. Lapse definition for the 3-min PVT was adjusted from the standard ≥ 500 ms definition to ≥ 355 ms. The number of lapses was considered as the primary PVT outcome metric.

Flexibility: The lower-limb posterior chain flexibility was measured through the sit-and-reach test [29]. The subjects were requested to carry out a maximal flexion of the spine so as to push the cursor located on a graduated scale on the top of the box as far as possible, using the index finger of each hand. The scale was graded from -20 to 30 cm with 0 corresponding to foot level and -20 cm corresponding to the maximal level of flexibility. The final position was to be maintained for at least 2 sec so that the measurement could be validated.

Vertical jump capacity: It was determined using the counter-movement jump (CMJ) test [30]. Flight time and jump height were measured using an Optojump® device (Microgate, Bolzano, Italy). The participants had to perform jumps from an upright standing position while performing a countermovement to reach a knee angle of about 90°. 3 trials were realized with the hands positioned on the waist and with a 20 sec pause between successive trials. The highest of the 3 jumps was selected for analysis.

Statistical analysis

The different scores at the questionnaires and scales (KSS, Pichot, HAD, POMS, VAS), the parameters for sustained attention, flexibility and vertical jump were analyzed using a Friedman ANOVA with repeated measures as were the nocturnal sleep parameters. In case of significance, a Wilcoxon test was performed to evidence pairwise differences. To examine the relationships between parameters, the Spearman's rank correlation coefficient was used. Results are described as means ± SEM for each assessment. All statistical differences were considered as significant for a p-value<0.05. All statistical analysis was performed using Statistica software® v.10 (Statsoft Inc, France).

Results

Nocturnal sleep

Significant increases for time in bed (TIB) ($\chi 2$=26.79; p<0.001), sleep period time (SPT) ($\chi 2$=26.85; p<0.001), and total sleep time (TST) ($\chi 2$=29.55; p<0.001) were observed (20% for TST during the first night at the resort (Night 1 compared to Night 0) and 6% more during the second night following hydrotherapy cares (Night 2 compared to Night 1) (Table 1).

Considering sleep stages (Table 1), N2 sleep duration significantly increased ($\chi 2$=14.71; p<0.05) in Night 1 (Z=2.59; p<0.01) and Night 2 (Z=2.80; p<0.01) in comparison with Night 0. N3 sleep duration also increased ($\chi 2$=18.63; p<0.01) in Night 2 (Z=2.19; p<0.05), Night 3 (Z=2.39; p<0.05) and Night 4 (Z=1.99; p<0.05) compared with Night 0. In contrast, no significant effect was observed on Sleep onset latency (SOL) ($\chi 2$=5.29; p=0.38), N1 sleep duration ($\chi 2$=4.14; p=0.53) and Rapid eye movement (REM) sleep ($\chi 2$=8.04; p=0.15). In addition, these changes appeared without any modification of sleep architecture as no significant effect was observed on sleep stages percent [N1 sleep percent ($\chi 2$=4.14; p=0.53), N2 sleep percent ($\chi 2$=6.20; p=0.29), N3 sleep percent ($\chi 2$=6.40; p=0.27), REM sleep percent ($\chi 2$=2.48; p=0.78)].

	Night 0	Night 1	Night 2	Night 3	Night 4	Night 5
TIB (min)	416 ± 19	475 ± 9*	497± 8*§	486 ± 11*	477 ± 9*	447 ± 9§
SPT (min)	405 ± 19	463 ± 10*	488 ± 10*§	477 ± 11*	465 ± 10	438 ± 11
TST (min)	358 ± 15	428 ± 13*	455 ± 11*§	443 ± 12*	429 ± 11*	391 ± 19§
SOL (min)	10.5 ± 1.9	11.8 ± 2.1	8.1 ± 2.7	9.1 ± 1.5	11.3 ± 5.2	8.8 ± 2.3
WASO (min)	48 ± 11	35 ± 8	33 ± 6	34 ± 8	36 ± 9	47 ± 12
SEI (%)	87 ± 3	90 ± 2	92 ± 1	91 ± 2	90 ± 2	87 ± 3
N1 (min)	25 ± 5	22 ± 3	25 ± 3	27 ± 4	22 ± 4	21 ± 2
(% TST)	5.8 ± 0.9	4.6 ± 0.7	5.0 ± 0.6	5.5 ± 0.8	4.6 ± 0.8	4.6 ± 0.5
N2 (min)	166 ± 15	217 ± 10*	214 ± 11*	200 ± 12	198 ± 13	191 ± 11
(% TST)	46 ± 3	51 ± 2	47 ± 2	45 ± 2	46 ± 3	49 ± 2
N3 (min)	77 ± 7	97 ± 11	99 ± 9*	104 ± 9*	102 ± 9*	78 ± 9
(% TST)	22 ± 3	23 ± 2	22 ± 2	23 ± 2	24 ± 2	20 ± 2
REM (min)	91 ± 7	92 ± 9	117 ± 10	113 ± 7	107 ± 9	102 ± 12
(% TST)	25 ± 2	21 ± 2	26 ± 2	25 ± 2	25 ± 2	25 ± 2

Table 1: Sleep parameters. At baseline (Night 0), the first night in the thalassotherapy resort (Night 1), the first, second, and third night after hydrotherapy cares (Nights 2, 3 and 4) and the night after week-end at home followed by three days at work (Night 5). TIB: time in bed, SPT: sleep period time, TST: total sleep time, SOL: sleep-onset latency, WASO: wake after sleep onset, SEI: sleep efficiency index, N1, N2, N3, REM (non-rapid eye movement and rapid eye movement) sleep stages. * p<0.05): significant difference with Night 0; § p<0.05: significant difference with Night 1. N=11, Means ± SEM. Nights in the resort are in gray.

Daytime sleepiness

Daytime subjective sleepiness was significantly influenced by the thalassotherapy stay ($\chi2$=29.94; p<0.001). More precisely, KSS scores decreased at T3 and T4 (Z=2.37; p<0.05 and Z=2.52; p<0.05, respectively) and were still reduced at T5 (Z=2.80; p<0.01), and T6 (Z=2.66; p<0.01) in comparison with T0 (Table 2). Moreover, the participants felt less sleepy at T2, T3, T4, T5 and T6 compared with T1 (p<0.05) (26% less at T2).

Mood states and fatigue

The total mood disturbance (TMD) score obtained in the POMS questionnaire significantly improved throughout the stay in the thalassotherapy resort ($\chi2$=40.58; p<0.001) (Table 2). We observed a progressive and persistent improvement in TMD until T6 in comparison with T0 (p<0.05) and T1 (-67% at T2 compared to T1). Until T6, negative items Confusion, Anger, Depression and Fatigue were lower than T0 (p<0.001) (Table 2). The scores for Confusion were also significantly lower at T3 (Z=2.66; p<0.01) and T4 (Z=2.24; p<0.05) than at T1. The scores for Depression were lower at T2 (Z=2.80; p<0.01), T3 (Z=2.37; p<0.05), T4 (Z=2.31; p<0.05) and T5 (Z=2.66; p<0.01) than at T1. The scores for Anger were also lower at from T2 (Z=2.10; p<0.05), T3 (Z=2.66; p<0.01), T4 (Z=2.66; p<0.01), T5 (Z=2.38; p<0.05) and T6 (Z=2.43; p<0.05) than at T1. The scores for Fatigue were significantly lower at T3 (Z=2.65; p<0.01), T4 (Z=2.37; p<0.05), T5 (Z=2.70; p<0.01), T6 (Z=2.84; p<0.01). As for vigor (Z=20.61; p<0.01), an improvement was observed at T3 (Z=2.24; p<0.05) and T5 (Z=2.93; p<0.01) in comparison with T0. Moreover, vigor scores were improved from T2 (Z=2.45; p<0.05) to T6 (Z=2.04; p<0.05) in comparison with T1.

The scores obtained in the fatigue Pichot questionnaire were significantly influenced by the thalassotherapy stay ($\chi2$=28.32; p<0.001). More precisely, post-hoc comparisons indicated that the participants felt less tired since T2 until T6 in comparison with T0 (p<0.05) (Table 2). Moreover, the scores at T2 (Z=2.44; p<0.05), T3 (Z=2.93; p<0.01), T4 (Z=2.70; p<0.01), T5 (Z=2.80; p<0.01), T6 (Z=2.80; p<0.01) were significantly lower than at T1 (-71% at T2).

Anxiety and depression

The scores for anxiety obtained in the HAD questionnaire were significantly changed by the stay in the thalassotherapy resort ($\chi2$=15.21; p<0.05) (Table 2). Post-hoc comparisons indicated that anxiety was reduced from T2 to T6 in comparison with T0 (p<0.05). Moreover, anxiety was also reduced at T2 (Z=2.03; p<0.05), T3 (Z=2.07; p<0.05), T5 (Z=2.19; p<0.05), T6 (Z=2.19; p<0.05) in comparison with T1 (-17% for T2). Depression scores were also significantly impacted by the thalassotherapy stay ($\chi2$=18.64; p<0.01). The Wilcoxon comparisons reported that depression scores were lower at T4 (Z=2.07; p<0.05), T5 (Z=2.49; p<0.05) and T6 (Z=2.24; p<0.05) in comparison with T1.

		T0	T1	T2	T3	T4	T5	T6
KSS	Daytime sleepiness	5.1 ± 0.5	5.3 ± 0.7	3.9 ± 0.6 §	3.8 ± 0.4* §	3.6 ± 0.4* §	3.2 ± 0.5* §	3.6 ± 0.4* §
POMS	Confusion	6.5 ± 0.7	4.9 ± 0.6*	3.8 ± 0.4*	3.3 ± 0.3* §	3.5 ± 0.5* §	3.6 ± 0.3*	3.5 ± 0.5*
	Anger	11.5 ± 2.3	8.8 ± 1.7*	4.6 ± 0.9* §	3.6 ± 0.7* §	4.6 ± 1.0* §	4.5 ± 1.1* §	5.0 ± 1.3* §
	Depression	3.8 ± 1.1	4.0 ± 1.2	1.4 ± 0.5* §	1.4 ± 0.4* §	1.2 ± 0.4* §	1.4 ± 0.4* §	1.9 ± 0.9*
	Fatigue	11.2 ± 1.3	8.7 ± 1.4	6.4 ± 1.6*	3.5 ± 0.5* §	3.1 ± 0.8* §	1.9 ± 0.7* §	2.0 ± 0.4* §
	Tension	8.1 ± 1.3	6.4 ± 0.8	5.3 ± 0.8	5.4 ± 0.5	5.4 ± 0.6	5.4 ± 1.2	4.7 ± 0.7
	Vigor	14.6 ± 1.1	13.6 ± 1.3	15.2 ± 1.5 §	17.7 ± 1.0* §	17.7 ± 1.1 §	18.8 ± 1.1* §	17.6 ± 1.8 §
	Total mood disturbances	26.5 ± 4.8	19.2 ± 4.5*	6.3 ± 4.0* §	-0.7 ± 1.3* §	0.0 ± 2.6* §	-2 ± 2.5* §	-0.5 ± 3.5* §
PICHOT	Fatigue	6.8 ± 0.8	5.3 ± 0.8	3.1 ± 1.0* §	1.7 ± 0.5* §	2.1 ± 0.7* §	1.5 ± 0.7* §	1.7 ± 0.5* §
HADS	Anxiety	6.3 ± 0.8	5.8 ± 0.8	4.8 ± 0.8* §	4.5 ± 0.7* §	4.4 ± 0.9*	4.3 ± 1.0* §	3.7 ± 0.7* §
	Depression	3.2 ± 0.6	3.9 ± 0.8	2.9 ± 0.8	2.8 ± 0.7	2.4 ± 0.7 §	2.0 ± 0.7 §	2.3 ± 0.7 §
VAS	General well-being	57 ± 5	55 ± 5	71 ± 4* §	76 ± 4* §	75 ± 5* §	76 ± 4* §	73 ± 4* §
	Soreness	39 ± 11	32 ± 10	23 ± 8	32 ± 11	18 ± 8*	14 ± 7* §	18 ± 9*
	Relaxation	38 ± 8	43 ± 7	65 ± 6* §	76 ± 4* §	72 ± 6* §	68 ± 7* §	74 ± 3* §

Table 2: Psychological parameters; Scores at baseline (T0), the first, second, third and fourth days in the thalassotherapy resort (T1, T2, T3, T4), after week-end at home (T5) and after week-end at home followed by three days at work (T6). *p<0.05): significant difference with Night 0; §p<0.05: significant difference with Night 1. N=11, Means ± SEM. Nights in the resort are in gray.

General well-being, relaxation and perceived soreness

The general level of well-being of the participants obtained using VAS scales was influenced by the thalassotherapy stay ($\chi2$=25.67; p<0.001). They felt significantly better (p<0.05) since T2, which lasted until T6 in comparison with T0 and T1 (Table 2) (+23% at T2 compared to T1). They also felt more relaxed ($\chi2$=32.53; p<0.001) and this, more precisely from T2 to T6 in comparison with T0 and T1 (p<0.05). Finally, the subjective level of soreness ($\chi2$=22.49; p<0.001) were significantly lower at T4 compared to T0, and stay lower until T6 (p<0.05). Moreover, perceived soreness scores were also lower at T5 than at T1 (Z=2.31; p<0.05).

Sustained attention

The number of lapses observed in the PVT-B test was significantly influenced by the thalassotherapy stay ($\chi2$=24.66; p<0.001). Post-hoc comparisons indicated that the participants had less lapses from T2 to T6, in comparison with T0 and T1 (p<0.05) (Table 3). The participants had less lapses at T2 compared to T1 (-59%).

	T0	T1	T2	T3	T4	T5	T6
PVT Number of lapses	7.4 ± 1.8	9.4 ± 1.7	3.9 ± 1.1*§	2.9 ± 0.6*§	3.7 ± 1.4*§	4.2 ± 1.0*§	4.4 ± 1.3*§
Lower limb flexibility cm	-5.2 ± 2.9	-6.2 ± 3.1	-6.9 ± 3.1*	-9.1 ± 2.8*	-10.0 ± 2.9*§	-10.1 ± 2.5*§	-11.2 ± 2.5*§
Vertical jump cm	26 ± 3	25 ± 3*	26 ± 3	26 ± 3	27 ± 3	27 ± 3	27 ± 2§

Table 3: Cognitive (sustained attention through the Psychomotor vigilance test, PVT) and physical parameters. At baseline (T0), the first, second, third and fourth days in the thalassotherapy resort (T1, T2, T3, T4), after week-end at home (T5), and after week-end at home followed by three days at work (T6). *p<0.05): significant difference with Night 0; §p<0.05: significant difference with Night 1. N=11, Means ± SEM. Nights in the resort are in gray.

Lower-limb flexibility

The level of dorsal flexion of the participants, measured using the Sit-and-reach test, was significantly impacted by the days of experiment ($\chi2$=34.86; p<0.001). In comparison with T0 and T1, our results indicated a flexibility improvement particularly at T4, T5 and T6 (p<0.05) (Table 3). The participants were 38% more flexible at T4 compared to T1.

Vertical jump capacity

The level of vertical jump varied throughout our experiment (χ^2=14.03; p=0.03). The participants performed better at T1 compared to T0 (Z=2,09; p<0.05) (Table 3).

Correlation analysis between parameters

The change of TMD between T0 and T4 was positively correlated with the change of the number of lapses (r=0.68). The more TMD score in the POMS decreases, the more important was the decrease in the number of lapses. The evolution of the self-reported general well-being between T0 and T4 was positively associated with the vertical jump capacity (r=0.83). The change of perceived soreness between T0 and T4 was positively associated with the change of fatigue in the Pichot's questionnaire (r=0.77). The more important was the decrease in subjective soreness, the more important was the decrease in fatigue complaint. No other significant correlation was observed.

Discussion

This study showed for the first time that three days of thalassotherapy combined to sleep management have immediate and delayed beneficial effects in healthy workers. Sleep management consisted of asking participants to increase the opportunity to sleep while staying in bed between 22:30 and 07:00 during the four nights in the resort.

We showed that TST was significantly higher during the four nights in the resort compared to the baseline night (Night 0) and we also showed an additional effect of cares the second night compared to the first. This additional effect was not observed at nights 3 and 4, probably because subjects get used to the care or because their need for sleep has lessened. The TST increase during the four nights in comparison with the baseline night was mainly associated to an increase duration of N2 sleep stage during the first two nights (1 and 2) and to an increase of N3 duration at nights 2, 3 and 4 (by nearly 30%), while the REM paradoxical sleep as well as the sleep architecture were unchanged. Other sleep parameters such as sleep-onset latency (SOL) and duration of brief bouts of wake, known as Wake after Sleep Onset (WASO), and sleep efficiency have not been statistically changed. The N3 sleep, also known as slow-wave sleep, represents the deepest sleep stage of non-REM sleep, and has been proven vital for health and well-being, as well as cognitive functions and brain plasticity [31].

In our study, the higher TST at the first night at the resort (Night 1 compared to Night 0) was not followed by reduced daytime sleepiness (i.e., KSS scores) the day after (at T1 compared to T0). However, when TST was at its highest level (at Night 2) because of the combined effect of beginning cares during the day and night-time sleep opportunity, the subsequent daytime sleepiness (at T2 testing) dropped and are further decreased at T3 and T4. Beneficial effects of the thalassotherapy stay including cares on daytime sleepiness were always present at T5 and T6 (after returning home for the weekend home and after 3 days of work).

The thalassotherapy stay including cares and higher opportunity of sleep significantly improved the total mood disturbance (TMD) score in the Profile of mood states (POMS-f) questionnaire, and this was maintained back to home and work. The POMS has been developed to quickly and reliably define and evaluate situational and short-term changes in mood states [25]. For example, there is evidence suggesting a consistent decline in mood states during sleep restriction or during high level athletic competition [32]. As regards to POMS subscales, anger, depression and fatigue scores, there was significant lowering effect of thalassotherapy conditions including cares but also the increase of night-time sleep opportunity, at the third and fourth days (T3 and T4) and the third day back to home. The subjective fatigue score was significantly lowered when assessed both by the POMS questionnaire and the Pichot scale. Additional beneficial effects of the thalassotherapy stay and cares were observed on self-reported anxiety, general well-being and relaxation respectively. The beneficial effects of balneotherapy on mood, well-being, motivation, fatigue, and quality of life have been repeatedly reported in healthy subjects [3,10,12]. In actively working seamen, Rapolienė, et al. [11] reported that two weeks and five times a week of balneotherapy decreased the number and intensity of stress-related symptoms, and pain and general, physical, and mental fatigue, and improved stress-related symptoms management, mood, activation, motivation, and cognitive functions. For these authors, the beneficial effects on relaxation, a sense of well-being, and a reduction of stress are likely related to changes in hormones like cortisol or the neurotransmitter serotonin system [33,34].

The daily cares combined with sleep management improved the cognitive capacity assessed through sustained attention as number of lapses were significantly lower at T2, T3 and T4 (compared to T0 and T1), and remained lower after week-end at home (T5) and after three days of consecutive work (T6). Adding night-time sleep opportunity (sleep intervention) was previously shown effective in improving alertness and performance in sustained attention using the PVT test in short sleeper workers [19,35]. Our results are the first to show that hydrotherapy cares have a beneficial effect on the sustained attention the very next day, which persisted the week after leaving the resort, while the TST returned to the baseline level. The PVT test has previously emerged as the dominant assay of vigilant attention in paradigms of sleep deprivation, as well as intervention with psychoactive, wake-promoting drugs, and finally, the test shows very minor learning effects making it suitable for regular repeated administration over the course of hours or days [36,37]. In addition, it has been evidenced that optimal performance (i.e., the fastest RTs) during the PVT is related to greater activation of a network of subcortical and cortical brain regions in well-rested individuals [38]. Interestingly, changes in the scores of sustained attention and TMD are positively correlated.

Beneficial effects of the thalassotherapy stay with sleep management are present on lower limb flexibility after three days of cares (T4) and were maintained at the fifth (T5) and sixth tests sessions (T6) back to home and then to work. Thalassotherapy cares involved hydrotherapy cares and manual modelling under affusions of the entire body. The sit-and-reach test is widespread use for the evaluation of physical flexibility in the sport and clinical environments. It evaluates hamstring flexibility, rather the whole-body motion, and represents a simple reproducible procedure easy to administer, requires minimal skills training and is particularly useful in large scale [29]. Among the objective physical parameters, the vertical jump was only significantly different at T6 (back to home and work) in comparison with T1. In untrained healthy men, 45 minutes of leg immersion in warm water (44°C) before a stretch-shortening exercise reduced the creatine kinase activity (indirect blood marker of exercise-induced muscle damage) and prevent prolonged decreases in jump height and maximal voluntary muscular force [39]. The limited effect of hydrotherapy cares on the jump capacity in our participants is probably related to the fact that we did not specifically explore it in response to an exercise protocol. In our study, the beneficial effect of thalassotherapy cares was mainly observed on muscle flexibility after three days cares and is interestingly maintained the week after, underlying a delayed beneficial response to muscular mobilization. This may be related in part to thermal water effects that promotes dilation of blood vessels, and increases blood oxygenation and metabolic rate [5]. These effects would increase oxygen supply to the skeletal muscles, which would facilitate muscular improvement such as flexibility of the musculotendinous unit. Nevertheless in our study, we assessed eleven healthy and actively working individuals, a relatively small number of subjects, thus these results deserve to be confirmed in a larger number of subjects. Future research should aim to replicate these findings adding a control condition and preferably with a crossover design.

This study's multiple approaches, using objective and subjective tools, was challenging and allowed new insights into the beneficial effects of 3 days of thalassotherapy cares combined with sleep management for mood states, well-being, health outcomes, and cognitive and physical capacities in the general working population. We suggested that hydrotherapy cares (3 days with two 2-hours sessions of cares) and sleep management resulting in increased total sleep time (TST) in the second night may explain immediate positive effects on self-reported psychological outcomes and objectively measured vigilance attention but also delayed positive effects on lower limb flexibility. It also would be interesting to evaluate interest of thalassotherapy in the prevention or management of professional burnout that we previously described as associated with anxiety and sleep disorders [40].

Acknowledgments

The authors would like to thank M. Serge Raulic, the Chief Executive Officer of the resort "Les Thermes Marins de Saint-Malo", M. Olivier Raulic, the Executive Officer, M. Jean-Michel Colleu, the Thalassotherapy Director, Ms. Véronique Le Gall, the Public Relations Director, and the Marine Hydrotherapy Service and members of the management.

Authors Contributions

The authors have made substantial contributions: conception and design of the study: Mounir Chennaoui, Clément Bougard and Didier Lagarde; acquisition, analysis and interpretation of data: Mounir Chennaoui, Clément Bougard, Pascal Van Beers, Mathias Guillard, Catherine Drogou; manuscript writing: Mounir Chennaoui, Danielle Gomez-Merino, Clément Bougard; final approval of the version to be submitted: all authors.

Funding

This research received no specific grant from any funding agency in the public, commercial or not-for-profit sectors.

Competing Interests

None.

References

1. Åkerstedt T, Wright KP (2009) Sleep loss and fatigue in shift work and shift work disorder. Sleep Med Clin 4: 257-271.
2. Peterson AL, Goodie JL, Satterfield WA, Brim WL (2008) Sleep disturbance during military deployment. Mil Med 173: 230-235.
3. Gutenbrunner C, Bender T, Cantista P, Karagülle Z (2010) A proposal for a worldwide definition of health resort medicine, balneology, medical hydrology and climatology. Int J Biometeorol 54: 495-507.
4. Becker ME (2009) Aquatic therapy: Scientific foundations and clinical rehabilitation applications. PMR 1: 859-872.
5. Franchimont P, Juchmes J, Lecomte J (1983) Hydrotherapy--mechanisms and indications. Pharmacol Ther 20: 79-93.
6. de Andrade SC, de Carvalho RF, Soares AS, de Abreu Freitas RP, de Medeiros Guerra LM, et al. (2008) Thalassotherapy for fibromyalgia: A randomized controlled trial comparing aquatic exercises in sea water and water pool. Rheumatol Int 29: 147-152.
7. Bender T, Karagülle Z, Bálint GP, Gutenbrunner C, Bálint PV, et al. (2005) Hydrotherapy, balneotherapy, and spa treatment in pain management. Rheumatol Int 25: 220-224.
8. Becker BE, Kasee Hildenbrand K, Whitcomb RK, Sanders JP (2009) Biophysiologic effects of warm water immersion. Int J Aquat Res Educ 3: 24-37.
9. Horne JA, Reid AJ (1985) Night-time sleep EEG changes following body heating in a warm bath. Electroencephalogr Clin Neurophysiol 60: 154-157.
10. Sekine MA, Nasermoaddeli A, Wang H, Kanayama H, Kagamimori S (2006) Spa resort use and health-related quality of life, sleep, sickness absence and hospital admission: The Japanese civil servants study. Complement Ther Med 14: 133-143.
11. Rapolienė L, Razbadauskas A, Sąlyga J, Martinkėnas (2016) A stress and fatigue management using balneotherapy in a short-time randomized controlled trial. eCAM 2016: 9631684.
12. Yang B, Qin QZ, Han LL, Lin J, Chen Y (2017) Spa therapy (balneotherapy) relieves mental stress, sleep disorder, and general health problems in sub-healthy people. Int J Biometeorol 62: 261-272.
13. Vitorino DF, Carvalho LB, Prado GF (2006) Hydrotherapy and conventional physiotherapy improve total sleep time and quality of life of fibromyalgia patients: Randomized clinical trial. Sleep Med 7: 293-296.
14. Latorre-Román PA, Rentero-Blanco M, Laredo-Aguilera JA, García-Pinillos F (2015) Effect of a 12-day balneotherapy programme on pain, mood, sleep, and depression in healthy elderly people. Psychogeriatrics 15: 14-19.
15. Blasche G, Leibetseder V, Marktl W (2010) Association of spa therapy with improvement of psychological symptoms of occupational burnout: A pilot study. Forsch Komplementmed 17: 132-136.
16. Bixler E (2009) Sleep and society: An epidemiological perspective. Sleep Med 10:S3-S9.
17. Rabat A, Gomez-Merino D, Roca-Paixao L, Bougard C, Van Beers P, et al. (2016) Differential kinetics in alteration and recovery of cognitive processes from a chronic sleep restriction in young healthy men. Front Behav Neurosci 23: 10:95.
18. Reilly T, Edwards B (2007) Altered sleep-wake cycles and physical performance in athletes. Physiol Behav 90: 274-284.
19. Swinbourne R, Miller J, Smart D, Dulson DK, Gill N (2018) The effects of sleep extension on sleep, performance, immunity and physical stress in rugby players. Sports (Basel) 6: 42.
20. Horne JA, Ostberg O (1976) A self-assessment questionnaire to determine morningness-eveningness in human circadian rhythms. Int J Chronobiol 4: 97-110.
21. Buysse DJ, Reynolds CF3rd, Monk TH, Berman SR, Kupfer DJ (1989) The pittsburgh sleep quality index: A new instrument for psychiatric practice and research. Psychiatry Res 28: 93-213.
22. Johns MW (1991) A new method for measuring daytime sleepiness: The Epworth sleepiness scale. Sleep 14: 540-545.
23. Ruehland WR, O'Donoghue FJ, Pierce RJ, Thornton AT, Singh P, et al. (2011) The 2007 AASM recommendations for EEG electrode placement in polysomnography: Impact on sleep and cortical arousal scoring. Sleep 34: 73-81.
24. Akerstedt T, Gillberg M (1990) Subjective and objective sleepiness in the active individual. Int J Neurosci 52: 29-37.
25. Cayrou S, Dickès P, Dolbeault S (2003) French version of the profile of mood states (POMS-f). Sci Sport 12: 83-88.
26. Pichot P, Brun JP (1984) Brief self-evaluation questionnaire for depressive, asthenic and anxious dimensions. Ann Med Psychol (Paris) 142: 862-865.

27. Zigmond AS, Snaith RP (1983) The hospital anxiety and depression scale. Acta Psychiatr Scand 67: 361-370.
28. Basner M, Dinges DF (2011) Maximizing sensitivity of the psychomotor vigilance test (PVT) to sleep loss. Sleep 34: 581-591.
29. Ayala F, Sainz de Baranda P, De Ste Croix M, Santonja F (2012) Reproducibility and criterion-related validity of the sit and reach test and toe touch test for estimating hamstring flexibility in recreationally active young adults. Phys Ther Sport 13: 219-226.
30. Glatthorn JF, Gouge S, Nussbaumer S, Stauffacher S, Impellizzeri FM, et al. (2011) Validity and reliability of optojump photoelectric cells for estimating vertical jump height. J Strength Cond Res 25: 556-560.
31. Rasch B, Born J (2013) About sleep's role in memory. Physiol Rev 93: 681-766.
32. Chennaoui M, Bougard C, Drogou C, Langrume C, Miller C, et al. (2016) Stress biomarkers, mood states, and sleep during a major competition: "success" and "failure" athlete's profile of high-level swimmers. Front Physiol 7: 94.
33. Toda M, Morimoto K, Nagasawa S, Kitamura K (2006) Change in salivary physiological stress markers by spa bathing. Biomed Res 27: 11-14.
34. Baroni S, Marazziti D, Consoli G, Picchetti M, Catena-Dell'Osso M, et al. (2012) Modulation of the platelet serotonin transporter by thermal balneotherapy: A study in healthy subjects. Eur Rev Med Pharmacol Sci 16: 589-593.
35. Kubo T, Takahashi M, Sato T, Sasaki T, Oka T, et al. (2011) Weekend sleep intervention for workers with habitually short sleep periods. Scand J Work Environ Health 37: 418-426.
36. Lim J, Dinges DF (2008) Sleep deprivation and vigilant attention. Ann N Y Acad Sci 1129: 305-322.
37. Arnal PJ, Sauvet F, Leger D, van Beers P, Bayon V, et al. (2015) Benefits of sleep extension on sustained attention and sleep pressure before and during total sleep deprivation and recovery. Sleep 38: 1935-1943.
38. Drummond SP, Bischoff-Grethe A, Dinges DF, Ayalon L, Mednick SC, et al. (2005) The neural basis of the psychomotor vigilance task. Sleep 28: 1059-1068.
39. Skurvydas A, Kamandulis S, Stanislovaitis A, Streckis V, Mamkus G, et al. (2008) A Leg immersion in warm water, stretch-shortening exercise, and exercise-induced muscle damage. J Athl Train 43: 592-599.
40. Metlaine A, Sauvet F, Gomez-Merino D, Elbaz M, Delafosse JY, et al. (2017) Association between insomnia symptoms, job strain and burnout syndrome: A cross-sectional survey of 1300 financial workers. BMJ Open 7: e012816.

5

Biomimetic Oral Appliance Therapy in Adults with Severe Obstructive Sleep Apnea

G Dave Singh[1,*], **Tara Griffin**[2] **and Samuel E Cress**[3]

[1]*BioModeling Solutions, Inc., 17933 NE Evergreen Parkway, Beaverton, USA*

[2]*Emerald Coast Dental Sleep Medicine, Panama City Beach, FL 32408, USA*

[3]*Craniofacial and Dental Sleep Medicine, Sugar Land, TX 77479, USA*

[*]**Corresponding author:** G Dave Singh, BioModeling Solutions, Inc., 17933 NE Evergreen Parkway, Suite 280, Beaverton, OR 97006, USA, E- mail: drsingh@drdavesingh.com

Abstract

Introduction: While Continuous Positive Airway Pressure (CPAP) is widely used to manage Obstructive Sleep Apnea (OSA), compliance can be problematic in some cases. These patients are often referred for Mandibular Advancement Devices (MADs) but there is less evidence of their efficacy in severe cases. We investigated the use of biomimetic oral appliance therapy (BOAT) to test the hypothesis that severe cases of OSA can be addressed using BOAT.

Materials and Methods: 15 consecutive adults aged >21 yrs with severe OSA that were unable to comply with CPAP according to a medical physician were treated using BOAT with or without primary mandibular advancement by a dentist with advanced training in dental sleep medicine. The mean Apnea-Hypopnea Index (AHI) of the sample was calculated prior to and after BOAT with no appliance in the mouth during the sleep studies. The findings were subjected to statistical analysis, using paired t-tests.

Results: Prior to treatment the mean AHI of the study sample was 45.9 hr^{-1} ± 10.5. A follow-up sleep study at 9.7 mos. ± 1.9 showed a 64% decrease in AHI to a mean value of 16.5 hr^{-1} ± 8.8 after BOAT ($p<0.01$) with no appliance in the mouth during the post-treatment sleep studies. Results for those without primary mandibular advancement were: 46.6 hr^{-1} ± 12.9 pre-treatment vs. 13.9 hr^{-1} ± 10.5 after BOAT ($p<0.01$); and for those treated with initial mandibular advancement: 45.2 hr^{-1} ± 8 pre-treatment vs. 19.5 hr^{-1} ± 6 after BOAT ($p<0.01$).

Conclusions: BOAT may be a useful method of managing severe cases of OSA in adults, and represents an alternative to CPAP and MADs. However, long-term follow up is needed to reach more definitive conclusions on these initial findings.

Keywords: Biomimetic; Oral appliance therapy

Introduction

Continuous Positive Airway Pressure (CPAP) is the treatment of choice in patients diagnosed with Obstructive Sleep Apnea (OSA). However, it is prone to intolerance, and compliance is typically less than optimal [1]. As an alternative, it was thought that mandibular advancement devices (MADs) would be an effective treatment in patients with mild to moderate OSA who have failed treatment with CPAP therapy. It was also assumed that MADs would not be as effective as CPAP, and that complications would not occur; but occlusal changes with MADs are more common than previously thought [2]. Despite these findings, MADs have become a common treatment for OSA, and their primary use is in patients with mild to moderate OSA. In fact, recent studies indicate that MADs are also effective in controlling OSA in patients with severe OSA [3]. In a study of adults intolerant to CPAP, the respiratory disturbance index (RDI) decreased by about 50% with a MAD in the patients' mouth during sleep [4]. But, the role of MADs in the treatment of severe OSA is still not well defined.

One study [5] investigated a thermoelastic MAD, and reported an increase in velopharyngeal airway size, as well as a reduction in the RDI, in patients with moderate to severe OSA when the device was worn while asleep at night. In view of these types of findings, the practice parameters of the American Academy of Sleep Medicine recommend MADs for mild to moderate cases of OSA, or for patients with severe OSA who are unable to tolerate or refuse treatment with CPAP [6]. However, other reports suggest that only 50% of the patients will be compliant with MAD therapy after about 3 years of use [7]. Therefore, we tested the hypothesis that severe cases of OSA can be addressed using biomimetic oral appliance therapy (BOAT; DNA appliance® system), which might mitigate long-term use and side effects of MADs, as no previous using this technique have been reported in the literature.

Methods and Samples

After obtaining informed consent, we included 15 consecutive adults that had been diagnosed with severe OSA following an overnight sleep study, but were unable to comply with CPAP according to a medical physician. The rights of the subjects were protected by following the Declaration of Helsinki. Inclusion criteria were: subjects aged >21 yrs. diagnosed with severe OSA following an overnight sleep study that had been interpreted by a physician; documented failure/intolerance to CPAP therapy; good oral appliance compliance; no history of hospitalization for craniofacial trauma or surgery; no congenital craniofacial anomalies, and dentate upper and lower arches. The exclusion criteria included: age <21 yrs.; lack of oral appliance compliance; active periodontal disease; tooth loss during treatment; poor oral hygiene, and systemic bisphosphonate therapy. The study protocol (#121310) was reviewed and approved by the institution's review board.

Following a confirmed diagnosis of severe OSA by a medical physician, careful history-taking and craniofacial examination was undertaken for each subject by a dentist with advanced training in dental sleep medicine, and each subject was treated using BOAT. BOAT differs from the conventional MADs as it aims to remodel the upper airway through combined maxillo-mandibular correction with or without primary mandibular repositioning. Therefore, a bite registration was obtained in the upright-sitting position with the jaw posture corrected in the antero-posterior and vertical axes specific for each subject, using a sibilant phoneme registration protocol or 'phonetic bite' [8]. Upper and lower polyvinylsiloxane impressions were also obtained. The upper model was then mounted on an articulator and the lower model was mounted relative to the upper model, using the bite registration captured. Blinded to two investigators (SC and GDS), a biomimetic oral appliance without primary mandibular repositioning (Daytime-Nighttime Appliance: DNA appliance®; Figure 1) was prescribed for half of the study population (8 subjects).

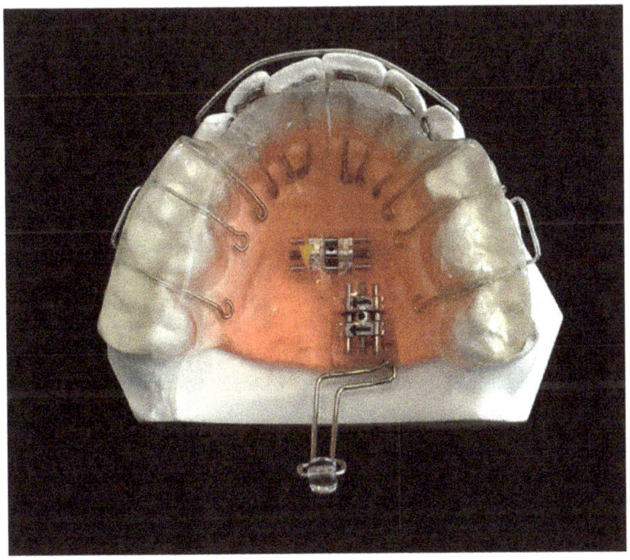

Figure 1: An upper biomimetic appliance (DNA appliance®) that was prescribed for the non-mandibular advancement half of the study population with: anterior 3D axial springs™, a beaded pharyngeal extension, a midline screw, bilateral occlusal coverage, retentive clasps, and a labial bow.

Blinded to two investigators (TG and GDS), a biomimetic oral appliance with mandibular repositioning (mandibular Repositioning Nighttime Appliance: mRNA appliance®; Figure 2) was prescribed for the other half of the sample (7 subjects). Therefore, all authors were blinded in terms of appliance allocation. BOAT is designed to address upper airway deficiencies and to correct maxillo-mandibular hypoplasia in both children and adults [9-17]. All biomimetic oral appliances used in this study had: 6 anterior 3-D axial springs™, a beaded pharyngeal extension, a midline screw, bilateral occlusal coverage, retentive clasps, and a labial bow (Figure 1), but only half of the biomimetic appliances incorporated a mandibular repositioning nighttime component (Figure 2).

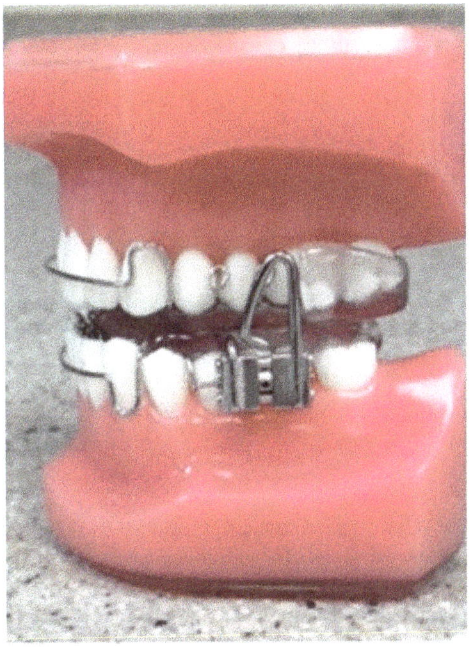

Figure 2: The mandibular repositioning nighttime appliance (mRNA appliance®) that was prescribed for the other half of the sample with: anterior 3-D axial springs™, a midline screw, bilateral occlusal coverage, retentive clasps, a labial bow and a lower mandibular advancement component.

All subjects were instructed to wear the appliances during the evening and at nighttime (for approx. 12-16 hrs. in total), but not during the day time and not while eating, partly in line with the circadian rhythm of tooth eruption [18], although this only occurs in children. Proffit [19] notes that an appliance needs to be worn for at least 8 hrs. in the mouth to have a clinical effect. Written and verbal instructions were given to all subjects.

BOAT requires professional adjustments approximately every 4 weeks, and all subjects reported for review each month. At each monthly follow-up, examination for the progress of craniofacial correction was recorded. Adjustments to the devices were performed to optimize their efficacy. Only gentle pressures were transmitted to the teeth and surrounding tissues and the functionality of the devices was checked with the subject activating a mild force on biting. The subjects were encouraged to maintain their treatment protocol as outlined at the beginning of treatment. Development of the lower arch was implemented using a separate lower appliance (Figure 3) to permit arch re-coordination. A lower appliance (Figure 3) was implemented between 1 to 3 months after the upper appliance unless the subject was wearing the biomimetic appliance design that incorporated the mandibular repositioning nighttime component at the outset (Figure 2). Every 3 months, the overnight sleep studies were repeated. The post-treatment sleep tests were done with no appliance in the mouth and were interpreted by a medical physician. The mean apnea-hypopnea index (AHI) of the study sample was calculated prior to and after BOAT, and the findings were subjected to statistical analysis, using paired t-tests.

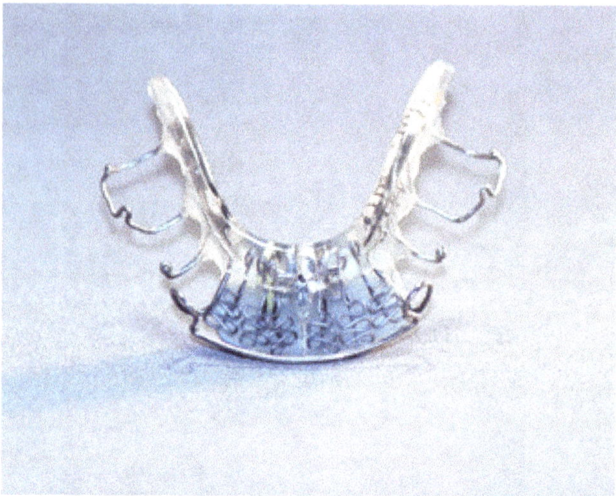

Figure 3: A lower biomimetic appliance (DNA appliance®) with anterior 3-D axial springsTM, a midline screw, retentive clasps and a labial bow that was prescribed for the non-mandibular advancement half of the study population.

Results

Of the total of 15 adults in this study (Table 1), 8 were treated without primary mandibular advancement (Table 1) and 7 were treated with initial mandibular advancement (Table 1). Prior to treatment the mean AHI of the total study subjects was 45.9 $hr^{-1} \pm 10.5$ with no appliance in the mouth when the sleep studies were done. A follow-up sleep study was done at a mean time interval of 9.7 mos. ± 1.9. At this time, the AHI decreased to a mean value of 16.5 $hr^{-1} \pm 8.8$ ($p<0.001$) after BOAT with nothing in the mouth when the post-treatment sleep studies were done. This finding represents a fall in the mean AHI by 64% for the total study sample.

For the subjects treated without primary mandibular advancement, there were 8 adults in this part of the study (Table 1). Prior to treatment the mean AHI of the subjects without primary mandibular advancement was 46.6 $hr^{-1} \pm 12.9$. The final sleep study was done at a mean time interval of 10.4 mos. ± 2.6. At this time, the AHI decreased significantly ($p<0.001$) to a mean value of 13.9 $hr^{-1} \pm 10.5$, which represents a fall in the mean AHI by 70% for this sample. Indeed, three subjects had an AHI of between 3 hr^{-1} to 5 hr^{-1} with no appliance in the mouth when the post-treatment sleep studies were done.

For the subjects treated with primary mandibular advancement, there were 7 adults in this part of the study (Table 1). There was no statistical difference in the initial AHI between this group and those without primary mandibular advancement. Prior to treatment the mean AHI of these study subjects was 45.2 $hr^{-1} \pm 8$. The final sleep study for this group was done after approximately 9 mos. At this time, the AHI decreased significantly ($p<0.001$) to a mean value of 19.5 hr^{-1} ± 6 after BOAT, which represents a fall in the mean AHI of 57% for this study sample. Therefore, it appears that the upper airway can be improved in adults with severe OSA by targeting craniofacial correction with or without primary mandibular advancement using BOAT.

	Total Sample				Non-mandibular advancement		Primary mandibular advancement	
	Pre AHI	Post AHI	Mths	Age	Pre AHI	Post AHI	Pre AHI	Post AHI
Mean	45.9	16.5	9.7	60.2	46.6	13.8	45.2	19.5
Std	10.5	8.8	1.9	5.6	12.9	10.5	7.9	5.9

Table 1: Summary of findings of subjects treated with BOAT with or without primary mandibular advancement. AHI: Apnea-Hypopnea Index, Std: Standard deviation.

Discussion

Although , long-term follow up using a larger sample size is needed to make more definitive conclusions on these initial findings, according to Guilleminault and Stoohs [20] there is a distinct interaction between craniofacial morphology and the upper airway, at least in pediatric patients. This present study suggests that combined maxillo-mandibular, biomimetic oral appliance therapy (BOAT) with or without primary mandibular advancement may be a useful method of managing severe cases of OSA in adults, and may represent a viable alternative to CPAP and MAD therapy. Lettieri et al. [21] compared the efficacy of adjustable and fixed MADs for the treatment of OSA. About 37% of their sample had severe OSA ($AHI \geq 30$) while sleeping with the device. With adjustable MADs the AHI was reduced to <5 hr^{-1} in about 57% cases compared to 47% with non-adjustable appliances. For both devices, success was more common in patients with less than severe OSA. Therefore, the severity of AHI should be considered when selecting the type of MAD. But in our present study, no differences in outcome were found when comparing a biomimetic appliance with or without primary mandibular advancement. Presumably, BOAT permits correction of craniofacial components that might not be addressed with MADs alone. In that respect, it would be interesting to analyze the results of the sleep studies performed at 3 months and 6 months, in order to estimate the progress of their improvement, but not all patients were available for this detailed assessment. However, further studies to replicate these current findings, including patients with different disease severity, allowing stratification that might be correlated with the two treatment protocols, are being planned for the future.

Anandam et al. [22] evaluated long-term cardiovascular mortality in patients with severe OSA treated with either CPAP or MAD therapy. They reported that the residual AHI for MAD-treated patients was higher than a CPAP-treated group, but concluded that both CPAP and MAD may be effective therapies to reduce the risk of cardiovascular fatalities in patients with severe OSA. Although CPAP is regarded as the first option for patients with severe OSA, one study [23] investigated whether patients with severe OSA could use a MAD as an alternative treatment to CPAP. In that study, the AHI decreased with MAD use from 30.7 hr^{-1} to 13.2 hr^{-1}, and they concluded that MADs completely reduce sleep disordered breathing in selected patients with severe OSA. Note that for the subjects treated without primary mandibular advancement in our present study, the mean AHI decreased from 46.6 hr^{-1} to a 13.9 hr^{-1} ($p<0.001$), with no appliance in the mouth for this sample. Similarly, for the subjects treated with primary mandibular advancement in our study the mean AHI decreased from 45.2 hr^{-1} to 19.5 hr^{-1} ($p<0.001$) with no appliance in the mouth. Therefore, BOAT appears to correct sleep disordered breathing in subjects with severe OSA possibly using a different corrective mechanism than MADs, such as craniofacial correction and non-surgical, upper airway remodeling or "Pneumopedics". This pneumopedic notion is supported by preliminary work that indicates midfacial bone volume [12] and nasal cavity volume [9] increases in adults undergoing BOAT, as well as morphologic changes in the upper airway [10,13,17], which we refer to as upper airway remodeling or pneumopedics. Pneumopedics may be regarded as an epigenetic phenomenon in the sense that morphologic changes are elicited in craniofacial locations remote from the site(s) of genetic change [24], as predicted by the spatial matrix hypothesis [25].

Phillips et al. [26] compared health outcomes after 1 month of CPAP and MAD therapy in patients with moderate-severe OSA. They reported that while CPAP was more efficacious than MADs in reducing the AHI, compliance was higher with MADs. Surprisingly perhaps, neither treatment improved blood pressure, in contrast to sleepiness and quality of life for both treatments. It was therefore concluded that the similar effectiveness for both treatment modalities may be explained by the greater efficacy of CPAP being balanced by better compliance with MADs. Similarly, Lam et al. [27] assessed the efficacy of MADs in patients with severe OSA and hypertension at 3 months and 1 year intervals. It was found that MADs reduced systolic blood pressure in subjects with hypertension and OSA. In those subjects with retrognathia, MADs reduced the AHI from 47.5 hr^{-1} to 13.1 after 1 year. These AHI results are similar to those noted in our present study; however, although we did not assess blood pressure or hypertension in this present study, our post-treatment sleep studies were performed with no appliance in the mouth while sleeping. Nevertheless, these differences provide further premises for future studies using BOAT. In addition, Tegelberg et al. [28] evaluated the effects of MAD treatment on cognitive functions in patients with moderate-to-severe OSA. After 6 months of MAD treatment, cognitive functioning improved and the AHI decreased with 54% of the patients showing normal breathing during sleep while wearing the MAD. Nevertheless, both treatment modalities presumably represent life-long use if the health outcomes noted above are to be maintained. While we did investigate cognitive function in this current study, BOAT may provide a novel protocol of managing severe cases of OSA and its clinical sequelae in adults, and thus represent an alternative to CPAP and MADs.

Acknowledgements

We would like to thank Vicky Autry CDT, ArtWires, LLC, Florida, USA, for fabricating the appliances used in this study.

References

1. Gulati A, Oscroft N, Chadwick R, Ali M, Smith I (2015)The impact of changing people with sleep apnea using CPAP less than 4h per night to a bi-level device. Respir Med 109: 778-783.
2. Ferguson KA (2003) The role of oral appliance therapy in the treatment of obstructive sleep apnea. Clin Chest Med 24: 355-364.
3. Ng A, Gotsopoulos H, Darendeliler AM, Cistulli PA (2005) Oral appliance therapy for obstructive sleep apnea. Treat Respir Med 4: 409-422.
4. Menn SJ, Loube DI, Morgan TD, Mitler MM, Berger JS, et al. (1996) The mandibular repositioning device: role in the treatment of obstructive sleep apnea. Sleep 19: 794-800.
5. Lowe AA, Sjöholm TT, Ryan CF, Fleetham JA, Ferguson KA, et al. (2000) Treatment, airway and compliance effects of a titratable oral appliance. Sleep 15: S172-178.
6. Chan AS, Lee RW, Cistulli PA (2007) Dental appliance treatment for obstructive sleep apnea. Chest 132: 693-699.
7. Clark GT (1998) Mandibular advancement devices and sleep disordered breathing. Sleep Med Rev 2: 163-174.
8. Singh GD, Olmos S (2007) Use of a sibilant phoneme registration protocol to prevent upper airway collapse in patients with TMD. Sleep Breath 11: 209-216.
9. Singh GD, Heit T, Preble D, Chandrashekhar R (2016). Changes in 3D nasal cavity volume after biomimetic oral appliance therapy in adults [Epub ahead of print].
10. Liao F, Singh GD (2015) Resolution of Sleep Bruxism using Biomimetic Oral Appliance Therapy: A Case Report. J Sleep Disord Ther 4: 1-5.
11. Singh GD, Griffin TM, Chandrashekhar R (2014) Biomimetic oral appliance therapy in adults with mild to moderate obstructive sleep apnea. Aust J Sleep Dis 1: 1-5.
12. Singh GD, Heit T, Preble D (2014) Changes in 3D midfacial parameters after biomimetic oral appliance therapy in adults. J Ind Orthod Soc 48: 104-108.
13. Singh GD, Cress SE (2013) Craniofacial Enhancement using a Biomimetic Oral Appliance: Case Report. Dent Today 329: 92-92.
14. Singh GD, Callister JD (2013) Use of a maxillary oral appliance for the resolution of obstructive sleep apnea. Cranio 31: 171-175.
15. Singh GD, Cress SE (2013) Case presentation: Effect of full mouth rehabilitation and oral appliance therapy on obstructive sleep apnea. Dialogue 2: 18-20.
16. Singh GD, Cress SE, McGuire MK, Chandrashekhar R (2012) Case report: Effect of mandibular tori removal on obstructive sleep apnea parameters. Dialogue 1: 22-24.
17. Singh GD, Wendling S, Chandrashekhar R (2011) Midfacial development in adult obstructive sleep apnea. Dent. Today 30: 124-127.
18. Proffit WR, Frazier-Bowers SA (2009) Mechanism and control of tooth eruption: overview and clinical implications. Orthod Craniofac Res 12: 59-66.
19. Proffit WR, Fields HW Jr, Sarver DM (2006) Contemporary Orthodontics. (4thedn), Elsevier, Philadelphia.
20. Guilleminault C, Stoohs, R (1990) Obstructive sleep apnea syndrome in children. Pediatrician 17: 46-51.
21. Lettieri CJ, Paolino N, Eliasson AH, Shah AA, Holley AB (2011) Comparison of adjustable and fixed oral appliances for the treatment of obstructive sleep apnea. J Clin Sleep Med 7: 439-445.
22. Anandam A, Patil M, Akinnusi M, Jaoude P, El Solh AA (2013) Cardiovascular Mortality in Obstructive Sleep Apnea Treated with Continuous Positive Airway Pressure or Oral Appliance: an Observational Study. Respirology. 8: 1184-1190.

23. Almeida FR, Mulgrew A, Ayas N, Tsuda H, Lowe AA, et al. (2013) Mandibular advancement splint as short-term alternative treatment in patients with obstructive sleep apnea already effectively treated with continuous positive airway pressure. J Clin Sleep Med 15: 319-324.
24. Parsons TE, Downey CM, Jirik FR, Hallgrimsson B, Jamniczky HA (2015) Mind the Gap: Genetic Manipulation of Basicranial Growth within Synchondroses Modulates Calvarial and Facial Shape in Mice through Epigenetic Interactions. PLoS ONE 10(2): e0118355. doi:10.1371/journal.pone.0118355
25. Singh GD (2004) Growth and treatment. Craniofacial Growth Series. Monograph 41: 197–239.
26. Phillips CL, Grunstein RR, Darendeliler MA, Mihailidou AS, Srinivasan VK, et al. (2013). Health outcomes of continuous positive airway pressure versus oral appliance treatment for obstructive sleep apnea: a randomized controlled trial. Am J Respir Crit Care Med 187: 879-887.
27. Lam B, Sam K, Lam JC, Lai AY, Lam CL, et al. (2011) The efficacy of oral appliances in the treatment of severe obstructive sleep apnea. Sleep Breath 15: 195-201.
28. Tegelberg A, Wilhelmsson B, Erixon-Lindroth N, Lindström LH (2012) Improved cognitive functions after treatment with an oral appliance in obstructive sleep apnea. Nat Sci Sleep 22: 89-96.

6

Can Research Confirm Psychopathological Subtypes and Relationship between Recurrent Mood Disorders and Personality Disorders?

Diego Cohen[1*] **and Ricardo Corral**[2]

[1]*Admission Unit, Hospital Borda, Ramón Carrillo 375 CABA, Argentina*

[2]*Department of research and education, Hospital Borda, Ramón Carrillo 375 CABA, Argentina*

[*]**Corresponding author:** Diego Cohen, Admission Unit, Hospital Borda, Ramón Carrillo 375 CABA, Argentina, E-mail: drdiegocohen@gmail.com

Abstract

The aim of this study is to estimate the frequency of personality disorders in patients with recurrent unipolar or bipolar affective disorders and the possible relationship of the categorical model with two dynamic psycho-pathological configurations. Forty-eight patients were studied using semi-structured interviews for assessing Axis I and Axis II disorders. We found that approximately 70% of patients had some types of personality disorder according to the DSM-IV TR classification model. The most frequent personality disorders were cluster C dependent personality disorder and cluster B borderline personality disorder. The most common affective disorders were depressive bipolar I subtype disorder and manic bipolar I subtype disorder. The high frequency of personality disorders in patients who are in partial or complete remission of recurrent affective disorders can be explained by a combination of two subtypes of psycho-pathological configurations (the anaclitic or introjective configurations are based on the Blatt model) and neuro-biological interactions.

Keywords: Affective disorders; Personality disorders; Comorbidity; Psycho-pathological models; Anaclitic-introjective

Introduction

The purpose of this study is to investigate whether there is a relationship between recurrent affective disorders classified as Axis I by Diagnostic and Statistical manual of Mental Disorders Fourth Edition (DSM-IV TM) and personality disorders classified as Axis II of the same manual [1]. This association has not been completely resolved as numerous studies have shown varying temporal associations (comorbidity) between recurrent affective disorders and personality disorders [2-6]. In psychiatry, the dimensional theory, which is used for assessments, considers personality disorders as clinical forms of recurrent affective disorders. This is especially true for borderline personality disorder (BPD). Other researchers consider it useful to promote BPD as Axis I of DSM-IV, anyway this approach could be not longer tenable because of DSM-5 section III dimensional model and no "split" between Axis I-Axis II [7-9].

Classification of temperament traits (neurobiological and affective components of personality disorders) creates even more confusion. According to the Akiskal model [10-14]; some personality disorder subtypes appear as forms of syndromic or subsyndromic variants of affective disorders. Personality disorders seem to be reduced to four basic temperaments: 1) depressive; 2) hyperthymic, in which a person has a tendency to be in a euphoric mood; 3) cyclothymic oscillations between depression and an upbeat mood; and 4) irritable-explosive. The dimensional model may be useful to reduce countless nosological clinical symptoms and to study neurochemical, neuropshysiological (adding sleep and circadian pattern abnormalities) and pharmacological basics. It also leads to poor psychopathological specificity. For instance, some researchers consider cyclothymia or hypomanic personality disorder as a personality disorder, while other researchers judge these as a level of mood disorder [11,15,16].

The relationship between psychopathological states and abnormal traits of character is not a new issue. It appears in both classical psychiatry and in its most dynamic versions. The history of psychiatry goes back to the Hippocratic school trying to relate the prevalence of humors (black, yellow, sanguine, phlegmatic bile) with temperament and personality. Phlegmatic temperament and its blood type were related to the predisposition for four diseases: mania, melancholia, phrenitis or paranoia [17]. Kraepelin described several affective states, known as manic-depressive psychosis. This classification laid the basis for recognizing psychopathological subsyndromal states based on observable fluctuations in motor activity, emotions and thoughts (cognitions). Kraepelin, quoted by Akiskal, considered these manifestations temperamental (1992). From a dynamic point of view, [18] found that patients suffering from melancholy after the end of the episode also showed an obsessive-compulsive character.

Freud studied melancholy and considered the existence of "a pathological predisposition" that led to melancholy instead of mourning. He proposed a narcissistic type of relationship with the object, which now may apply to patients from cluster B (American Psychiatric Association, 1994) [1]. Freud seemed to relate melancholy with obsessional neurosis due to the degree of ambivalence present in both conditions and referred to it as " obsessive depression" [19].

Recent studies [5,20] have evaluated that BPD is a personality disorder that shows higher percentage of comorbidity with type I and type II bipolar disorder (BD I and II) compared to the other disorders of axis II (19.4% vs. 7.4% respectively). Moreover, the emergence of "new episodes" of type I and II BD occurs more frequently in BPD compared to other personality disorders (OPD) with percentages reaching 8.2% vs. 3% respectively. More proof of the disagreement among researchers, Kernberg [16] proposed that during bipolar illness (though bipolar subtype was not mentioned), patients may suffer from borderline personality organization (BPO), psychosis, neurosis and even a normal personality. One of the authors of this study (DC) found that, in clinical psychiatry, one of the most difficult differential diagnosis is between BPO hypomanic/cyclothymic subtypes and type I or II bipolar disorder with severe impulsivity, affective instability and chaotic relationships that continue after remission of each acute episode [21].

This research is a preliminary attempt to establish correlations between cyclic affective disorders and all axis II disorders. Establishing the relationship between character traits and psychopathological conditions may be important from the following points of view: 1) prediction; 2) form and duration of psychotherapeutic and psychopharmacological treatment; 3) prevention of complications during treatment (suicide, psychotic episodes, severe regressions); and 4) the treatment of patients with a diagnosis on Axis I usually have more complications when accompanied by an Axis II disorder [22].

Methods

The following is a prospective, observational and cross-sectional study of patients diagnosed with bipolar disorder in two health centers in the city of Buenos Aires: Borda Hospital and Italian Hospital between September 2009 and June 2010.

Inclusion criteria: 1) patients of either sex between 18 and 65 years old; and 2) patient still undergoing outpatient treatment with a presumed diagnosis of recurrent affective disorders (unipolar, bipolar, mixed and rapid cycling). Exclusion criteria: 1) patients with evidence or clinical history of organic mental disorder according to DSM-IV TM; 2) patients who presented with substance and/or alcohol use disorder at the time of the study diagnosis; 3) patients diagnosed with dysthymia and 4) patients who refused to complete the informed agreement. Patients with incomplete questionnaire data (n=2) were removed from the statistical analysis.

The Structured Clinical Interview for DSM-IV Axis I Disorders User´s Guide Clinical, Version (SCID I) was used as a screening and diagnostic tool. In the second phase of the study, the Structured Clinical Interview for DSM-IV axis II Personality Disorders (SCID-II) was used in order to typify the possible personality disorder (both interview were translated to Spanish and validated version applied) [23,24]. At the time of assessment, all demographics and medication information were recorded on a separate sheet.

Each interview was conducted by psychiatrists trained in the use of assessment tools and experienced in treating patients with personality disorder. The interviews were supervised by a principal investigator to avoid misunderstandings and to make the final forms.

Variables considered in the analysis were: age, gender, type of Axis I disorder (recurrent depressive disorder; bipolar disorder type I, most recent manic or depressive episode; bipolar disorder type II, most recent hypomanic or depressive episode; bipolar disorder type I, unspecified; and recurrent unipolar disorder), type of Axis II disorder and pharmacologic treatment (this last variable was not illustrated and subsequently was not part of the research objectives).

The data were entered in an Excel Microsoft 2000 spreadsheet (version 9.0.2812) and were analyzed using the statistical package Epi Info 2000 version 1.1.2 (CDC and WHO). For all variables, the distribution of frequencies and/or percentages was established relative to the total number of cases. Statistical analysis consisted of a quantitative analysis from measures of central tendency and dispersion, yielding proportions, averages, ranges, medium or standard deviation as appropriate for each variable studied. Smith Statistical Package (v. 2.80, 2005) was used for analysis of confidence intervals.

Results

The study group included 48 patients, of whom 50% (n=24, CI=0.35 to 0.64) were female and 50% (n=24, CI=0.35 to 0.64) were male. The patients were aged between 23 and 65 years with a mean of 47 ± 13.42 years.

Diagnosis	Frequency
BPD. Depressive Type I (N=17) IC=0.21-0.49	35.41%
BPD. Manic Type I. (N=13) IC=01.14-0.40	27.00%
BPD. Mix Type I. (N=4) IC=0.0022-0.16	8.00%
BPD. Type I Hypomaniac. (N=1) IC=0.021-0.06	2.00%
BPD. Type I Not Specified. (N=1) IC=0.021-0.06	2.00%
BPD. Depressive Type II. (N=5) IC=0.014-0.19	10.41%
BPD. Type II Hypomaniac. (N=3) IC=-0.215	6.25%
DPD. Recurring. (N=4) IC=0.0022-0.16	8.00%

Table 1: Percentage of patients with recurrent affective disorders.

Of the patients, 35.41% (n=17, CI=0.21 to 0.49) were diagnosed as type I BD with the most recent episode being a depressive state. Twenty-seven percent (n=13, CI=0.14 to 0.40) received a diagnosis of BD I with the most recent episode being a manic state. Only 8% (n=4, CI=0.0022 to 0.16) presented with the most recent episode being a mixed state. Finally, only one patient displayed with the most recent episode being hypomanic and one patient had an unspecified episode (CI=-0.021-0.06 for each). Of the patients, 10.41% (n=5, CI=0.014 to 0.19) were diagnosed as type II BD with the most recent episode being depressive and three patients most recently had a hypomanic episode

(CI=-0.085 to 0.13). Eight percent (n=4, CI=0.0022-0.16) received a diagnosis of recurrent depressive disorder (unipolar depression). Data can be viewed in Table 1 and graphic bar 1 (Figure 1).

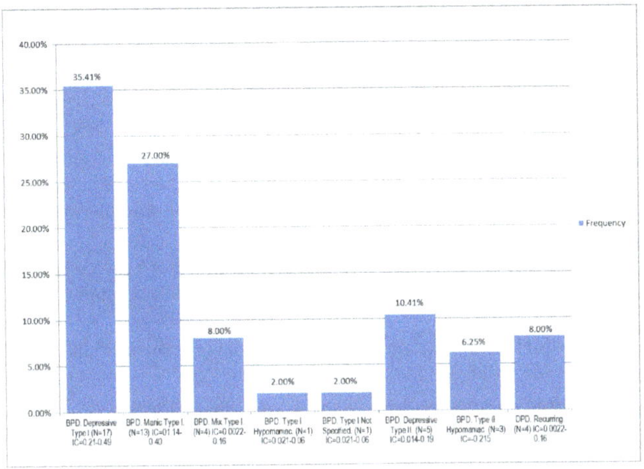

Figure 1: Percentage of patients with recurrent affective disorders.

Regarding personality disorders, nearly 23% (n=11, CI=0.33 to 0.62) did not display a personality disorder, while 77% were positive for any personality disorder (n=37, CI=0.64 to 0.89). About 27% of the patients positive for axis II disorders (n=10, CI=0.12 to 0.42) had comorbidity with other disorders on axis II.

Diagnosis	Frequency
Without PD (N=11) IC=0.33-0.62	22.90%
With PD (N=37) IC=0.64-0.89	77.10%
Dependent (N=8) IC=0.077-0.35	21.00%
Limit (N=6) IC=0.037-0.28	16.00%
Histrionic (N=4) IC=0.031-0.21	11.00%
Obsessive Compulsive (N=4) IC=0.031-0.21	11.00%
Narcissistic (N=2) IC=-0.15	5.40%
Avoidant (N=1) IC=-0.1	2.70%
Schizotypal (N=1) IC=-0.1	2.70%
Not Specified (N=1) IC=-0.1	2.70%

Table 2: Estimated percentage of patients with personality disorder in patients who had recurrent affective disorders.

Among those who had only one diagnosis, the majority presented with a dependent personality disorder (21%, n=8, CI=0.077 to 0.35), followed by 16% with BPD (n=6, CI=0.037 to 0.28), 11% each with histrionic and obsessive compulsive disorder (n=4, CI=.031 to .21) and finally 5.4% with narcissist disorder (n=2, CI=-0.02 to 0.13). Only one patient had avoidant or schizotypal or unspecified disorder (n=1, CI=-0.02 to 0.08). Data can be viewed in Table 2 and graphic bar 2 (Figure 2).

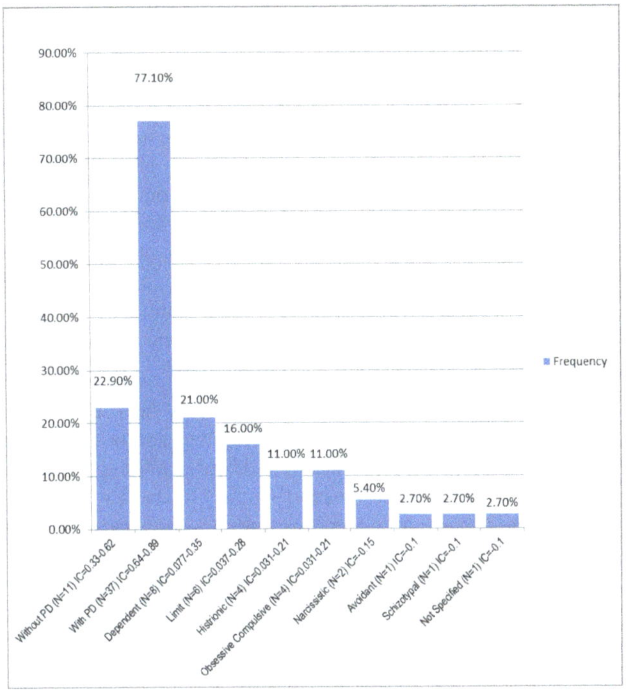

Figure 2: Estimated percentage of patients with personality disorder in patients who had recurrent affective disorders.

Discussion

A high percentage of personality disorders were found in patients who were in complete or partial remission of recurrent affective disorders according to DSM-IV TM diagnostic criteria. This data is generally consistent with current literature reviews. A high degree of variability in the rates of comorbidity is similar to our findings with the largest association in cluster C Axis II disorders. This is especially true for dependent personality disorder and BPD (Table 2 and graphic bar of Figure 2). This association may have a variety of predisposing factors including: a) neurobiological (including the well-known sleep disorganization in affective disorders); b) genetic (as a diathesis toward affective, impulsive and interpersonal relationships or as a personality trait among various affective disorders); c) psychosocial; d) life special cycle period in women like postpartum [25] and d) a combination resulting in the interaction of these factors [26]. We hypothesize that points b, c and could be related to BD in parents and the tendency of their offsprings to show more sleep problems, aggressive behavior, ADHD diagnosis and emotional reactivity all features that could also be related to personality disorders traits in adolescence, the known onset of BD [27].

In the subgroup of patients with mood disorders without personality disorders (a figure close to 25% in our research) it could be considered part of the neurobiological dominance hypothesis. Affective disorders could be an example of severe emotional deregulation and sometimes cover the cognitive dimension. So the older term "manic-depressive psychosis" is still useful [28].

In this paper, we suggest the high correlation responds to a high index of Axis I- Axis II association. From a theoretical point of view, a relationship can be established between the depression model investigated by Blatt [29] and subtypes of personality disorders. Blatt considers two essential psychopathological configurations, which are presented in a continuous of immaturity towards higher levels of personality integration. These configurations are the anaclitic and the introjective types.

In the first type, the central conflict is about the nature and quality of interpersonal relationships. Anaclitic psychopathology derives mainly from difficulties in achieving and maintaining deep and meaningful relationships. Critical is finding appropriate objects that give integration to the self ("libido is seeking for object rather than instinctual gratification", [30]. According to Blatt, this psychopathological predisposition can span from undifferentiated schizophrenia to personality disorders such as dependent, borderline and anaclitic depression (abandon depression) [31].

In this study, approximately 48% of patients have the anaclitic configuration with respect to personality disorders and in a majority of the cases it is associated with some mood disorder. We suggest that the personality disorder in this situation would also be associated with biological predisposition. The disruption of attachment (the neurobiological underpinning of relationships) or their inevitable transformations leads these patients to more depression or as a defense have manic/ hypomanic episodes. In the latter situation, there is a tendency to confirm, at least theoretically Kleinian hypothesizes the occurrence of mania as a defense against depression and object dependency [18,19,32,33] anticipates this configuration and its relationship to the blues. He considers three fundamental premises in this condition: 1) object loss; 2) ambivalence; and 3) the regression of the libido to the self. In short, according to Blatt's model, the anaclitic configuration (including a form of depression) is characterized by: feelings of hopelessness, emptiness and abandon anxieties with desperate desire to maintain physical/emotional contact with objects.

Instead, in the introjective type of organization has a particularly intense interest about defining personal and individual achievement and the maintenance of highly differentiated limits of self-respect. It correlates to Blatt's subtype, the DSM-IV obsessive-compulsive personality disorder and the narcissistic personality disorder subtype. In our study, the prevalence of these clinical forms was lower (11% and 4, 5 % respectively).

In summary, our study confirms high rates of association between Axis I mood disorders and Axis II disorders (psycho-pathological trait). The separation between the axes should be reconsidered beyond neurobiological etiologies. Recurrent affective disorders are associated with non-integrated forms of relationships with significant others, along with difficulties in maintaining self-esteem and problems with self/other differentiation (anaclitic and introjective pathology respectively). These results should be taken as preliminary findings mainly due to: 1) low number of cases studied, b) cross sectional rather than longitudinal observation, 3) absence of randomization, 4) no control group, 5) the proposed Blatt model would not explain all manic/hypomanic episodes unless they can be considered as a defense against depression or painful and unsuccessful attempts to restart the relation with the object in front of a threat of abandonment in anaclitic organization.

Acknowledgment

To Martín Ruiz, M.D., Cintia Pereira, Psych and Carolina Vairo for patients provition.

References

1. Strawbridge WJ, Deleger S, Roberts RE, Kaplan GA (2002) Physical activity reduces the risk of subsequent depression for older adults. Am J Epidemiol 156: 328-334.
2. Benazzi F (2008) A relationship between bipolar II disorder and borderline personality disorder? Prog Neuropsychopharmacol Biol Psychiatry 32: 1022-1029.
3. Fan AH, Hassell J (2008) Bipolar disorder and comorbid personality psychopathology: a review of the literature. J Clin Psychiatry 69: 1794-1803.
4. Koenigsberg HW, Harvey PD, Mitropoulou V, Schmeidler J, New AS, et al. (2002) Characterizing affective instability in borderline personality disorder. Am J Psychiatry 159: 784-788.
5. Paris J, Gunderson J, Weinberg I (2007) The interface between borderline personality disorder and bipolar spectrum disorders. Compr Psychiatry 48: 145-154.
6. Stone MH (2006) Relationship of borderline personality disorder and bipolar disorder. Am J Psychiatry 163: 1126-1128.
7. American Psychiatric Association: Diagnostic and Statistical Manual of Mental Disorders, fifth Edition: Arlington,VA, American Psychiatric Association 2013.
8. New AS, Triebwasser J, Charney DS (2008) The case for shifting borderline personality disorder to Axis I. Biol Psychiatry 64: 653-659.
9. Siever LJ, Davis KL (1991) A psychobiological perspective on the personality disorders. Am J Psychiatry 148: 1647-1658.
10. Akiskal HS (1991) Chronic depression. Bull Menninger Clin 55: 156-171.
11. Akiskal HS (1992) Delineating irritable and hyperthymic variants of the cyclothymic temperament: Reassessing personality disorder constructs. Journal of Personality Disorders 6: 326-342.
12. Akiskal HS (1994) The temperamental borders of affective disorders. Acta Psychiatr Scand Suppl 379: 32-37.
13. Akiskal HS (2001) Dysthymia and cyclothymia in psychiatric practice a century after Kraepelin. J Affect Disord 62: 17-31.
14. Akthar S (1995) Quest for Answers. Northvale, Jason Aronson.
15. Kernberg OF (1987) Trastornos Graves de la Personalidad. México, Manual Moderno.
16. Maj M, Sartorius N (2002) Depressive Disorders. (2ndedn) Chichester, England, John Wiley & Sons.
17. Abraham K (1994). Psicoanálisis Clínico. Buenos Aires, Lumen-Hormé.
18. Freud S (1996) Duelo y Melancolía. (1915 [1917]). Madrid, Biblioteca Nueva.
19. Gunderson JG, Weinberg I, Daversa MT, Kueppenbender KD, Zanarini MC, et al. (2006) Descriptive and longitudinal observations on the relationship of borderline personality disorder and bipolar disorder. Am J Psychiatry 163: 1173-1178.
20. Judd LL, Paulus MJ, Schettler PJ, Akiskal HS, Endicott J, et al. (2000) Does incomplete recovery from first lifetime major depressive episode herald a chronic course of illness? Am J Psychiatry 157: 1501-1504.
21. Zanarini MC, Frankenburg FR, Dubo ED, Sickel AE, Trikha A, et al. (1998) Axis I comorbidity of borderline personality disorder. Am J Psychiatry 155: 1733-1739.
22. First MB, Spitzer RL, Gibbon M, Williams JB (1999) Guía del usuario para la entrevista clínica estructurada para los trastornos del eje I del DSM-IV versión clínica (SCID-I). Barcelona, Masson.
23. First MB, Spitzer RL, Gibbon M, Williams JB (1999) Guía del usuario para la entrevista clínica estructurada para los trastornos de la personalidad del eje II del DSM-IV (SCID-II). Barcelona, Masson.
24. Stevens AWM, Goosens PJJ, Hoogendoom AW, Knoppert-van der Klein EM, Honig A, et al. (2014). The effect of sleep disturbance during pregnancy and perinatal period on postpartum psychopathology in women with bipolar disorder. J Women's Health Care, 3: 1-6.
25. McCrae P, Costa P (2006) Personality in adulthood. New York, The Guilford Press.

26. Maoz H, Goldstein T, Axelson DA, Goldstein BI, Fan J, et al. (2014) Dimensional psychopathology in preschool offspring of parents with bipolar disorder. J Child Psychol Psychiatry 55: 144-153.
27. Marneros A, Goodwing F (2005) Bipolar Disorders. Cambridge, University Press.
28. Blatt S (2008) Polarities of experience. Washington DC, American Psychiatric Association.
29. Fairbairn WRD (2001) Estudio psicoanalítico de la personalidad. Buenos Aires, Lumen-Hormé.
30. Masterson J (1993) The Emergin Self. New York, Brunner/Mazel.
31. Gabbard GO (2005) Psychodynamic Psychiatry in clinical practice, Washington DC, American Psychiatric Association.
32. Klein M (1984) Love, Guilt and Reparation and other works 1921-1945. New York, The Free Press.
33. Karam EG, Salamoun MM, Yeretzian JS, Mneimneh ZN, Karam AN, et al. (2010) The role of anxious and hyperthymic temperaments in mental disorders: a national epidemiologic study. World Psychiatry 9: 103-110.

CBT-Based Group Intervention for Insomnia - A Non-Randomized Trial in Primary Care

Magnus Falk* **and Hagesund E**

Division of Community Medicine, Primary Care, Department of Medicine and Health Sciences, Linköping University, Linköping, Sweden

***Corresponding author:** Magnus Falk, Division of Community Medicine, Primary Care, Department of Medicine and Health Sciences, Linköping University, S-581 83, Linköping, Sweden, E-mail: magnus.falk@regionostergotland.se

Abstract

Insomnia is a major health problem, commonly leading to pharmacological treatment. During recent years, behavioural therapies have gained stronger therapeutic position, not least cognitive behavioural therapy (CBT). The aim was to investigate the effect of a CBT-based group intervention for insomnia in primary care, by means of self-reported sleep quality and duration. In addition, cortisol in saliva, as a biological marker of stress was tested. Methods: Fifty participants with primary insomnia, attending primary care, were enrolled, 35 receiving the intervention, and 15 serving as control. The intervention group was recruited during the first two study years, and controls during a following third year, without randomization. The intervention included eight CBT-based group sessions, each two-hour long and led by a psychologist, with 4-6 participants in each group. Controls were handled in accordance with ordinary clinical routine, including pharmacological intervention.

Sleep onset time, duration and quality were assessed before and after the intervention, by patients filling-out the Pittsburgh Sleep Quality Index (PSQI). Insomnia severity was assessed by the Insomnia Severity Index (ISI). Also, cortisol in saliva levels were monitored. Results: In the intervention group, significant shortening of mean sleep onset time, from 60-27 min ($p<0.05$) was observed, and a prolongation of mean sleep duration time, from 298-358 min ($p<0.05$), in neither case seen in the control group, although between-group difference was not statistically significant. Both PSQI and ISI means scores were significantly improved in the intervention group, from 12.1 to 7.9 ($p<0.05$) and from 19.4 to 12.5 ($p<0.01$), respectively, in the latter case significantly more so than in the control group ($p<0.05$). No effect on cortisol levels was detected, in either group. In conclusion, the tested eight-session CBT-based group intervention for insomnia appears to reduce severity and duration of insomnia, and to shorten time before falling asleep, when provided in primary care.

Keywords: Insomnia severity; Sleep duration; Cognitive behavioural therapy; Primary care; Group therapy

Introduction

Insomnia is a major health problem in western societies. In Sweden a prevalence of up to 30% among women and 20% among men has been reported [1]. Also, the proportion of younger adults (20-30 years of age) appears to be increasing, and was doubled during the two last decades of the 20th century. In Sweden, with a total population of about 9.5 million inhabitants, around 4.5 million yearly prescriptions of different sleep medicines, by medical doctors, are performed [2]. Sleeping disorders stand for substantial suffer for the individual involved, as well as for excessive costs for the society.

Apart from pharmacological treatment, behavioural therapies have gained a stronger position in treating insomnia during recent decades, not least cognitive behavioural therapy (CBT) [3,4]. Studies comparing the effectiveness of CBT and pharmacologic treatment have shown CBT to be more effective in the longer perspective, to higher extent leading to persistent improvement of both sleep quality and difficulties in falling asleep [3,4]. Also, negative aspects of pharmacological treatment include unwanted side effects (such as day drowsiness, delayed reaction time and others) and for some substance groups risk for drug dependence, effects that may be avoided by using behavioural therapies instead. Although not all substance groups are associated with biological dependence, an element of psychological drug dependence may still appear.

A negative aspect of CBT and other behavioural therapies is that they are rather time consuming for the provider, putting high demands on necessary resources. Therefore, adequate accessibility may be difficult to achieve. For that reason alternative models to the traditional individual therapist-to-patient concept have been tried, including group-delivered and internet based CBT, both of which have shown promising results [5], as well in comparison with individual CBT as with pharmacological treatment.

A possible positive additive effect of group intervention, reported in previous studies, is the benefits gained from interaction with the other group participants [5-7]. For a majority of patients with insomnia, primary care is likely to be the natural primary instance to seek help if suffering from insomnia, and is thus of interest and importance when exploring effective ways to provide adequate treatment that meet the an apostrophe is lacking in patient's needs.

The aim of the present study was to investigate the effect of a CBT based group intervention for insomnia in primary care, by means of self-reported sleep quality and duration. In addition, cortisol in saliva, as a biological marker of stress, was tested before and after the intervention.

Materials and Methods

The study was performed at four primary health care (PHC) units in the city of Linköping, Southeastern Sweden, during January 2009 to December 2011. At all four units a CBT-based group intervention for insomnia was implemented, giving the caregiver the possibility to refer patients with insomnia for inclusion in the study.

To be included the patients had to be aged >18 years and to suffer from insomnia, diagnosed by either a medical doctor or a psychotherapist at any of the involved PHC units. The insomnia could be newly debuted or having existed for a longer time (months to years), but should have persisted for at least one month, and could be either idiopathic or associated with perceived stress, mental exhaustion or overload. Ongoing pharmacological treatment for insomnia was no hinder for inclusion. However, if the patient had no ongoing sleep medication and was enrolled for the CBT group intervention, concomitant pharmacological treatment should not be initiated.

Insomnia directly associated with different pain conditions was an exclusion criterion, as was other diseases commonly followed by secondary sleeping disorder, including narcolepsy, obstructive sleep apnea syndrome (OSAS), restless legs syndrome, alcohol overconsumption, depression, primary anxiety conditions and depression. In addition to a clinical judgment of depression, all patients to be included were to fill-out the MADR-S (Montgomery-Åsberg Depression Rating Scale) form in order to exclude possible cases of depression not primarily identified by the doctor or the psychotherapist.

Participants for inclusion in the study group (given the intervention) were recruited consecutively during the first two years of the study. During the following final year, participants were instead recruited for inclusion in a control group, by the same inclusion criteria. Thus, no randomization between intervention and control was performed.

The CBT group intervention

Each group consisted of four to six patients. The CBT group intervention was led by a psychologist/psychotherapist (one of the authors, E.H.), and included eight two-hour long group sessions, the first four sessions held once a week, and the last four sessions two weeks apart.

The more frequent meetings during the first part of the intervention aimed to promote motivation and to enhance the process of change, while the latter part gave more time for exploring new habits, and to establish new ways of how to think and relate towards sleep. In case of drop-outs, no new participants were included in each group after initialization. The group sessions comprised a knowledge part, based on information on sleep related factors, a follow-up part with review of completed home tasks, and a final part introducing new tasks for completion until next session.

During the first half of the intervention, the goals were to map and describe the participants' sleep disturbances, and to identify possible underlying reasons or circumstances contributing to maintaining them. To their assistance, the participants recorded sleep diaries, behaviour and activity diaries, thoroughly registering daily life activities.

In the second half of the intervention, individual goals and targets regarding measures that could contribute to improved sleep were set, and the sleep diaries used as a basis for group discussion and evaluation of effect. Finally, an individual maintenance plan, in which each participant described what they considered as the most important steps in their process of change, a document intended for them to be able to get back to in case the sleeping problem should return.

Control group

The participants in the control group consisted of patients who were prescribed a sleep medication for insomnia, either if the prescription was new for the patient (i.e. the patient had no ongoing sleep medication) or if a change in a previously prescribed sleep medication was decided (increase of dose or change to/addition of another medication).

Measurements

Prior to the CBT group intervention, the participants graded their sleep time and quality by filling-out the Pittsburgh Sleep Quality Index (PSQI) form [8,9], and estimated the severity of their sleeping problems by filling-out the Insomnia Severity Index (ISI) [10]. In both cases, measurement was then repeated directly (within maximum one week) and two months after the final group session, i.e. after having completed the intervention.

Apart from sleep estimation, cortisol in saliva was also measured before and directly after the intervention, as a possible biomarker of stress. Since the normal biological pattern for blood cortisol (reflected also in saliva) is a natural peak in the morning, at about half an hour after awakening, the saliva test was at each occasion taken twice: 1) directly after awakening, and 2) half an hour after awakening. An absence of a ≥50% increase in saliva cortisol level from the initial to the half-hour measurement was seen as an indication of possible stress [11,12].

The test was taken by the participants themselves, using the SalivaBio Oral Swab sample equipment (Salimetrics Inc., London, UK) by placing a saliva collection swab sublingually for two minutes, and then closing it in the sample tube. The samples were then to be brought to the PHC unit laboratory within three days, and should if not brought in during the same day be kept in refrigerator. After arrival to the laboratory, the test was centrifuged and frozen at -20° Celsius until analysis.

Results

Fifty-six participants were initially enrolled in the study, 41 in the intervention group and 15 in the control group. Of the participants in the intervention group, six interrupted the intervention after one or two group sessions and were thus excluded from the study. Of the remaining 35 participants in the intervention group, 28 were women and seven were men, and in the control group the corresponding gender distribution was eleven women and four men.

The mean age was 54 years, ranging between 21 to 85 years. Main characteristics of the study population is shown in Table 1.

	Intervention group (n=35)	Control group (n=15)	Total (n=50)
Gender (n): Female	28	11	39
Male	7	4	11
Mean age (years): Total	54	54	54
Females	55	54	55
Males	48	56	51
Baseline sleep characteristics:	Mean value (±SD)	Mean value (±SD)	Mean value (±SD)
Mean estimated time before falling asleep (minutes)	60 (±50)	58 (±65)	59 (±54)
Mean estimated total sleep time (minutes)	298 (±62)	325 (±54)	306 (±61)
Mean PSQI score	12.1 (±2.2)	11.2 (±2.7)	11.8 (±2.3)
Mean ISI total score	19.4 (±3.7)	17.3 (±4.7)	18.7 (±4.1)

Table 1: Main study population characteristics, by means of age and gender distribution, and characteristics of sleep estimates at baseline.

Sleep onset and duration

In Figure 1, the mean value of the participants estimated time before falling asleep, before and after the intervention, is presented. In the CBT intervention group, there was a significant shortening of the mean time interval ($p<0.05$). In the control group there was also a shortening of the mean time interval, however not as pronounced, and not statistically significant. Although there was a marked difference in mean time before falling asleep at follow up between the two groups, this showed not to be statistically significant.

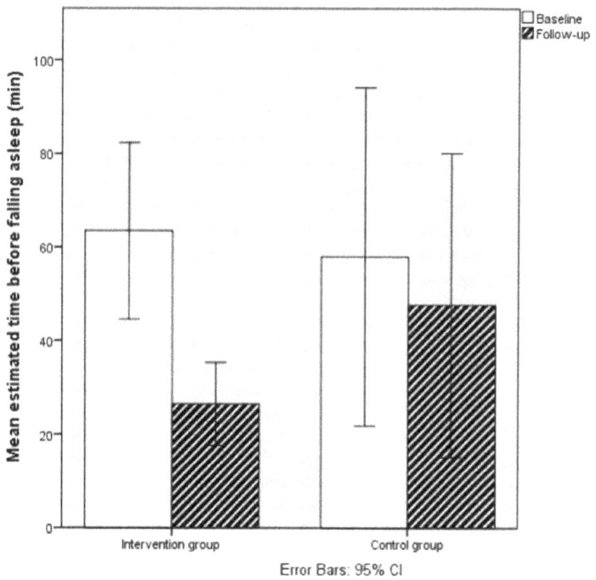

Figure 1: Comparison of mean estimated time before falling asleep, before and after the intervention, and between the intervention and control group, based on responses to the Pittsburgh Sleep Quality Index (PSQI).

Figure 2 shows the mean value of the participants' estimated total sleeping time, before and after the intervention. In the CBT intervention group, the participants reported significantly prolonged duration of night sleep at follow-up ($p<0.05$). A corresponding, less pronounced and non-significant prolongation of sleeping time was seen in the control group. Neither was the difference between the groups statistically significant.

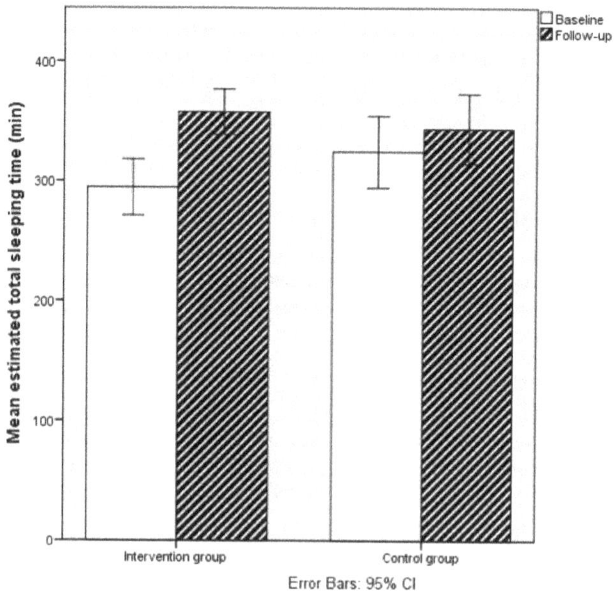

Figure 2: Comparison of mean estimated total sleeping time, before and after the intervention, and between the intervention and control group, based on responses to the Pittsburgh Sleep Quality Index (PSQI).

Sleep quality

The mean PSQI scores before and after the intervention is shown in Figure 3. In both the intervention and control group, the participants reported a significant improvement of sleep quality, reflected in a lowered PSQI score (p<0.05). Although seemingly somewhat more pronounced change in the CBT intervention group, the difference between the groups was not statistically significant.

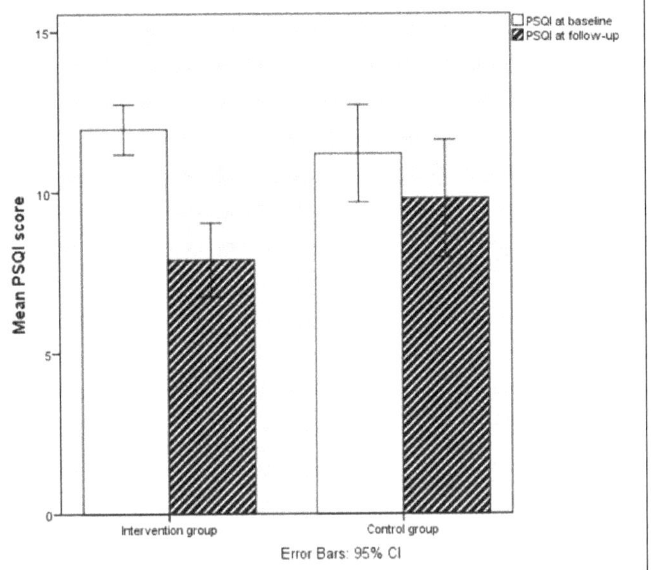

Figure 3: Comparison of sleep quality, in terms of mean Pittsburgh Sleep Quality Index (PSQI) scores, before and after the intervention, and between the intervention and control group.

Insomnia severity

The mean ISI scores before and after the intervention are shown in Figure 4. In the CBT intervention group, the participants reported a significantly lowered severity degree after the intervention (p<0.01). No corresponding difference was seen in the control group, and when comparing the ISI scores at follow-up, the ISI scores were significantly lower in the CBT intervention group than in the control group (p<0.05).

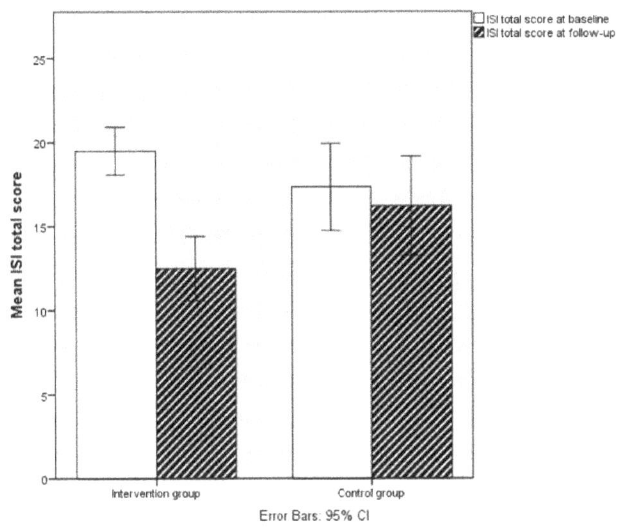

Figure 4: Comparison of insomnia severity, in terms of mean total Insomnia Severity Index (ISI) scores, before and after the intervention, and between the intervention and control group.

Regression analysis

In Table 2, odds ratios (OR) for improvement of sleep onset and duration, sleep quality (by means of PSQI score) and insomnia severity (by means of ISI score), when analyzed in a binary logistic regression model, using group, gender, age and baseline outcome within each field as covariates, in order to adjust for possible confounding effects of these. As seen in the table, being in the intervention group was the only variable significantly associated with improvement of any of the fields, namely insomnia severity, for which the OR against the control group was 15.5 (1.4-172.3 95% C.I.).

	Shortened sleep onset time OR (95% C.I.)	Prolonged total sleep time OR (95% C.I.)	Improved PSQI score OR (95% C.I.)	Improved ISI score OR (95% C.I.)
Group (intervention group)	3.1 (0.6-16.5)	3.5 (0.8-16.4)	4.9 (0.8-20.9)	15.5 (1.4-172.3)
Gender (female)	0.4 (0.04-3.2)	5.9 (1.1-30.6)	0.8 (0.1-5.3)	1.3 (0.15-11.9)
Age (increasing)	1 (0.9-1.1)	1 (0.9-1.1)	1 (1.0-1.1)	1 (0.9-1.1)
Baseline value (less favourable)	1.1 (1.0-1.1)	1 (0.9-1.9)	1.2 (0.8-1.7)	1.3 (1.0-1.7)

Table 2: Odds ratios (OR) and its 95% confidence intervals (C.I) for improvement of sleep onset and duration, and PSQI and ISI scorings, according to group (intervention/control), gender, age and baseline measurement outcome within each field, based on binary logistic regression analysis.

Cortisol in saliva

Expectedly, cortisol levels in saliva varied highly between individuals, ranging from 3 to >800 nmol/L (maximum measurement level). No significant difference between baseline and follow-up mean cortisol levels in either of the two groups could be observed. At baseline, 13 of 30 participants in the intervention group and six of twelve in the control group did not react with a with a ≥50% increase in saliva cortisol from awakening-test to test to half-hour test (the remaining eight participants had missing or incomplete saliva tests). At follow-up, the corresponding distribution was 15 of 30, and 3 of seven, respectively (tests missing or incomplete for 13 participants), showing no statistical significance in this respect.

Discussion

In this study we have shown that a CBT-based group intervention for insomnia in primary care may be effective in improving individual sleep duration and quality. This is in line with what has been found in previous research, from which CBT for insomnia has strong evidence. The major advantage of the intervention in the previous study is the fact that it is group based, both making it more resource effective (with six patients in a group attending six group sessions equaling one visit for six patient receiving individual therapy), and also using the therapeutic benefits of group dynamics and sharing of experiences by other group participants.

The most pronounced sleeping improvements observed in the study were reduction of the estimated time before falling asleep and lowering of perceived insomnia severity. In the latter case, ISI decreased by about a third, a change that was not only markedly more pronounced than in the control group, but also of statistical significance when comparing the two groups. Estimated mean time before falling asleep more then halved in the intervention group, a result that also differed markedly from that of the control group, although not statistically significant. Lack of sufficient power due to the relatively low sample size, especially in the control group, is likely to be contributory to this.

Although viewed as a common and major public health problem in many countries, insomnia is still probably under-diagnosed [3]. It is known to be associated with increased morbidity in terms of both physical and psychological illness [13-15] and substantial impairment of quality of life [16,17] for those affected. Ciccone et al. illustrated that improvement of sleep quality can be associated with reversibility of related co-morbidity even on a micro morphological level, in this particular case for OSAS patients (having an established increased risk for cardiovascular disease) receiving Continuous Positive Airway Pressure (CPAP) treatment, for which significant improvement on endothelial function could be detected [17]. Moreover, insomnia is likely to have important impact on work capacity and sick leave, as suggested by DiBonaventura et al. [18]. Thus, both from an individual patient perspective, as well as on a community level, strategies for healthcare providers to adequately handle sleep disorders should be essential and of high priority. The heterogeneity of the general population brings a need for alternate treatment possibilities, of which a group based CBT approach may be one suitable alternative, depending on local resources and competence. The findings in our study provide some evidence for the method to be chosen when available.

Study limitations

The study has some major limitations, of which the small sample size must be considered to be the most important one. Especially this accounts for the control group, making reliable comparisons difficult to attain. Difficulties in recruiting participants to the control group was the main reason for this, together with a limitation of capacity to prolong the control group sample interval. The same recruitment difficulty may also have affected the results by means of possible selection bias, as is probably the case also in the study group. Another important limitation, also probably further contributing to this, is the circumstance that the study was non-randomized. However, the intention of the chosen study design was to mimic the clinical routine in the primary care context, as it is performed in reality, and to compare the intervention with how the patients would have been treated in the normal case, without the opportunity to provide the tested group intervention. This would not have been achieved if the participants had been randomized to any kind of alternative "placebo" or similar control intervention. However, conclusions from the study results should be drawn with caution, and to confirm the presented findings, further studies in a larger population would be needed.

Conclusion

In conclusion, the tested eight-session CBT group based intervention for insomnia appears to reduce severity and duration of insomnia, and to shorten time before falling asleep, when provided in primary healthcare.

References

1. Swedish Council of Health Technology Assessment. Treatment of insomnia. National report.
2. The National Board of Health and Welfare. Drug register.
3. Morin CM, Benca R (2012) Chronic insomnia. Lancet 379: 1129-41.
4. Morin CM (2014) Cognitive-behavioral approaches to the treatment of insomnia. J Clin Psychiatry 65 Suppl 16: 33-40.
5. Blom K, Tarkian Tillgren H, Wiklund T, Danlycke E, Forssén M, et al. (2015) Internet vs. group-delivered cognitive behaviour therapy for insomnia: A randomized controlled non-inferiority trial. Behav Res Ther 70: 47-55.
6. Taylor R, Reeder C (2015) Intensive individual and group cognitive behavioural therapy for obsessive-compulsive disorder. Am J Psychother 69: 269-84.
7. Echeburúa E, Sarasua B, Zubizarreta I (2013) Individual versus individual and group therapy regarding a cognitive-behavioral treatment for battered women in a community setting. J Interpers Violence 29:1783-1801.
8. Keklund G, Åkerstedt T (1997) Objective components of individual differences in subjective sleep quality. J Sleep Res 6: 217-20.
9. Landry GJ, Best JR, Liu-Ambrose T (2015) Measuring sleep quality in older adults: a comparison using subjective and objective methods. Front Aging Neurosci 7: 166.
10. Bastien CH, Vallières A, Morin CM (2001) Validation of the Insomnia Severity Index as an outcome measure for insomnia research. Sleep Med 2: 297-307.
11. Maina G, palmas A, Filon FL (2008) Relationship between self-reported mental stressors at the workplace and salivary cortisol. Int Arch Occup Environ Health 81: 391-400.
12. Fekedulegn DB, Andrew ME, Burchfiel CM (2007) Area under the curve and other summary indicators of repeated waking cortisol measurements. Psychosom Med 69: 651-9.
13. Ford DE, Kamerow DB (1989) Epidemiologic study of sleep disturbances and psychiatric disorders. An opportunity for prevention? JAMA 262: 1479-84.
14. Foley DJ, Monjan AA, Brown SL, Simmonsick EM, Wallace RB, et al. (1995) Sleep complaints among elderly persons: an epidemiologic study of three communities. Sleep 18: 425-32.
15. Foley D, Ancoli-Israel S, Britz P, Walsh J (2004) Sleep disturbances and chronic disease in older adults: results of the 2003 National Sleep Foundation Sleep in America Survey. J Psychosom Res 56: 497-502.

8

Concepts of Neurophysiological Factors in the Central Regulatory Mechanism of Non-Rapid Eye Movement Sleep

Boniface EE*

Department of Physiology, School of Basic Medical Sciences, College of Medical Sciences, University of Benin, Benin City, Edo State, Nigeria

***Corresponding Author:** Ezenwanne E Boniface, Department of Physiology, School of Basic Medical Sciences, College of Medical Sciences, University of Benin, Benin City, Nigeria, E-mail: ezenwanneeeb@yahoo.co.uk

Abstract

Objective: It is now fully ascertained that the generation of non-rapid eye movement sleep (NREM) involves vital brain processes achieved through complex interactions of underlying neurophysiological factors, including those of the mechanism for the production of the behavioral expressions of NREM sleep. These central processes in the mechanism of NREM sleep are still far from clear and are subject of much speculations and even controversy. It was the aim of this review to identify and assemble those factors in brain function that informed current research postulations of workers in the subject of the production of NREM sleep.

Methods: Information gathering adopted in this review included, articles and published research works, seminars and conference articles on sleep, information from current textbooks in neuroscience on sleep, lecture notes in behavioral neurophysiology and biology, and articles and reports on sleep accessed from the Internet using search engines such as Google, PubMed etc., were all sources of information consulted.

Results: The significance of specific neurotransmitter systems – Serotonin, GABA and Adenosine, in the proposed central mechanism for the production and behavioral expressions of NREM sleep have been clearly highlighted in this review. Facts noted in this review successfully sensitized the attention of research to the growing profile of the more recently identified Metabolic Energy substrates Drive in the proposed possible central mechanism for the generation of NREM sleep stage.

Conclusion: Research postulations and proposals assembled in this review appear generally to support the notion that different brain processing networks and neurochemical units are probably involved in the production of NREM sleep and other distinct states of sleep. It is therefore concluded from this review that probably different neuronal pathways and systems make up specific vital brain processes for the production and expressions of NREM sleep stage, and these central processes are still far from fully understood with certainty.

Key words:

NREM Sleep; Neurophysiological factors; Central regulatory mechanism

Introduction

Sleep as a subject, has undergone several definitions and re-definitions in the past years, with different groups of workers coming up with different approaches to the subject. Neuroscientists studied sleep as part of psychology and medicine. Meanwhile, the initial problem started with the fact that sleep was viewed and defined as a state of consciousness and not a physiological state. The problem of ascertaining a comprehensive definition of sleep became even more complicated because there was no clear demarcation or understanding of the minimum set of events that constitute sleep and distinguishes it from other states of partial or non consciousness. Nevertheless, the study of sleep appeared to receive a big boost with advances in technology from the second half of the twentieth century. The major contributors to the modern concepts of the subject of sleep and waking states evolved from the discovery of electroencephalogram in 1929 by Hans Berger, and the landmark discovery of the Ascending Reticular Activating system. Thus, sleep was then seen as a behavioral state in the animal, and was known to be present in all species of animals including fetuses, birds, fish, reptiles and amphibians. In one earlier concept, sleep was regarded as the natural state of bodily rest during which the brain is resting, as part of the daily routine in everyone. This earlier concept gave birth to some erroneous concepts which regarded sleep as the state of natural unconsciousness from which an individual (or the animal) can be aroused. Nevertheless, among the more modern proposals was the definition which regarded sleep as the deactivation of the cerebral cortex and thalamus, expressed by the near lack of response to sensory inputs during sleep [1]. However, this definition suffered some defects of neurophysiological facts and was later invalidated because it was a known fact that both regions of the brain (cortex and thalamus) are active in some phases of sleep; in fact, only the thalamus may be assumed to be deactivated in the sense of transmission of sensory information to the cortex. The effort to ascertain a more comprehensive definition of sleep was apparently addressed through the observation method of the overall brain activity in characteristic electroencephalogram (EEG) patterns during sleep [2], and these concepts later gave way to the definition which regarded sleep as a naturally recurring state of relatively suspended sensory and motor activity in the animal, characterized by total or partial unconsciousness and nearly complete inactivity of voluntary muscles

[3]. This later explanation appears to be even more scientific and the more comprehensive and adequate for the purpose of the present discussion on the subject of none-rapid eye movement (NREM) sleep in this review.

It is now known that sleep is not a merely passive state in which the brain is resting or quiescent. It has become clear that cortical functions in sleep are characteristically dynamic and complicated condition during which the brain is quite active, and that certain vital processes in brain function are driven by certain stages of sleep. For example, there are observations attributed to specific stages of sleep which included: decrease of sympathetic activity and increase of parasympathetic activity in NREM sleep (3), increase in heart rate and blood pressure accompanied by decrease in homeostatic responses and muscle tone in rapid eye movement (REM) sleep [4].

Normal sleep is partitioned into the cyclic alternations of NREM sleep and REM sleep stages, clearly indicating that each sleep stage repeats itself in a characteristic pattern in the course of a night's sleep. Thus, this recurring phenomenon in which each sleep stage repeats itself in the course of the night, is clear demonstration that sleep is not merely a state of neural inactivity in which the brain is quiescent. Research findings have shown that non-rapid eye movement sleep (NREM) occupies about 75-80% of total sleep period in the human. Several studies have also shown that Slow-Wave sleep (SWS) is made up of the deepest stage of NREM sleep, and is often referred to as the deep sleep. Although muscles are not paralyzed as in REM sleep, research findings have confirmed that the highest arousal thresholds (i.e. difficulty of awakening) are generally observed in the stage 3 of the NREM sleep, and because muscles are generally not paralyzed, sleepwalking is possible in a person in NREM sleep. Reports from recent studies indicate that Slow-Wave sleep (SWS) is a highly active state of the brain, unlike the state of quiescence of the brain as previously thought. Although it has been widely reported that NREM sleep is characterized by decreased global and regional cerebral blood flow, data from brain Imaging Studies indicate that blood flow to parahippocampal gyrus increases during NREM sleep. Among several brain activities that have been studied to date, sleep spindles and K-complexes have been shown to be unique to NREM sleep, and up to date there is no reliable answer or clear understanding of what these waves activities mean. There are indications from recent study and reports which show that regional brain activities are influenced by the waking experiences of the recent past in some stages of NREM sleep [5]. It has also been observed that mental activities that take place during NREM sleep are generally thought-like. Furthermore, increased secretions of growth hormone in some parts of the brain have been demonstrated during NREM sleep, and this was shown to be indicative that there are increases in the firing rate and metabolism in these cortical cells [5]. These aforementioned facts offered the background and the basis for the follow-up working hypothesis to address the speculations that the memory encoding regions of the brain (i.e. information encoding and recall capacity of the hippocampus) are generally activated, and not functionally dormant during NREM/Slow-Wave sleep stage as previously thought [5].

Proposals and Research Hypotheses

Neurotransmitter systems implicated in NREM sleep

It has been noted that the anterior hypothalamus and adjacent forebrain areas are important in the production of NREM sleep, as are the thalamus, dorsal raphe and nucleus tractus solitarius. Serotonin and GABA are now believed to play important roles in the regulatory mechanisms of NREM sleep, and they are known to be densely located in these regions. There is enough evidence to suggest that serotonin (5-HT) found in raphe neurons of the brainstem are involved in the central mechanism of sleep onset (Stage 1 of NREM sleep). Thus, the discharge of the serotonin secreting neurons was linked to the onset of NREM sleep. It was noted that insomnia occurred when the serotonergic cells in dorsal raphe nucleus was lesioned, while MAO Inhibitors (specific for 5-HT) enhanced NREM sleep [6]. In another report, it was noted that substances within the biosynthetic pathways of serotonin (such as tryptophan and vitamin B6) facilitated sleep onset (i.e., Stage 1 of NREM sleep) [7].

Several recent studies have shown that the inhibitory neurotransmitter, GABA, is released in highest amounts during NREM sleep [8]. GABA secreting neurons have been demonstrated throughout the basal forebrain, hypothalamus, thalamus, brainstem and cortex. Workers have shown conclusively that the ventrolateral preoptic (VLPO) cells contain GABA and Galanin, and that these transmitters play important role in the mammalian brain by attenuating the ascending monoaminergic arousal system activity during sleep [8]. Thus, it is obvious from these findings that the ventrolateral preoptic (VLPO) neurons are sleep promoting by some reciprocal inhibitory interactions and activity with the waking systems. It was then hypothesized that the reciprocal inhibitory exchanges between the major ascending monoaminergic (arousal) neuronal group and the sleep-inducing VLPO neurons act on a feedback loop model; when the monoamine nuclei discharge intensively during wakefulness, they inhibit the VLPO group, and when the VLPO neurons fire rapidly during sleep, this blocks the discharge of the monoamine cells group. Thus, the two halves of the circuit strongly inhibit each other to produce two stable discharge patterns-On or Off [8]. The research hypothesis demonstrated in this proposed sleep model may have helped to clarify why the sleep-awake transitions are relatively abrupt, and changes between sleep and arousal occur infrequently and rapidly.

There are pieces of evidence to show that hypnotics such as benzodiazepines (diazepam or triazolam) and barbiturates tend to work by potentiating GABA mediated inhibitory processes, thus, causing hyperpolarizations and reduced cell firing. These drugs shut down neurons in the reticular activating system, thereby inhibiting transmissions projected to the cortex and thalamus. In the overall, hypnotics have been noted to increase total sleep time, decrease sleep latency, decrease the duration of stages 3 and 4 of NREM sleep and decrease the number of awakenings [9]. Withdrawal from these drugs (hypnotics) resulted into insomnia and REM sleep rebound fairly quickly [9].

Brain areas implicated in the mechanism of NREM sleep

Hypothalamus: During the period of initial speculations on the actual role of the hypothalamus in the production of NREM sleep, workers proposed a Two-Process Model of sleep regulation to explain the homeostatic and circadian drives for sleep [10]. In the functional organization of this setting which is also under the control of hypothalamus (HT) and suprachiasmatic nucleus (SCN), the two process sleep model was of parallel mechanisms described as Process S (homeostatic) and Process C (circadian), respectively. The homeostatic component is believed to be driven by a substrate or protein which registers a homeostatic "need to sleep" during periods of extended wakefulness that is subsequently relieved during sleep. It was hypothesized that the sleep model is driven by the pressure build-up of adenosine accumulation and the circadian rhythm of 24 hr cycle in the body. According to this proposal, the slow wave density of adenosine increases through the night and then drops off at the beginning of dawn, while the circadian rhythm is like a sinusoid; the pressure to sleep (towards the onset of NREM sleep) was maximum when the difference between the two was highest. However, a few years later another group of workers proposed a completely different sleep model known as Opponent Process Model [11]. In the working hypothesis of this later sleep model, these workers observed that the two parallel mechanisms as earlier described in the Borbely's Two-Process Model of sleep [10], actually opposed each other in the production of NREM sleep. Thus, according to this Opponent Process Sleep Model, the SCN enhances wakefulness and opposes the homeostatic rhythm, and the homeostatic rhythm is regulated via a complex multisynaptic pathway in the hypothalamus to shut off wakefulness system [11]. Thus, both systems mutually produce the critical effects characteristic of NREM sleep and wakefulness. However, it is noteworthy that the underlying mechanisms in these proposed sleep models are still far from clear. Nonetheless, it was suggested that both sleep models actually have some validity to them [10,11]. Meanwhile, a much later theory also maintained that the inhibition of NREM sleep by REM sleep could play significant role, hence, the two sleep processes or mechanisms add flexibility to the simple circadian rhythm and could have evolved as an adaptive measure.

Thalamus: Most of the known brain activities in sleep have been attributed to the thalamus and there appears to be pockets of evidence to suggest that a thalamic mechanism may play a critical role in Slow-Wave sleep. Pursuant to this idea, a group of workers proposed a Thalamic Pacemaker hypothesis which holds that two primary oscillations of slow spindles and delta waves are generated by both the thalamus and cortex reciprocally in NREM sleep [12]. Since sleep spindles can be generated only by the thalamus, it proves this to be very significant because inputs from the thalamus is critical in sleep onset (NREM sleep Stage 1); it was noted that when the change is from tonic to the phasic mode of the pacemaker oscillations in the neural circuit, it denotes the linking of parts of the cortex in the co-ordination of sleep onset (NREM sleep Stage 1).

Brain Stem Systems: In one of the research proposals, it was hypothesized that the reticular activating system through three groups of neuronal systems in the brainstem-pedunculopontine nucleus, locus ceoruleus and raphe nucleus-act via two pathways, mainly: the cholinergic pathway which clears the system for the thalamocortical transmission [13] and, the monoaminergic pathway which by projecting to the hypothalamus and cerebral cortex, shuts down the arousal systems to activate the NREM sleep phase [14]. Considerable evidence suggest that the neural systems concerned with sleep and waking states are in the brainstem, and several studies have shown that there are neural elements in the brain stem which inhibit neuronal communications to turn off the arousal systems during sleep. A research sleep model proposal was later put forward by some workers, known as Sleep Process S [15], and this model later formed the basis for the Sleep-Generating Systems Hypothesis of the brainstem reticular formation. In this model, Sleep Process S is regulated by neurons that shut down the arousal systems of the brain stem, thus, allowing the brain to fall asleep (NREM Stage 1). There was the suggestion that many of the neurons that initiate NREM sleep by inhibiting the arousal systems are also found in the preoptic area of the hypothalamus and loss of these nerve cells lead to profound insomnia [15]. There are also proposals that provided evidence to the fact that among the mechanisms of the sleep-generating neurons in the brainstem are: activation of inputs from the lower brainstem centers that relay information about the state of the body including emotional and cognitive areas; activation of inputs from the circadian system which allows the awake-sleep system to synchronize with the day-night cycle, but also to override this cycle when it is necessitated by the needs; activation of the cholinergic pathways to the thalamus for the characteristic EEG patterns [16]. Another group of workers also noted the possibility of the state of parasympathetic dominance during NREM sleep [17].

Energy molecules drive hypotheses

In general, sleep is considered a behavioral state in the animal, governed by some central control mechanisms. There is accumulating evidence which suggest that NREM sleep might be a fundamental property of local neuronal networks since it can be initiated at lower brain assemblies, and only later may become consolidated by general cortical mechanisms. It has been observed that in humans, NREM sleep in each local cortical column can be initiated by metabolically driven changes from manufactured molecules of sleep-regulating substances produced by neuronal activity during wakefulness-like activity. It is thought that the process may involve increased electrical activity, blood flow, extracellular levels of ATP, extra and intracellular levels of adenosine, all of which decrease the intracellular ATP level, and this may drive individual columns to enter a sleep-like activity state [7]. It was further noted that once a sleep state was reached this process would be reversed and the cortical columns become prepared for wakefulness [7] The possible role of astrocytes as potential mediators in the adenosine sleep mechanism was also proposed [18]. It was suggested that adenosine, while acting in the basal forebrain, is a key mediator of homeostatic control of sleep expression [6]. Some of these proposals and conclusions were based on the earlier suggestion that increased adenosine release accompanies the accumulation of the need to sleep [19]. Thus, based on simple energy demand, and since the cerebral cortex-thalamus unit is a large part of the human and mammalian brain, it was considered that an awake state for long periods of time was obviously apparently very expensive, hence, energy economy by the brain during NREM sleep is one of the prevalent hypotheses to explain the pressure for going into the NREM sleep [20].

It has been observed that during periods of wakefulness, glycogen (the body's principal store of energy) becomes exhausted [21] It was also observed that as glycogen is broken down into adenosine, extracellular levels of adenosine begin to accumulate in the basal forebrain [22], leading to the replenishment and recovered sleep [21,23]. Experimental sleep models have shown that the injection of adenosine or an adenosine A1 receptor agonist into rat's basal forebrain or cat's VLPO, respectively, promoted sleep by inhibiting multiple awake-promoting regions of the brain or by exciting sleep promoting cells groups [24,25]. Recent evidence have confirmed that the sleep-promoting effects of adenosine is further enhanced through its actions at the A1 receptors production cites [18].

Theories of NREM sleep

A number of theories were put forward by workers in the effort to conceptualize some of the central neuronal factors in NREM sleep, but with very little data. Unfortunately and surprisingly also, most of these theories failed to address the issue of ascertaining the actual mechanism involved in the generation of NREM sleep, and production of the behavioural expressions. Most of the theories were mainly revised proposals and redefinitions expressed in the speculations that sought to explain or reposition the benefits of NREM sleep. For example, it was hypothesized that slow wave sleep has restorative effects since it appears to be a period of rest for the brain [26]. In another proposal, some workers further noted that brain areas that are very active during wakefulness show an increase in slow wave sleep with a rise in certain growth hormones that have been shown to increase during period of NREM sleep [26,27].

Conclusion

Although the processes of sleep and waking states have generally been attributed to the thalamus, hypothalamus, brainstem structures and their interaction with the cortex, advances in knowledge of the neurophysiology of distinct brain systems clearly indicate that central processes in the mechanism of various sleep stages in a subject have become even more complex than previously conceived and are still far from full understanding.

Recent insights into the neurophysiological patterns in various sleep stages indicate that different brain processing networks and neurochemical systems are probably involved in the different sleep states. Thus, it is possible that specific neuronal pathways and transmitter systems that make up the ascending arousal systems and centered in the hypothalamus, interact with sleep active neurons in the VLPO area to produce NREM sleep and other distinct sleep states with characteristic abrupt transitions.

NREM sleep is associated with synchronized EEG patterns in which unique and specific neurophysiological events take place (e.g., Sleep spindles, K complexes, Slow-wave activity etc.). It is possible that the thalamus and cerebral cortex are absolutely necessary for the expression of the most significant bioelectrical and behavioral events of NREM sleep, whilst other structures like the basal forebrain, cerebellum and brainstem, may modulate NREM sleep but are not necessary for the actual generation of the bioelectrical and behavioral events accompanying the expressions of NREM sleep.

It is the expectation that future steps in understanding the neural processes in brain circuitary underlying the production of NREM sleep may lead to less speculations on the actual mediatory roles of Serotonin, Adenosine and GABA in the production of NREM sleep, and provide greater insight into the underlying mechanisms to identify discrete neuronal substrates involved in the generation of NREM sleep. It is hoped that information assembled in this review may serve as important information source for researchers and various neuroscientists engaged in the efforts to obtain a clearer understanding of the central factors in the neuronal mechanism of NREM sleep.

References

1. Magnin M, Rey M, Bastuji H, Guillemant P, Mauguiere F, et al. (2010) Thalamic deactivation at sleep onset precedes that of the cerebral cortex in humans. Proc Natl Acad Sci U S A 107: 3829-3833.
2. Dement W, Kleitman N (1957) Cyclic variations in EEG during sleep and their relation to eye movements, body motility and dreaming. Electroencephalogr Clin Neurophysiol 9: 673-690.
3. Macmillan Dictionary for Students, Macmillan Pan Ltd. (1981) New York, Simon & Schuster Books, USA, pp: 936.
4. Somers VK, Dyken ME, Mark AL, Abboud FM (1993) Sympathetic-Nerve ativity during sleep in normal subjects. N Engl J Med 328: 303-307.
5. Tononi G, Cirelli C (2005) Sleep function and synaptic homeostasis. Sleep Med Rev 10: 49-62.
6. Maquet P (2010) Understanding non-rapid eye movement sleep through neuroimaging. World J Biol Psychiatry 11: S9-S15.
7. Jones BE (2000) Basic mechanisms of sleep-awake states, In: Principles and Practice of Sleep Medicine. Philadelphia: W.B. Saunders & Co, USA, pp: 121-140.
8. Krueger JM, Rector DM, Roy S, van Dongen HP, Belenky B, et al. (2008) Sleep as a fundamental property of neuronal assemblies. Nat Rev Neurosci 9: 910-919.
9. Schwartz JRL, Roth T (2008) Neurophysiology of sleep and wakefulness: basic science and clinical Implications. Curr Neuropharm 6: 367-378.
10. Gailard JM, Nicholson AN, Pascoe PA (1989) Neurotransmitter systems, In: Principles and Practice of Sleep Medicine. Kryger MH, Roth T, Dement WC (eds), W.B. Saunders and Co., Philadelphia, pp: 202-212.
11. Borbely AA (1982) A two process model of sleep regulation. Human Neurophys 1: 195-204.
12. Edgar DM, Dement WC, Fuller CA (1993) Effect of SCN lesions on sleep in squirrel monkeys: evidence for opponent processes in sleep-wake regulation. J Neurosci 13: 1065-1079.
13. McCormick DA, Bal T (1997) Sleep and arousal: Thalamocortical mechanisms. Annu Rev Neurosci 1997; 20: 185-215.
14. Mesulam MM (1995) Cholinergic pathways and the ascending reticular activating system of the human brain. Ann N Y Acad Sci 757: 169-179.
15. Saper CB, Chou TC, Scammell TE (2001) The sleep switch: Hypothalamic control of sleep and wakefulness. Trends Neurosci 24: 726-731.
16. Saper CB, Scammell TE, Lu J (2005) Hypothalamic regulation of sleep and circadian rhythms. Nature 437: 1257-1263.
17. Rebecca T (2008) Theories of Sleep.
18. Andreasen NC, Black DW (2006) Introductory Textbook of Psychiatry. Arlington: American Psychiatric Publishing, Inc, USA.
19. McCarley W (2007) National Institute of Neurological Disorders and Stroke. Brain basics: Understanding sleep.
20. Benington JH, Kodaly SK, Keller HC (1995) Stimulation of A1 adenosine receptors mimics the encephalographic effects of sleep deprivation. Brain Res 692:79-85.
21. Mignot E, Huguenard JR (2009) Resting our cortices by going down to sleep. Neuron 63: 719-721.
22. Kong J, Shepel PN, Holden CP, Maciewicz M, Pack AI, et al. (2002) Brain glycogen Decreases With increased periods of wakefulness implications for homeostatic drive to sleep. J Neurosci 22: 5581-5587.
23. Porkka-Heiskanen T, Strecker RE, McCarley TW (2000) Brain site-specificity of extracellular adenosine concentration changes during sleep deprivation and spontaneous sleep: an in vivo microdialysis study. Neurosci 99: 507-517.
24. Chepel PN, Ramonet D, Stevens P, Geiger JD (2005) Purine level regulation during energy depletion associated with gated excitatory stimulation in brain. Neurol Res 27; 139-148.
25. Scammell TE, Estabrooke IV, McCarthy MT, Chemelli RM, Yanagisawa M, et al. (2000) Hypothalamic arousal regions are activated during modafinil-induced wakefulness. J Neurosci 20: 8620-8628.
26. Strecker RE, Morairty S, Thakkar MM, Porkka-Heiskanen T, Basheer R, et al. (2000) Adenosinergic modulation of basal forebrain and preoptic/antetior hypothalamic neuronal activity in the control of behavioral state. Behav Brain Res 115: 183-204.
27. Siegel JM, Moor R, Thannickal T, Nienhuis R (2001) A brief History of hypocretin/oexin and narcolepsy. Neuropsychopharmacol 25: S14-S20.

CPAP with Pressure Relief during Exhalation (C-Flex+) is as Effective as CPAP in the Treatment of Obstructive Sleep Apnea

Monika Krawietz[1], Carmen Garcia[1], Carsten Pilz[1], Martin Glos[1], Beate Diecker[1], Ingo Fietze[1] and Thomas Penzel[1,2*]

[1]*Charité University Medicine Berlin, Berlin, Germany*

[2]*International Clinical Research Center, St. Anne's University Hospital Brno, Brno, Czech Republic*

Abstract

Purpose: Continuous positive airway pressure (CPAP) is the accepted therapy for obstructive sleep apnea (OSA). An expiratory pressure relief technology called C-Flex has been developed to improve the comfort of CPAP therapy. It provides a 2 mbar lower exhalation pressure and an additional flow-based pressure relief at the beginning of exhalation. The following study was conducted to investigate whether C-Flex was as effective as CPAP in treating OSA, and the patients' preference.

Methods: 60 newly diagnosed patients with OSA completed this double-blind controlled crossover-study. Patients were randomized to one night of C-Flex and one of CPAP under full attended polysomnography (PSG). A comfort visual analog scale (VAS) ranging from 0 to 10, with 10 being the highest comfort, was completed by all patients immediately after each PSG.

Results: There was no significant difference between the therapy modes in the apnea/hypopnea index (median 1.5 events/hour (h) with C-Flex (interquartile range (IQR) 0.7 to 3.6) *vs.* 1.7 events/h with CPAP (IQR 0.8 to 3.8), p=0.178). The sleep efficiency, sleep architecture and nocturnal oxygenation were also comparable. Most patients preferred C-Flex over CPAP (65%, p<0.001). C-Flex earned significantly higher ratings in the VAS (8.1 (7.2 to 9.0) *vs.* 7.0 (5.1 to 8.8), p<0.001).

Conclusion: C-Flex was as effective as CPAP therapy in treating OSA and patients preferred this mode of therapy.

Keywords: Obstructive sleep apnea; Continuous positive airway pressure; CPAP; Expiratory pressure relief; C-Flex+

Introduction

Obstructive sleep apnea (OSA) is a common sleep-related breathing disorder with a prevalence of 10% in women and 20% in men in high-income countries [1]. Repeated collapses of the pharynx lead to reductions or cessations of air flow [2]. These collapses can be caused by a small upper airway lumen, dysfunctional dilating muscles and unstable respiratory control [1].

The most important risk factor for developing an obstructive sleep apnea is obesity. Approximately 70% of the patients are obese [2]. Other risk factors include increasing age, male gender, craniofacial predisposition, and postmenopausal status in women [1,2].

The pathophysiology of OSA is not completely understood; however, there are proposed associations with increased activity of the sympathetic nervous system, activation of inflammatory pathways, endothelial dysfunction, abnormal coagulation, and metabolic dysregulation leading to insulin resistance and impaired lipid metabolism [3].

The health risks related to the presence of OSA are serious and many patients suffer from hypersomnia which can cause occupational problems [4] or increased chances for car accidents [5]. Severe obstructive sleep apnea leads to an increased risk of cardiovascular events especially stroke [6]. Untreated sleep apnea is also thought to be associated with hypertension [7] and atrial fibrillation [8].

OSA is also thought to be related to higher rates in depression [9]. Even increased cancer mortality has been suggested [10]. Sequelae generally appear to increase according to the severity of the sleep apnea, which is measured by the apnea/hypopnea index (AHI).

The reference standard for the diagnosis is attended cardiorespiratory polysomnography (PSG) [11]. The state-of-the-art treatment of moderate to severe OSA is the administration of continuous positive airway pressure (CPAP) with individually titrated pressure settings [12,13]. CPAP provides a pneumatic splint of the nasopharyngeal airways [14]. CPAP therapy improves the vascular function [15] and shows a reduced risk for cardiovascular events in long-term studies [16]. It also improves the objective and subjective criteria of daytime sleepiness, especially in patients with severe OSA and high levels of daytime sleepiness [17]. A major problem with CPAP is the low adherence rate. In a long-term study of a Swiss population, only 55% of the patients prescribed CPAP still used their device after 5 years. The same study also showed improved adherence with newer CPAP technologies and increased service and technical support [18]. Several new features were developed to provide more comfort during therapy as an attempt to improve adherence [19]. In general the risk of pharyngeal collapse is higher during inspiration and lower during expiration. Therefore, a high pressure is not necessary during expiration [20]. A new pressure regulating mode had been introduced to lower pressure dynamically during expiration. C-Flex+ (Philips Respironics,

***Corresponding author:** Thomas Penzel, Sleep Medicine Center, Charité - University Medicine Berlin, Berlin, Germany, E-mail: thomas. penzel@charite.de

PA, USA) is a comfort feature applying the prescribed therapy pressure during inspiration and providing a 2 mbar pressure reduction during expiration in a dynamic way. There is a further pressure relief at the beginning of expiration based on pressure measurement as sensed by the machine. For the patient there is no difference handling a device with plain CPAP mode or with the additional C-Flex+ mode. In summary the added feature is a software inside the CPAP machine which senses the pressure and modifies the applied pressure of the machine to imitate a more 'natural' pressure form to improve patient comfort and thereby therapy adherence. The additional cost for the machine with C-Flex+ mode differs much between countries. While it is marginal in some countries, the difference is considerable in other countries depending on national policies. The pressure curve of the dynamic C-Flex+ compared to CPAP is shown in (Figure 1).

We conducted a study to systematically assess whether C-Flex+ was as effective as CPAP in treating OSA.

The primary endpoint for the study was the AHI. The secondary endpoints were the nocturnal oxygen saturation, total sleep time, sleep efficiency, sleep architecture (N1, N2, N3 and REM sleep), average pressure output and the patients' preference.

Methods

93 CPAP-naive patients were enrolled in a prospective, double-blind, randomized, controlled study. The patients were referred to the sleep laboratory of the Charité Universitätsmedizin Berlin Campus Virchow with suspected OSA for a diagnostic attended PSG and treatment if required. The study was approved by the Ethics Committee of the Charité Universitätsmedizin Berlin. All patients were informed on the study purpose and provided written consent to participate.

Following diagnostic PSG, several patients were excluded because they did not fulfill eligibility criteria for the study . After a conventional attended titration night to determine the adequate therapy pressure, patients were randomized to one night of C-Flex+ and one night of conventional CPAP under full attended polysomnography (PSG). A comfort visual analog scale (VAS) was completed by the patients immediately after each PSG. After the last night patients were asked to decide which night (therapy) they preferred to evaluate the perceived comfort of the pressure curve. The study design is shown in (Figure 2).

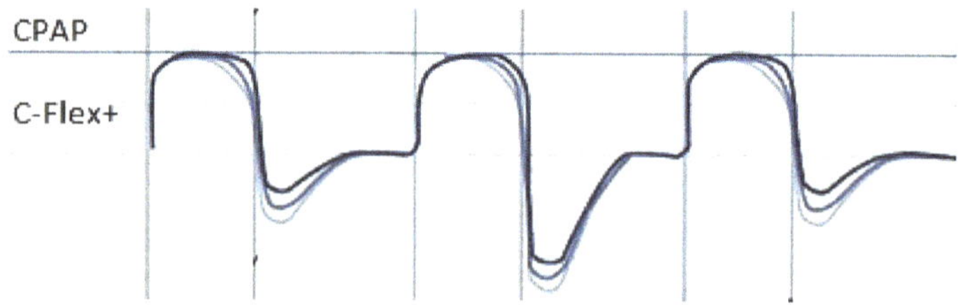

Figure 1: CPAP and C-Flex+ mode pressure curves over time [21]. The curves do show three subsequent inspirations and expirations. At the beginning of each expiration the particular relief drop in pressure is clearly observed.

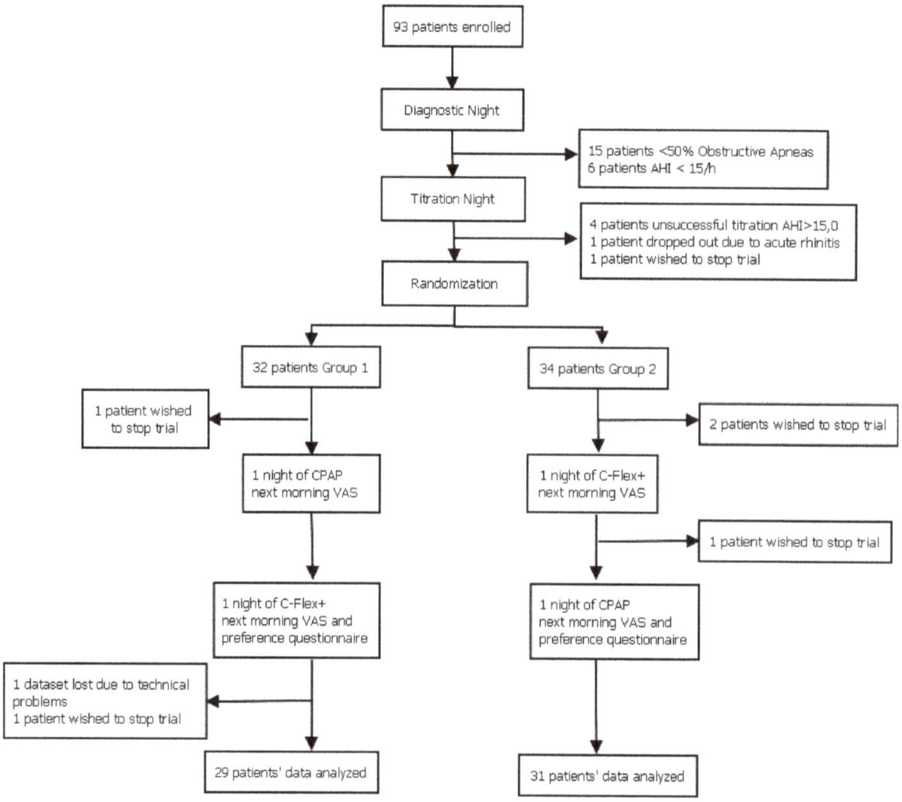

Figure 2: Flow chart of the study.

Only adult patients older than 21 years with a confirmed AHI > 15/hour (h) and > 50% obstructive apneas were included. They had to be able to provide consent as well as to follow the investigator's instructions concerning the CPAP device. Exclusion criteria were the inability to tolerate CPAP during the daytime session, failure of CPAP to adequately treat OSA during titration night (AHI > 15,0 under determined optimal pressure), medical contraindications to CPAP therapy such as sinusitis or surgery during the last 90 days, facial dermatitis or other skin lesions, untreated sleep disorders other than OSA like insomnia, periodic limb movements (PLM), restless legs syndrome (RLS), treated insomnia, intake of drugs affecting the central nervous system, previous experiences with CPAP, shift workers, participation in other clinical research during the last 4 weeks, or the patient requesting to withdraw from the study.

The data analyses were conducted with IBM SPSS Statistics Version 21. Differences between the treatments were analyzed using the Wilcoxon-signed-rank-test because the data were not distributed normally. Chi-square-test was applied to compare the patients' preferences.

Results

Sixty patients (48 males and 12 females) completed the study. For the baseline characteristics, see table 1. Based on the results of the titration night, the mean CPAP pressure was 8.7 ± 1.5 cmH_20.

As compared to the diagnostic night, both treatment interventions significantly improved the AHI, the obstructive, central and mixed apnea indexes, hypopneas index, minimum oxygen saturation and desaturation index (all $p<0.001$).The outcomes of both nights are listed in Table 2 and Figure 3

C-Flex+ earned significantly higher ratings by the VAS as compared to CPAP. 39 patients (65%) preferred C-Flex+, 12 patients (20%) preferred CPAP and 9 patients (15%) rated both C-Flex+ and CPAP equally comfortable ($p<0.001$). The rating values are shown in Figure 4.

Discussion

This study showed that C-Flex+ and conventional CPAP were equally effective with respect to respiratory parameters and sleep architecture. The primary endpoint, the AHI, was significantly

Parameters	Median (Interquartile Range,IQR)
Age (years)	53.2 (46.8-59.7)
Height (m)	1.78 (1.70-1.86)
Weight (kg)	99.0 (84.3-115.8)
BMI (kg/m²)	31.6 (29.1-36.0)
AHI (events/h)	38.0 (27.5-61.4)
ESS (points/24)	12 (8 – 16)
BMI=Body-Mass-Index, ESS=Epworth Sleepiness Scale	

Table 1: Patient characteristics at baseline visit.

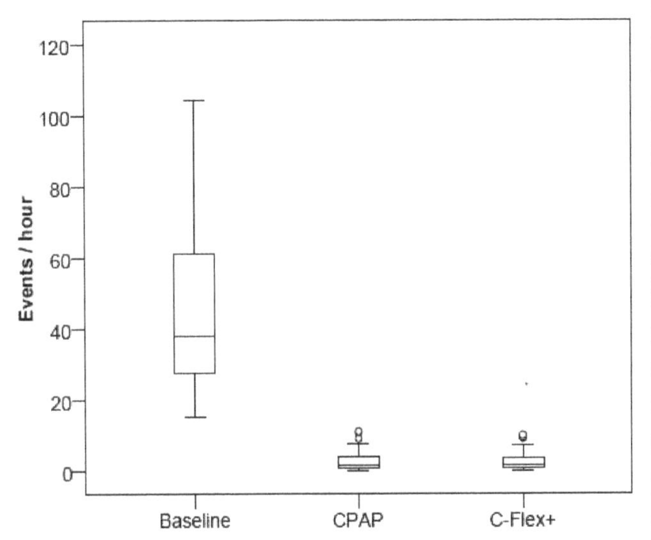

Figure 3: AHI at baseline, with CPAP and C-Flex+
Wilcoxon signed-rank test, both p<0.001 compared to baseline, no significant differences between the two modes. The circles symbolize outliers.

Parameter	Baseline	CPAP	C-Flex+	p Value
Apnea Index	23.1 (16.3-47.3)	0.9 (0.3-1.7)	0.3 (0.1-0.7)	<0.001
Obstructive Apnea Index	22.6 (11.5- 42.3)	0.2 (0.0-0.9)	0.0 (0.0-0.2)	<0.001
Central Apnea Index	0.9 (0.2-0.5)	0.4 (0.1-0.9)	0.2 (0.0-0.5)	0.034
Mixed Apnea Index	0.4 (0.0-3.4)	0.0 (0.0-0.0)	0.0 (0.0-0.0)	n.s.
Hypopnea Index	10.4 (4.3-16.7)	0.6 (0.3-1.8)	1.0 (0.4-2.5)	n.s.
Apnea / Hypopnea Index	38.0 (27.5- 61.4)	1.7 (0.8-3.8)	1.5 (0.7-3.6)	n.s.
Minimum Saturation in %	80.0 (70.0-84.0)	91.0 (90.0-93.0)	90.0 (88.0-93.0)	n.s.
Oxygen Desaturation Index>4%	26.6 (17.8-49.4)	1.5 (0.6-3.9)	2.5 (1.1-5.0)	0.003
Mean Heart Rate	70.1 (65.5-78.6)	70.3 (64.7-75.0)	73.0 (65.3-78.5)	0.044
Total Sleep Time in min	-	375.0 (333.8-397.8)	373.0 (341.0-405.8)	n.s.
Sleep Efficiency in %	-	86.8 (81.1-91.4)	88.4 (81.5-91.8)	n.s.
N1 in %	-	15.2 (12.0-23.6)	14.8 (10.2-19.6)	0.008
N2 in %	-	38.7 (34.5-45.8)	39.5 (33.0-50.0)	n.s.
N3 in %	-	20.5 (15.5-27.6)	23.6 (15.2-27.8)	n.s.
REM in %	-	19.9 (15.8 -25.1)	22.0 (16.3-25.0)	n.s.
Arousal Index	-	11.2 (7.8-17.3)	11.9 (9.2-18.0)	n.s.
RERA Index	-	0.4 (0.0-1.0)	0.5 (0.2-1.3)	n.s.
Movement ArousalIndex	-	2.6 (1.3-6.2)	3.2 (1.6-4.9)	n.s.
PLM Arousal Index	-	1.0 (0.0 -2.8)	1.4 (0.0-3.1)	n.s.

n.s.= not significant, N=NREM, Non Rapid Eye Movement, REM = Rapid Eye Movement, RERA = Respiratory Effort-Related Arousals,
Wilcoxon signed-rank test p-values refer to the differences between CPAP and C-Flex+.
Parameters marked with "-" were not determined

Table 2: PSG data of CPAP and C-Flex+, Median (IQR in parentheses)

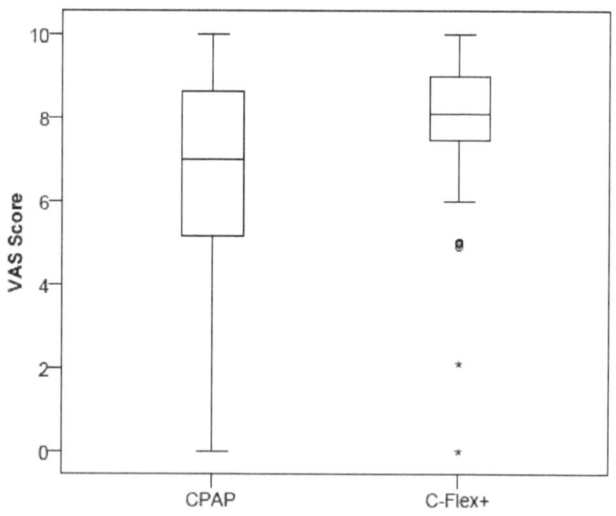

Figure: 4: Score in VAS with CPAP and C-Flex+ therapy showed that patients liked C-Flex+ more.
Wilcoxon signed-rank test, p<0.001. The circles indicate outliers and the stars indicate extreme outliers.

improved by both modes as expected. Between the two modes no significant difference could be detected concerning the AHI. By looking at the individual values we found that in three out of 60 patients the AHI was >4 events/hour higher with C-Flex+ compared to CPAP. This could be due to natural variability between nights or due to the more variable pressure with C-Flex+ mode.

Concerning most of the secondary endpoints there were no significant differences as well, though some differences nearly reached statistical significance.

In direct comparison with C-Flex+ there were significantly fewer total, obstructive and central apneas/h than with CPAP. There were no significant differences in mixed apneas/h, total sleep time, sleep efficiency and arousal index. There was significantly less stage NREM 1 (Non- Rapid Eye Movement) sleep with C-Flex+. With C-Flex+ there were significantly more oxygen desaturations > 4% /h and the heart rate was significantly higher compared to CPAP. Although these differences reached statistical significance there is minimal clinical significance of one additional desaturation per hour and a higher heart rate of less than three beats per minute, on average. The additional desaturation observed may be due to the same effect as reported with AHI: it could be either night-to-night variability or it could be due to the higher pressure fluctuations observed with the C-Flex+ pressure mode. For the heart rate values, CPAP lowered the mean heart rate significantly compared to baseline (p<0.03) whereas the mean heart rate with C-Flex+ compared to baseline heart rate did not show significant differences. Overall the differences in oxygen desaturation index (ODI) and in mean heart rate were statistically significant but cannot be considered as clinically relevant. Additional studies may clarify these findings.

However, these findings are surprising because most studies concerned with the predecessor comfort feature C-Flex (CPAP with expiratory pressure relief), did not find any significant differences between C-Flex versus conventional CPAP during attended PSG [22-28]. Only one study, conducted by Nilius et al., found statistically, but not clinically significant, differences in the number of central apneas/h with C-Flex (1.2 ± 2.5 versus 0.7 ± 1.0, p = 0.04) [20]. In contrary, our study showed a significantly lower central apnea index with C-Flex+ as compared to conventional CPAP.

In our study a significantly greater proportion of patients rated C-Flex+ as more comfortable than CPAP therapy. Two of the studies assessing C-Flex observed a significant preference for C-Flex as well [22,23]. A third one investigating the preference could not find a significant difference in the rating of the two [20].

However, based on data from this study, one cannot determine whether C-Flex+ leads to better long-term adherence. Studies assessing C-Flex showed that higher patient comfort ratings did not automatically lead to better adherence to treatment [22,23]. But Pépin et al. demonstrated that patients who showed low adherence to their CPAP device significantly improved their usage when changed to C-Flex [29] .

Therefore it would be desirable to perform a long-term study to see how C-Flex+ influences the adherence. If long-term studies investigating adherence to C-Flex+ are conducted they should have a duration of at least 3 months. Aloia et al. showed increasing differences in adherence between CPAP and C-Flex over this period of time. As time passed, fewer people in the CPAP group used their device while the people in the C-Flex group continued to use their therapy [24]. To check whether the incidence of cardiovascular consequences or even the cancer mortality changes with C-Flex+ compared to CPAP large trials and long-term observations are required.. This will require to establish a registry of CPAP and C-Flex+ users for well served regions.

In our study C-Flex+ proved to be as efficient as CPAP in treating sleep disordered breathing and can be an effective alternative for CPAP. Although we saw some statistical differences between C-Flex+ and CPAP, the differences did not have clinical relevance as both interventions adequately treated sleep -disordered breathing. Therefore C-Flex+ can be established as an alternative for CPAP therapy.

Acknowledgments

This study was partially supported by a grant from Philips Home Healthcare Solutions.

References

1. Jordan AS, McSharry DG, Malhotra A (2014) Adult obstructive sleep apnoea. Lancet 383: 736-747.
2. Malhotra A, White DP (2002) Obstructive sleep apnea. Lancet 360: 237-245.
3. McNicholas WT (2007) Cardiovascular outcomes of CPAP therapy in obstructive sleep apnea syndrome. Am J Physiol Regul Integr Comp Physiol 293: 1666-1670.
4. Ulfberg J, Carter N, Edling C (2000) Sleep-disordered breathing and occupational accidents. Scand J Work Environ Health 26: 237-242.
5. Tregear S, Reston J, Schoelles K, Phillips B (2009) Obstructive sleep apnea and risk of motor vehicle crash. Systematic review and meta-analysis. J Clin Sleep Med 5: 573-581.
6. Dong JY, Zhang YH, Qin LQ (2013) Obstructive sleep apnea and cardiovascular risk: meta-analysis of prospective cohort studies. Atherosclerosis 229: 489-495.
7. Parati G, Lombardi C, Hedner J, Bonsignore MR, Grote L, et.al. (2012) Position paper on the management of patients with obstructive sleep apnea and hypertension: joint recommendations by the European Society of Hypertension, by the European Respiratory Society and by the members of European COST (COoperation in Scientific and Technological research) ACTION B26 on obstructive sleep apnea. J Hypertens 30: 633-646.
8. Digby GC, Baranchuk A (2012) Sleep apnea and atrial fibrillation; 2012 update. Curr Cardiol Rev 8: 265-272.

9. Peppard PE, Szklo-Coxe M, Hla KM, Young T (2006) Longitudinal association of sleep-related breathing disorder and depression. Arch Intern Med 166: 1709-1715.

10. Nieto FJ, Peppard PE, Young T, Finn L, Hla KM, et al. (2012) Sleep-disordered breathing and cancer mortality. Results from the Wisconsin Sleep Cohort Study. Am J Respir Crit Care Med 186: 190-194.

11. Douglas NJ, Thomas S, Jan MA (1992) Clinical value of polysomnography. Lancet 339: 347-350.

12. Giles TL, Lasserson TJ, Smith BH, White J, Wright J, et.al. (2006) Continuous positive airways pressure for obstructive sleep apnoea in adults. Cochrane Database Syst Rev 3: CD001106.

13. McDaid C, Durée KH, Griffin SC, Weatherly HL, Stradling JR, et.al. (2009) A systematic review of continuous positive airway pressure for obstructive sleep apnoea-hypopnoea syndrome. Sleep Med Rev 13: 427-436.

14. Sullivan CE, Issa FG, Berthon-Jones M, Eves L (1981) Reversal of obstructive sleep apnoea by continuous positive airway pressure applied through the nares. Lancet 1: 862-865.

15. Cross MD, Mills NL, Al-Abri M, Riha R, Vennelle M, et.al. (2008) Continuous positive airway pressure improves vascular function in obstructive sleep apnoea/hypopnoea syndrome: a randomised controlled trial. Thorax 63: 578-583.

16. Doherty LS, Kiely JL, Swan V, McNicholas WT (2005) Long-term effects of nasal continuous positive airway pressure therapy on cardiovascular outcomes in sleep apnea syndrome. Chest 127: 2076-2084.

17. Patel SR, White DP, Malhotra A, Stanchina ML, Ayas NT (2003) Continuous positive airway pressure therapy for treating sleepiness in a diverse population with obstructive sleep apnea: results of a meta-analysis. Arch Intern Med 163: 565-571.

18. Schoch OD, Baty F, Niedermann J, Rüdiger JJ, Brutsche MH (2014) Baseline Predictors of Adherence to Positive Airway Pressure Therapy for Sleep Apnea: A 10-year Single-Center Observational Cohort Study. Respiration 87: 121-128.

19. Garvey JF, McNicholas WT (2010) Continuous positive airway pressure therapy: new generations. Indian J Med Res 131: 259-266.

20. Nilius G, Happel A, Domanski U, Rühle KH (2006) Pressure-relief continuous positive airway pressure vs constant continuous positive airway pressure: a comparison of efficacy and compliance. Chest 130: 1018-1024.

21. Philips Homehealth [Internet]. System One REMstar Pro, Flex-Technologie [cited 2013 Oct 23]. Available from: http://www.healthcare.philips.com/de_de/ homehealth /sleep/ SystemOne_Hintergrundinfos/flextechnologie.wpd

22. Wenzel M, Kerl J, Dellweg D, Barchfeld T, Wenzel G, et.al. (2007) Expiratory pressure reduction (C-Flex method) versus fix CPAP in the therapy for obstructive sleep apnoea. Pneumologie 61: 692-695.

23. Leidag M, Hader C, Keller T, Meyer Y, Rasche K (2008) Mask leakage in continuous positive airway pressure and C-Flex. J Physiol Pharmacol 59: 401-406.

24. Aloia MS, Stanchina M, Arnedt JT, Malhotra A, Millmann RP (2005) Treatment adherence and outcomes in flexible vs standard continuous positive airway pressure therapy. Chest 127: 2085-2093.

25. Marshall NS, Neill AM, Campbell AJ (2008) Randomised trial of compliance with flexible (C-Flex) and standard continuous positive airway pressure for severe obstructive sleep apnea. Sleep Breath 12: 393-396.

26. Dolan DC, Okonkwo R, Gfullner F, Hansbrough JR, Strobel RJ, et.al. (2009) Longitudinal comparison study of pressure relief (C-Flex) vs. CPAP in OSA patients. Sleep Breath 13: 73-77.

27. Smith I, Lasserson TJ (2009) Pressure modification for improving usage of continuous positive airway pressure machines in adults with obstructive sleep apnoea. Cochrane Database Syst Rev 4:CD003531.

28. Bakker J, Campbell A, Neill A (2010) Randomized controlled trial comparing flexible and continuous positive airway pressure delivery: effects on compliance, objective and subjective sleepiness and vigilance. Sleep 33: 523-529.

29. Pépin JL, Muir JF, Gentina T, Dauvilliers Y, Tamisier R, et.al. (2009) Pressure reduction during exhalation in sleep apnea patients treated by continuous positive airway pressure. Chest 136: 490-497.

Effect of an Anti-Supine Shirt for Treatment of Supine-related Obstructive Sleep Apnea

Melissa Brijbassi[1,2], Takatoshi Kasai[1,2], Luigi Taranto Montemurro[1,2] and T Douglas Bradley[1,2*]

[1]*Sleep Research Laboratory of the University Health Network Toronto Rehabilitation Institute, Toronto, Canada*

[2]*Centre for sleep Medicine and Circadian Biology, University of Toronto, Toronto, Canada*

***Corresponding author:** T Douglas Bradley, Toronto General Hospital, University Health Network 9N-943,200 Elizabeth Street Toronto, ON, M5G 2C4 Canada, E-mail: douglas.bradley@utoronto.ca

Abstract

Background and Objective: To evaluate the effects of a t-shirt designed to prevent patients from sleeping supine (anti-supine shirt) on the frequency of apneas and hypopneas per hour of sleep (apnea-hypopnea index) in patients with supine-related obstructive sleep apnea.

Methods: Twenty-seven consecutive patients found to have supine-related obstructive sleep apnea on a diagnostic polysomnogram were prescribed an anti-supine shirt and then underwent a follow up polysomnogram while wearing this shirt. We then compared the amount of supine sleep time and apnea-hypopnea index between the baseline and follow-up polysomnograms.

Results: A comparison between the baseline and follow-up polysomnograms revealed that there was no significant difference in total sleep time (from 297.2 ± 76.5 to 289.8 ± 101.6 min, p=0.654), but there was a significant reduction in the amount of supine sleep time while wearing the anti-supine shirt (from 149.2 ± 82.9 to 21.3 ± 52.9 min, p<0.001). This was accompanied by a 55% reduction in the total apnea-hypopnea index (from 23.8 ± 8.0 to 10.7 ± 14.7, p<0.001)

Conclusions: The anti-snore shirt reduced the severity of supine-related obstructive sleep apnea by reducing the amount of time spent sleeping supine.

Keywords: Sleep apnea; Posture; Supine; Positional therapy; Anti-supine shirt

Abbreviations

AHI: Apnea-Hypopnea Index, BMI: Body Mass Index, NREM: Non-Rapid Eye Movement, REM: Rapid Eye Movement

Introduction

Obstructive sleep apnea (OSA) is a common disorder affecting approximately 5 to 10% of the adult population [1,2] Approximately 60% of patients with OSA have a significant postural component in which the frequency of apneas and hypopneas per hour of sleep (apnea-hypopnea index or AHI) is at least twice as high in the supine as in the non-supine position [3-7]. In such patients, the supine position not only increases the AHI, but also increases the degree of associated oxygen desaturation and frequency of brady- and tachyarrhythmias [8].

Some patients experience more apneas and hypopneas while supine because the tongue and soft palate are displaced posteriorly due to the effect of gravity, causing narrowing of the upper airway (UA) [4,5,8]. This combined with a reduction in genioglossus muscle tone at sleep onset increases the propensity for the tongue to relapse into the UA and cause obstruction [6,8-12]. In addition, the nasal mucosa tends to become edematous while in the supine position thereby increasing upstream inspiratory airflow resistance that further increases UA collapsibility [13].

Since OSA is often supine-related, and since continuous positive airway pressure (CPAP) is poorly tolerated by a substantial proportion of patients with OSA [14] therapies have been developed to prevent patients from sleeping supine. Anti-supine interventions include wearing a pyjama top with a tennis-ball sewn onto the back or wearing a belt or shirt with balls or cylinders attached to the back. However, there are few published studies that have evaluated the effects of such interventions on OSA severity. Furthermore, most studies have evaluated a non-standardized commercially unavailable device. Therefore, our study was conducted to assess the effects of a standardized commercially available anti-supine sleep shirt on sleeping position and AHI in patients with supine-related OSA.

Materials and Methods

Subjects

Inclusion criteria were: 1) men and women at least 18 years of age referred to the sleep laboratory because of a clinical suspicion of sleep apnea based on a history of habitual snoring and at least one of nocturnal dyspnea, morning headaches, or excessive daytime sleepiness, 2) supine-related OSA defined as a total AHI of at least 10, 3) an AHI in the supine position at least twice that in the non-supine position, and 4) no previous treatment for OSA.

Polysomnography

All subjects underwent overnight polysomnography (PSG) for an assessment of sleep apnea using standard techniques and scoring criteria for sleep stages and arousals from sleep [15,16]. All subjects slept on a single pillow with the bed flat. Thoracoabdominal motion was monitored by respiratory inductance plethysmography and nasal airflow by nasal pressure cannulae. Arterial oxyhemoglobin saturation (SaO_2) was monitored by oximetry. Apneas were defined as a greater than 90% reduction and hypopneas as a 50% to 90% reduction in airflow from baseline lasting at least 10 sec. They were classified as obstructive if there was out-of-phase thoracoabdominal motion, or airflow limitation on nasal pressure [17]. Sleeping position was determined by video monitoring throughout the PSG. The AHI was quantified. Variables analyzed included total AHI, total sleep time (min), stages N1, N2, N3 and rapid eye-movement (REM) sleep time (min), supine sleep time (min), AHI in supine and non-supine positions, REM and non-REM related AHI, the total arousal index (arousals per hr of sleep), respiratory arousal index (respiratory-related arousals per hour of sleep), and the mean and minimum SaO_2 during sleep.

Protocol

Subjects underwent overnight attended PSG in the sleep laboratory. Those with supine-related OSA with a total AHI ≥ 10 were offered positional therapy with an anti-supine shirt (Rematee AntiSnore Shirt, Vancouver, BC, Canada) consisting of a cotton T-shirt with three styrofoam cylinders inserted in three pouches across the mid-back (Figure 1). These cylinders are designed to prevent patients from sleeping on their back. Subjects who obtained the anti-supine shirt wore it for 2 to 4 weeks at home to allow acclimatization, following which they underwent a second PSG while wearing the anti-supine shirt to assess its effect on sleeping position, AHI, and sleep structure. The protocol was approved by the research Ethics Board of Toronto Rehabilitation Institute, and all subjects provided written consent prior to participation.

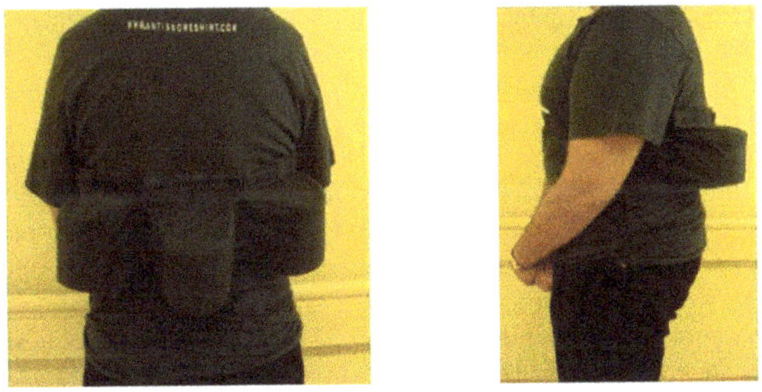

Figure 1: Photographs of the anti-supine shirt: rear view (left panel) and side view (right panel) illustrating three pouches on the back of the t-shirt containing cylinders of styrofoam that are designed to keep patients off their backs during sleep.

Statistical Analysis

We compared the sleep variables described above between the baseline and follow-up PSGs using paired t-tests and Wilcoxon-Signed-Ranks test for parametric and non-parametric data, respectively. Correlations were examined using the Pearson correlation coefficient. These variables were analyzed using a statistical package (SPSS version 11.0, Chicago, IL) and data are presented as mean ± SD. A p-value<0.05 was considered significant.

Results

Patient characteristics

Twenty-seven patients, 25 men and 2 women whose characteristics are shown in Table 1, participated. The AHI was much higher supine than non-supine. Figure 2 shows that compared to baseline, supine sleep time decreased significantly while wearing the anti-supine shirt (p<0.001).

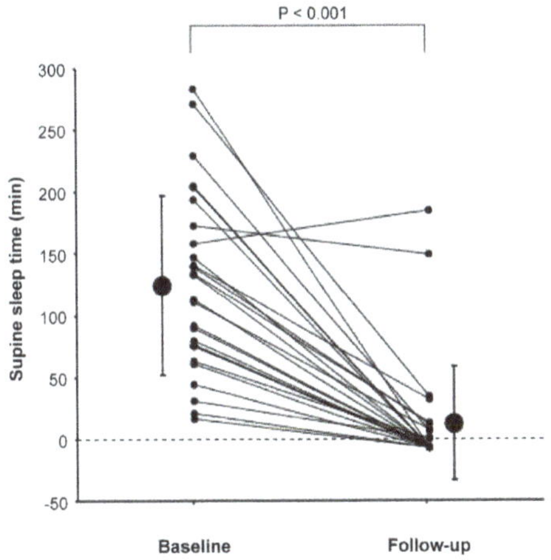

Figure 2: The anti-supine shirt significantly decreased supine sleep time from 149.2 ± 82.9 min at baseline to 21.3 ± 52.9 min at follow-up (P<0.001).

As expected, non-supine sleep time increased while wearing the anti-supine shirt (p<0.001, Table 1). This was associated with a significant (55%) reduction in the AHI (p<0.001, Figure 3) with a significant increase in minimum SaO_2 (p<0.001) but no significant increase in mean SaO_2 during sleep (Table 1).

N=27	Baseline	Follow-up	P-value
BMI (kg/m^2)	27.8 ± 4.0	27.9 ± 3.9	0.127

Total Sleep Time (min)	297.2 ± 76.5	289.8 ± 101.6	0.654
Sleep Efficiency (%)	74.9 ± 17.0	67.9 ± 21.1	0.041
Sleep Onset Latency (min)	17.1 ± 19.3	17.8 ± 26.7	0.904
Supine sleep time (min)	149.2 ± 82.9	21.3 ± 52.9	<0.001
Supine AHI (events/hour)	49.5 ± 23.6	16.4 ± 27.8	<0.001
Non-supine sleep time (min)	145.6 ± 64.1	267.8 ± 100.9	<0.001
Non-supine AHI	10.4 ± 33.6	10.2 ± 14.2	0.171
Total AHI	23.8 ± 8.0	10.7 ± 14.7	<0.001
Total Arousal Index (arousals/hour)	30.3 ± 15.1	27.2 ± 17.7	0.302
Total Respiratory Arousal Index (respiratory arousals/hour)	14.9 ± 7.9	6.3 ± 9.2	0.001
Sleep time in REM (min)	42.6 ± 27.1	49.2 ± 31.2	0.328
Sleep time in NREM (min)	254.6 ± 54.9	241.2 ± 76.7	0.253
Sleep time in N1 (min)	28.0 ± 16.3	23.8 ± 14.4	0.265
Sleep time in N2 (min)	174.9 ± 46.7	171.3 ± 66.5	0.722
Sleep time in N3 (min)	51.7 ± 21.0	46.0 ± 31.3	0.352
Mean O_2 Saturation during sleep	94.1 ± 2.8	94.7 ± 1.6	0.092
Minimum O_2 Saturation during sleep	83.0 ± 6.8	88.3 ± 4.4	<0.001

Table 1: Different characteristics of 27 patients (Values were expressed as mean ± SD).

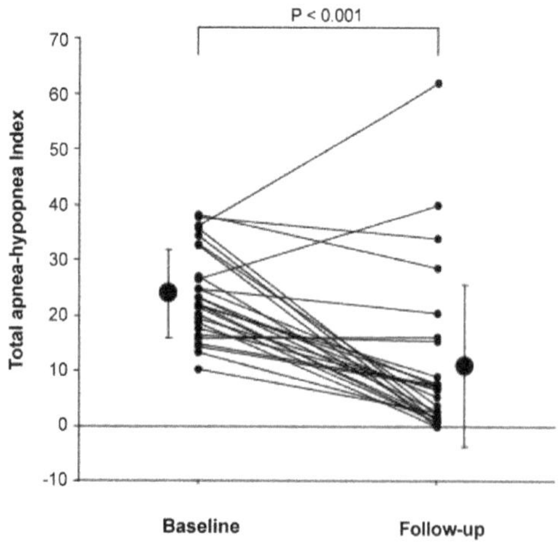

Figure 3: The anti-supine shirt significantly decreased the total AHI from 23.8 ± 8.0 at baseline to 10.7 ± 14.7 at follow-up (P<0.001).

This was not accompanied by any decrease in BMI. The change in the AHI while wearing the anti-supine shirt did not correlate significantly with the change in supine sleep time (r=0.109, p=0.589). Neither total sleep time nor the time in any of the sleep stages changed significantly between the baseline and intervention studies. However, sleep efficiency decreased significantly during the follow-up PSG (p=0.041). The respiratory-related arousal index decreased significantly.

In 20 out of 27 patients, the total AHI fell to less than 10 with the anti-supine shirt indicating virtual abolition of OSA. In this subset of patients, the supine sleep time decreased from 137.3 ± 82.4 to 5.6 ± 11.5 mins (p<0.001) and their AHI decreased from 22.4 ± 7.1 to 3.7 ± 3.1 (p<0.001) in association with an increase in their minimum SaO_2 from 84.4 ± 5.2 to 89.7 ± 3.9% (p=0.003), while mean SaO_2 was unchanged. Similar to the entire group, these 20 patients did not experience any significant change in total sleep time, N3 sleep time or total arousal frequency, and their sleep efficiency tended to decrease (from 72.6 ± 18.4 to 65.8 ± 22.6%, p=0.057). However, in contrast to the entire group, REM sleep time increased significantly from 39.7 ± 27.6 to 48.8 ± 33.2 mins (p=0.024). In 19 patients the AHI fell by greater than 50%. In 17 patients, supine sleep time fell to 0 minutes while wearing the anti-supine shirt. Although in 9 out of the 10 remaining patients supine sleep time fell, in one patient supine sleep time increased (from 187.9 to 218.7 min).

There were three patients in whom the total AHI increased at follow-up. One gained weight between the baseline and follow-up PSG (from 99.8 to 103.4 kg) and had an increase in the non-supine AHI from 7.7 to 40.0 despite complete abolition of supine sleep time (from 175.0 to 0 min). In the second, almost all respiratory events during the baseline PSG occurred during REM sleep while supine. During the follow-up PSG while wearing the anti-supine shirt, many respiratory events remained during REM sleep even though he did not sleep supine so that the REM sleep AHI remained unchanged (from 36.3 to 35.1) while his non-supine AHI increased from 8.2 to 16.0. The third had severe OSA on the baseline PSG (total AHI of 36.2; supine AHI of 76.3; and non-supine AHI of 2.5) and experienced marked increases in the total AHI to 62.0, supine AHI to 95.2, and non-supine AHI to 60.0 despite a marked reduction in supine sleep time (from 159.6 to 22.1 minute) and without any weight gain.

Discussion

Our study has given rise to two main findings. First, the anti-supine shirt significantly reduced supine sleep time, and second, it significantly reduced the AHI by 55% in association with an increase in the minimum SaO_2 during sleep. However, these changes were not accompanied by any improvement in sleep structure, and indeed there was a slight but significant reduction in sleep efficiency. The reason for this is not clear, but it is possible that discomfort associated with wearing the anti-supine shirt contributed. In addition, the degree of the reduction in AHI did not correlate with the degree of reduction in the time spent sleeping supine. This was because the amount of supine sleep time and the supine AHI varied widely among patients, and in many patients there were still events occurring in the non-supine position that contributed to the total AHI. However, among the subset of 20 patients in whom the AHI decreased to below 10 while wearing the anti-supine shirt, the amount of REM sleep increased significantly, suggesting when the anti-supine shirt abolished OSA, it did cause some improvement in sleep structure.

In approximately 60% of patients, OSA is supine-related [4,18]. However, only a very limited number of studies have evaluated the effects of positional therapy on severity of sleep apnea in such patients, and the anti-supine device used was generally not standardized or commercially available. The effects of these interventions on OSA severity varied widely.

Oksenberg et al. [3] examined the effects of a non-commercially available device consisting of a tennis ball in a pocket sewn onto the back of a belt worn around the chest in 12 patients with supine-related OSA. Patients had PSGs performed before and 2 months after wearing the belt. In association with a decrease in supine sleep time, the AHI decreased from 46.5 ± 19.9 to 17.5 ± 19.4 ($p<0.002$) in association with an improvement in minimum SaO_2. Seven patients (58%) had a reduction in their AHIs to <10. In two patients, supine sleep time did not decrease, and in one of these (8%), the AHI increased similar to the three subjects in our study whose AHI increased while wearing the anti-supine shirt.

Loord et al. [13] tested the effects of another non-commercially available device consisting of a vest with straps attached to a board with a pillow on top making it impossible to lie supine, but allowing movement from side to side. Twenty-three patients had home cardiopulmonary recordings without sleep monitoring before and after wearing the device for three months. The AHI decreased from 21.8 to 14.3 ($p=0.02$). In 13/18 subjects, the AHI decreased and in 11 it decreased to less than 10. However, in five patients (28%) the AHI increased. In addition, five subjects initially dropped out because of discomfort suggesting that it was not as well tolerated as the anti-supine shirt used in our study.

The only randomized trial of anti-supine therapy compared to an untreated control group was an abstract by Barnes et al. [19]. They conducted a four-week randomized trial to test the effects of a non-commercially available anti-supine device on severity of supine-related OSA. The device consisted of a belt worn around the upper chest with a pouch holding a single ball in the middle of the back. In 86 patients with supine-related OSA and a mean AHI of 20.9 ± 9.4, they found that although the device reduced supine sleep time, this was not accompanied by any decrease in the AHI or improvement in subjective sleepiness, quality of life, mood, or cognitive function. It is unclear why the device failed to cause a significant decrease in the AHI similar to that observed in our study.

In another study, 38 patients with a mean AHI of 13 were randomized to a night with a commercially available positional device called the Zzoma Positional Sleeper and a night on CPAP [20]. The positional device decreased supine sleep time from 40% to 0% of total sleep time in association with a significant reduction in median AHI (from 11 to 2, $p<0.001$). However, CPAP caused a greater fall in the median AHI to 0. Compared to our study, in which the AHI fell from 23.8 to 10.7, patients had a much lower AHI. Accordingly, the clinical significance of this reduction in AHI is unclear. Skinner et al. [21] compared a non-commercially available thoracic anti-supine band, to CPAP in a randomized double cross-over trial with one month in each treatment arm using home cardiopulmonary monitoring without sleep recordings. Results were similar to ours with an 82% reduction in supine time and a mean decrease in the AHI from 22.7 to 12.0. However, postural therapy was not as effective as CPAP which reduced the AHI to 4.9. Similar to our study, treatment success, defined as an AHI of <10, was achieved in 13 of 18 (72%) subjects while wearing the anti-supine band.

Jokic et al. [22] also compared the effects of a non-commercially available backpack with a 10 inch soft ball inside to treatment with CPAP in 13 patients with supine-related OSA using PSG. Patients were randomized to two weeks in each treatment group. They reported that positional treatment reduced supine sleep time and caused a reduction in the AHI from 17.9 to 9.5, but CPAP caused a greater fall in the AHI to 3.4.

In summary, with the exception of the abstract of Barnes et al. [19], the above studies reported that the use of a variety of anti-supine devices reduced supine sleep/recording time in association with a reduction in the AHI. The nature of the devices, the severity of the OSA, and the magnitude of the effect of the anti-supine interventions on AHI varied from study to study, indicating inconsistencies among them. Since most of these interventions were neither standardized, nor commercially available, it is difficult to make comparisons among them and to make assumptions about the efficacy of anti-supine interventions in general. The only study besides ours to employ a commercially available anti-supine device was that of Permut et al. [20] in which a thoracic belt was used. However, OSA was very mild in their patients making it difficult to assess the clinical significance of their findings. Our study tested the effects of a standardized, commercially available anti-supine t-shirt. Unlike the anti-supine belts described in most other studies, it is probably more comfortable to wear and should be less likely to slip out of position during the night.

Three patients from our study had an increase in AHI while wearing the anti-supine shirt. In all cases the non-supine AHI increased. In one subject, weight gain between the baseline and follow-up study may have contributed to this increase in AHI. In a second patient, REM-related OSA might have been the main issue rather than supine-related OSA, since OSA on the baseline PSG occurred mainly while in REM during which he was supine throughout. However, in the third patient, the reason for the increase in AHI is not clear, but could simply have been due to spontaneous variability in severity of OSA as previously reported [23-25]. The practical implication of this observation is that one cannot assume that prevention of supine sleep will cause resolution of OSA in all patients found to have predominantly supine-related OSA on a diagnostic PSG. Therefore, a follow-up PSG while wearing an anti-supine device should probably be performed routinely to ensure that it is effective.

Our study has a few limitations. First, it was not randomized. Nevertheless, the highly significant reductions in supine sleep time and AHI on the anti-supine shirt are most likely due to this intervention since it is designed to prevent lying on one's back and since the results are consistent with those of several previous studies using similar interventions [3,13,20-22]. In addition, because this was designed as a physiological study rather than a clinical trial, we did not assess clinical outcomes such as daytime sleepiness and quality of life.

In conclusion, this study provides evidence that the anti-supine shirt we tested significantly reduces supine sleep time and the AHI: in 20 of 27 patients, it reduced the AHI to <10. Although we did not measure whether this anti-supine shirt reduced patients' symptoms of OSA, some studies that have evaluated anti-supine therapy for OSA reported increased awake time on the maintenance of wakefulness test and reduced Epworth scores, indicating increased alertness and reduced daytime sleepiness [20]. Nevertheless, our study shows that anti-supine therapy does not reduce severity of OSA in all patients with supine-related OSA. Accordingly, when prescribing such therapy, one should consider performing a follow-up PSG on the device to determine whether or not it alleviates OSA. Our study suggests that an anti-supine shirt can be a reasonable alternative to CPAP for the therapy of supine-related OSA, particularly in view of its much lower cost, its convenience, and problems with CPAP compliance. Randomized trials of anti-supine interventions will be required to assess compliance and long-term effects on OSA severity and clinical outcomes.

Acknowledgment

This study was supported by operating grant MOP-82731 from the Canadian Institutes of Health Research. T. Kasai was supported by an unrestricted research fellowship from Fuji Respironics Inc., L. Taranto Montemurro by fellowships from the Chair of Respiratory Medicine, University of Brescia, Brescia, Italy and from Toronto Rehabilitation Institute who receives funding under the Provincial Rehabilitation Research Program from the Ministry of Health and Long-Term Care in Ontario, and T. D. Bradley by the Clifford Nordal Chair in Sleep Apnea and Rehabilitation Research.

References

1. Stradling JR, Davies RJ (2004) Sleep. 1: Obstructive sleep apnoea/hypopnoea syndrome: definitions, epidemiology, and natural history. Thorax 59: 73-78.
2. Young T, Peppard PE, Gottlieb DJ (2002) Epidemiology of obstructive sleep apnea: a population health perspective. Am J Respir Crit Care Med 165: 1217-1239.
3. Oksenberg A, Silverberg D, Offenbach D, Arons E (2006) Positional therapy for obstructive sleep apnea patients: A 6-month follow-up study. Laryngoscope 116: 1995-2000.
4. Oksenberg A, Silverberg DS, Arons E, Radwan H (1997) Positional vs nonpositional obstructive sleep apnea patients: anthropomorphic, nocturnal polysomnographic, and multiple sleep latency test data. Chest 112: 629-639.
5. Oksenberg A, Khamaysi I, Silverberg DS, Tarasiuk A (2000) Association of body position with severity of apneic events in patients with severe nonpositional obstructive sleep apnea. Chest 118: 1018-1024.
6. Walsh JH, Leigh MS, Paduch A, Maddison KJ, Armstrong JJ, et al. (2008) Effect of body posture on pharyngeal shape and size in adults with and without obstructive sleep apnea. Sleep 31: 1543-1549.
7. Richard W, Kox D, den Herder C, Laman M, van Tinteren H, et al. (2006) The role of sleep position in obstructive sleep apnea syndrome. Eur Arch Otorhinolaryngol 263: 946-950.
8. Isono S, Tanaka A, Nishino T (2002) Lateral position decreases collapsibility of the passive pharynx in patients with obstructive sleep apnea. Anesthesiology 97: 780-785.
9. Mezzanotte WS, Tangel DJ, White DP (1996) Influence of sleep onset on upper-airway muscle activity in apnea patients versus normal controls. Am J Respir Crit Care Med 153: 1880-1887.
10. Kobayashi I, Perry A, Rhymer J, Wuyam B, Hughes P, et al. (1996) Inspiratory coactivation of the genioglossus enlarges retroglossal space in laryngectomized humans. J Appl Physiol (1985) 80: 1595-1604.
11. Douglas NJ, Jan MA, Yildirim N, Warren PM, Drummond GB (1993) Effect of posture and breathing route on genioglossal electromyogram activity in normal subjects and in patients with the sleep apnea/hypopnea syndrome. Am Rev Respir Dis 148: 1341-1345.
12. Ayappa I, Rapoport DM (2003) The upper airway in sleep: physiology of the pharynx. Sleep Med Rev 7: 9-33.
13. Loord H, Hultcrantz E (2007) Positioner--a method for preventing sleep apnea. Acta Otolaryngol 127: 861-868.
14. Pepin JL, Leger P, Veale D, Langevin B, Robert D, Levy P (1995) Side effects of nasal continuous positive airway pressure in sleep apnea syndrome. Study of 193 patients in two French sleep centers. Chest 107:375-381.
15. (1992) EEG arousals: scoring rules and examples: a preliminary report from the Sleep Disorders Atlas Task Force of the American Sleep Disorders Association. Sleep 15: 173-184.
16. Rechtschaffen A, Kales AA manual of standardized terminology, techniques and scoring for sleep stages of human subjects. Los Angele, Calif: UCLA Brain Information Service/Brain Research Institute, 1968.
17. Redolfi S, Yumino D, Ruttanaumpawan P, Yau B, Su MC, et al. (2009) Relationship between overnight rostral fluid shift and Obstructive Sleep Apnea in nonobese men. Am J Respir Crit Care Med 179: 241-246.
18. Cartwright RD (1984) Effect of sleep position on sleep apnea severity. Sleep 7: 110-114.
19. Barnes M, Berlowitz D, Collins AL (2010) Prevention of supine sleep does not effectively treat obstructive sleep apnea. Am J Respir Crit Care Med 181:A5561.
20. Permut I, Diaz-Abad M, Chatila W, Crocetti J, Gaughan JP, et al. (2010) Comparison of positional therapy to CPAP in patients with positional obstructive sleep apnea. J Clin Sleep Med 6: 238-243.
21. Skinner MA, Kingshott RN, Filsell S, Taylor DR (2008) Efficacy of the 'tennis ball technique' versus nCPAP in the management of position-dependent obstructive sleep apnoea syndrome. Respirology 13: 708-715.
22. Jokic R, Klimaszewski A, Crossley M, Sridhar G, Fitzpatrick MF (1999) Positional treatment vs continuous positive airway pressure in patients with positional obstructive sleep apnea syndrome. Chest 115: 771-781.
23. Pittsley M, Gehrman P, Cohen-Zion M, Stepnowsky C, Marler M, et al. (2005) Comparing night-to-night variability of sleep measures in elderly African Americans and Whites. Behav Sleep Med 3: 63-72.
24. Chediak AD, Acevedo-Crespo JC, Seiden DJ, Kim HH, Kiel MH (1996) Nightly variability in the indices of sleep-disordered breathing in men being evaluated for impotence with consecutive night polysomnograms. Sleep 19: 589-592.
25. Gibson GJ (2005) Obstructive sleep apnoea syndrome: underestimated and undertreated. Br Med Bull 72: 49-65.

11

Effect of Body Position on Respiratory Muscle Activity in Subjects with Upper Costal or Costo-diaphragmatic Breathing Type

Rodolfo Miralles[1*], **Isabel Celhay**[1], **Rosa Cordova**[1, 2, 3], **Hugo Santander**[1], **Saúl Valenzuela**[1,2], **Aler Daniel Fuentes**[1,2], **Mario Felipe Gutiérrez**[1,2] **and Ricardo Bull**[1]

[1]*Oral Physiology Laboratory, Biomedical Sciences Institute, Faculty of Medicine, University of Chile, Santiago, Chile*

[2]*Institute for Research in Dental Sciences, Faculty of Dentistry, University of Chile, Santiago, Chile*

[3]*Faculty of Medicine, Diego Portales University, Santiago, Chile*

[*]**Corresponding author:** Rodolfo Miralles, Oral Physiology Laboratory, Biomedical Sciences Institute, Faculty of Medicine, University of Chile, Independencia 1027, Postal Code 838-0453, Independencia, Santiago, Chile; E-mail: rmiralle@med.uchile.cl

Abstract

Effect of body position on electromyographic (EMG) activity has been studied in the cranio-cervical-mandibular muscles, but its effect on the activity of respiratory muscles in subjects with different breathing types has not yet been elucidated. This study included two groups of twenty male subjects each, one with upper costal and the other with costo-diaphragmatic breathing type. EMG activity was recorded using bipolar surface electrode technique. Electrodes were placed on the sternocleidomastoid (SCM), diaphragm (DIA), and external intercostal (EIC) and Latissimus dorsi (LAT) muscles.

EMG activity was recorded in standing and lateral decubitus positions, during the following tasks: (1) Normal quiet breathing; (2) speaking the word "Mississippi"; (3) forced deep breathing. EMG activity of DIA and EIC muscles was higher in the standing than in the lateral decubitus position during all tasks in both breathing groups ($p<0.05$), excepting DIA activity during task 2 in the costo-diaphragmatic group. EMG activity of LAT muscle was higher in the standing than in the lateral decubitus position during task 3 in both breathing groups ($p<0.05$). EMG activity of DIA activity was higher in subjects with upper costal than in subjects with costo-diaphragmatic breathing type in the standing position during all tasks and also in the lateral decubitus position during tasks 1 and 2 ($p<0.05$).

EMG activity of ECM, EIC and LAT muscles was not significantly different between both breathing types in the studied body positions. The higher EMG activity observed in the standing than in the lateral decubitus positions in both breathing groups, suggests differences in the respiratory effort depending on the body position. The higher EMG activity observed in DIA muscle of subjects with upper costal than costo-diaphragmatic breathing types, suggests differences in the respiratory effort depending on the breathing type.

Keywords: Electromyographic activity; Standing position; Lateral decubitus position; Upper costal breathing; Costo-diaphragmatic breathing

Introduction

The acquisition and processing of oxygen is the primary task of any air-breathing vertebrate. Chewing, walking, reproducing and thinking are all fine, but first one must breathe [1]. There is no higher priority for the body than to breathe [2]. Respiratory muscle contraction is a continual process that ventilates the alveoli and it is usually under automatic control by respiratory centres in the ponto-medullary region of the brainstem [3].

Several breathing types have been defined depending on the expansion of the abdomino-thoracic region during inspiration at rest [4-6]: i) Costo-diaphragmatic breathing, ii) Upper costal breathing, and iii) Mixed breathing.

Obligatory muscles of respiration, e.g. diaphragm (DIA), scalene, parasternal and external intercostal (EIC) muscles, contract in every breath cycle during quiet breathing. Additional accessory respiratory muscles, e.g. sternocleidomastoid (SCM) and trapezius muscles, contract when the demand in the respiratory system changes, such as forced deep breathing [7-9].

In addition, the latissimus dorsi (LAT) muscle appears to have an inspiratory action in patients experiencing respiratory difficulty, e.g., hyperpnea, emphysema, and asthma [10,11], and with increased inspiratory load [12]. Electromyographic (EMG) activity of SCM, DIA, EIC and LAT muscles have been compared between subjects with costo-diaphragmatic or upper costal breathing in the standing position.

Higher EMG activity of DIA and EIC muscles was observed during different tasks in the upper costal group, whereas EMG activity of SCM and LAT was similar between both groups [13,14]. To the best of our knowledge no study has compared EMG activity of respiratory muscles, in the lateral decubitus position, between subjects with different breathing types. It is unknown if subjects with upper costal breathing also present higher EMG activity than subjects with costo-diaphragmatic breathing, in the lateral decubitus position.

Therefore, the aim of the present work is to compare EMG activity of respiratory muscles between subjects with upper costal or costo-diaphragmatic breathing types in the standing and in the lateral decubitus positions.

Methods

Ethical approval

All experimental procedures were conducted in accordance with the Helsinki Declaration of 1975, as revised in 1983 and approved by The Ethics Committee of the Faculty of Dentistry, University of Chile. Written informed consents were obtained from all participant subjects.

Subjects

This study included two groups of 20 male subjects each, one with upper costal and the other with costo-diaphragmatic breathing. The breathing type of the subjects was determined by two authors (RM and RC) and the agreement of both examiners was needed for subject classification. Consistency in the clinical diagnosis across the examiners was high, and when there was no agreement, the subject was not included.

Each subject was asked to remain standing, looking straight ahead, with their feet 10 cm apart, and to breathe normally for 2 minutes as a baseline. First, the examiners placed the left hand on the upper chest and the right hand on the upper back; next, they placed the left hand on the upper abdomen and the right hand on the lower left costal region.

After checking 10 inspirations on each step of the clinical examination, the subject was classified to be of the upper costal breathing type if, during inspiration at rest, the superior thoracic expansion was predominant, and the costo-diaphragmatic breathing type when the abdominal and lateral costal expansion was predominant [13,14].

Those subjects who did not show a clear predominance of superior thoracic expansion or abdominal and lateral costal expansion (mixed breathing type), were excluded from the study. The participants were students enrolled at the Dental or Medical School of the University of Chile, to complete 40 subjects who met the inclusion criteria mentioned below.

All subjets selected had complete natural dentition (excluding the third molars), no history of orofacial pain or craniomandibular-cervical disorders, no heart or respiratory disease. Subjects recruited were only male to avoid difficulties with breast size, asymmetry of breasts and the use of a bra related to female subjects during EMG recording. None of the subjects was on medication that could have influenced muscle activity.

Electromyography

Bipolar surface electrodes (BioFLEX, BioResearch Associates, Inc., Brown Deer, WI, and USA) were placed on the SCM, DIA, EIC and LAT muscles. Impedance was decreased by careful skin shaving and abrasion with alcohol.

The electrodes were placed as follows [13,14]: on SCM muscle (middle portion), in the anterior border 1 cm above and below the motor point; on DIA muscle, 1 cm below the xiphoid process; on EIC muscle, between the 6th and 7th ribs on the imaginary vertical line that passes through the nipple; and on LAT muscle, in the projection of the 12th rib or lumbar vertebra L1 following the thoracolumbar fascia edge.

The electrodes were unilaterally placed on the left side, because for EMG recording in the lateral decubitus position, all subjects were asked arbitrarily to lay on his right side. Surface ground electrode was attached to the forehead. EMG activity was recorded using a 4-channel computerized instrument in which the signals were amplified (Model 7P5B preamplifier, Grass Instrument Co., Quincy, MA, USA) and filtered (10 Hz high pass and 2 kHz low pass), with a common mode rejection ratio higher than 100 dB.

The output was filtered again (notch frequency of 50 Hz), full-wave rectified and then integrated (time constant of 0.1 s), and recorded online on a computer exclusively dedicated to acquisition and processing of EMG signals. EMG signal was acquired at a sample rate of 200 Hz (50 Hz each channel) with a 12 bits A/D converter (MAX191) connected to the computer through an RS-232 port. The system was calibrated before each record.

EMG activity was recorded in the following body positions:

Standing position; maintaining a stance with the feet 10 cm apart, eyes open, looking straight ahead. The self-balanced position was obtained by having each subject stand with his visual axis on the horizontal, with no external intervention or modification of his posture [13,14].

Right lateral decubitus position; head, neck and body horizontally aligned, checked by an external operator located approximately 3 m from the bed [5]. The head and neck of each subject were supported by a Sleep Easy Pillow (Interwood Marketing Groups, Ontario, Canada).

The subject placed his hands in front of the chest and slightly flexed his legs. A mattress (Rosen Runnair Physio-Actions, Temuco, Chile) was used. Lateral decubitus position was chosen because it is an habitual sleeping position and also it is possible to stay several hours a day in that position. At lateral decubitus position, room light was turn off and the subjects kept his eyes closed.

Each subject underwent three unilateral EMG recordings of left SCM, DIA, EIC and LAT muscles under the following experimental conditions:

Task 1: normal quiet breathing

Task 2: speaking the word "Mississippi"

Task 3: forced deep breathing

Before EMG recording, an examiner explained all tasks to each subject, in order he would be able to perform each one correctly. The order of the tasks was randomized. During task 1 the subject had his jaw in the resting posture.

During task 2 the subject pronounced the word "Mississippi". This phonetic method was chosen for being a functional activity commonly used by dentists in most oral reconstructive procedures [15]. During task 3, each subject was asked to breathe in total lung capacity, holding the breath for 10s.

This period was selected to ensure maximum and sustained muscle activity without producing a respiratory function disorder. Tasks 1 and 2 also lasted 10 seconds based on the duration of task 3. A 20 s resting period was allowed between each EMG recording in each task.

To obtain the average value of each curve, measurements were taken every 0.1 s from the beginning to the end of the recording, using a computer program. The mean value of the three curves obtained at each task and for each subject was used. Variability of EMG data during the tasks was assessed by the coefficient of variability.

The values obtained were 38.5% in the SCM muscle, 11.8% in the DIA muscle, 11.6% in the EIC muscle, and 20.1% in the LAT muscle.

Body mass index (BMI) was obtained for each subject by dividing the weight (kg) by the square of the height (m^2). Age and BMI were used to check for possible influence on EMG activity recorded in each muscle (Table 1).

Subjects	Costo-diaphragmatic breathing type				Upper costal breathing type				
	Age	Weight (Kg)	Height (m)	BMI	Subjects	Age	Weight (Kg)	Height (m)	BMI
1	21	76	1.75	24.82	1	25	60	1.74	19.82
2	22	80	1.76	25.83	2	24	76	1.81	23.20
3	21	68	1.7	23.53	3	24	73	1.77	23.30
4	24	67	1.8	20.68	4	19	65	1.66	23.59
5	24	64	1.76	20.66	5	20	73	1.76	23.57
6	22	70	1.7	24.22	6	19	71	1.73	23.72
7	23	73	1.67	26.18	7	20	94	1.8	29.01
8	24	69	1.7	23.88	8	18	90	1.81	27.47
9	23	72	1.79	22.47	9	19	70	1.75	22.86
10	26	74	1.8	22.84	10	19	70	1.64	26.03
11	25	85	1.75	27.76	11	18	58	1.64	21.56
12	19	64	1.74	21.14	12	18	69	1.73	23.05
13	22	78	1.75	25.47	13	19	65	1.75	21.22
14	19	60	1.68	21.26	14	19	70	1.71	23.94
15	19	68	1.73	22.72	15	20	69	1.73	23.05
16	18	100	1.8	30.86	16	22	63	1.76	20.34
17	20	69	1.71	23.60	17	19	55	1.68	19.49
18	18	82	1.76	26.47	18	21	75	1.86	21.68
19	20	80	1.83	23.89	19	22	90	1.7	31.14
20	21	64	1.75	20.90	20	22	70	1.68	24.80
Mean	21.6	73.2	1.7	24.0	Mean	20.4	71.3	1.7	23.6
SD	2.4	9.3	0.0	2.6	SD	2.1	10.2	0.1	2.9

Table 1: Characteristics of subjects studied.

Statistics

Data were analyzed using SYSTAT 13 program (Systat Software Inc. (SSI), San Jose, CA, USA).

EMG activity presented non-normal distribution ($p<0.05$; Shapiro-Wilk test); therefore, Wilcoxon rank-sum test for dependent samples was used to compare the activity of each muscle between body positions during tasks, and Mann-Whitney U-test was used to compare the activity of each muscle between both groups during tasks.

A value of $p<0.05$ was considered statistically significant. Age data presented a non-normal distribution ($p<0.05$; Shapiro-Wilk test); therefore Mann-Whitney U-test was used for the comparison between samples studied. BMI data presented a normal distribution ($p>0.05$; Shapiro-Wilk test); therefore t-test was used for the comparison between samples studied.

Results

Mean age values ± (SD) of both groups were 20.4 ± (2.1) and 21.6 ± (2.4) for upper costal and costo-diaphragmatic breathing types, respectively. No significant difference was observed between both groups ($p>0.05$, Mann-Whitney U-test). Mean BMI values ± (SD) of both groups were 23.6 ± (2.9) and 24.0 ± (2.6) for upper costal and costo-diaphragmatic breathing types, respectively. No significant difference was observed between both groups ($p>0.05$, t-test for independent samples).

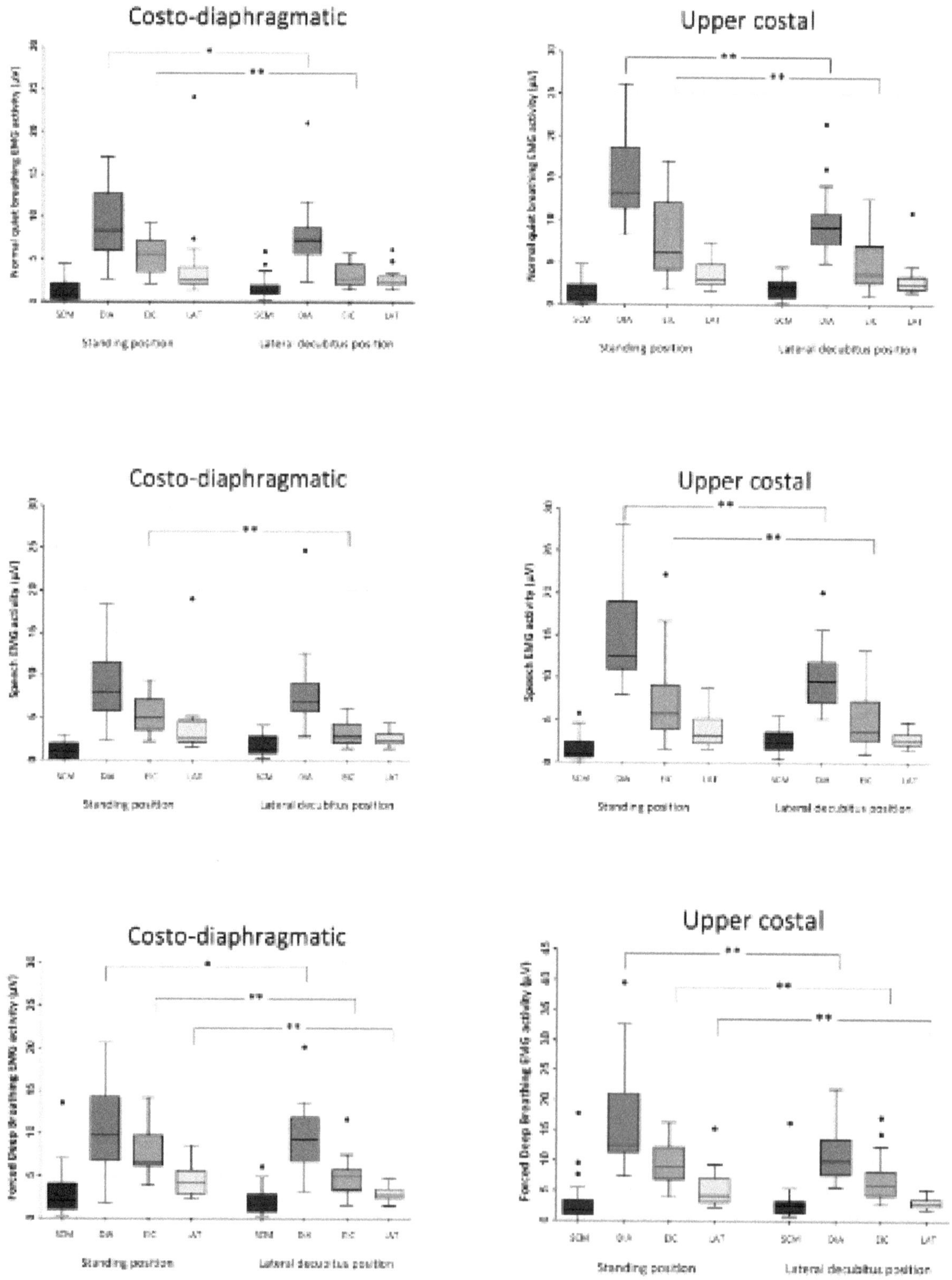

Figure 1: Box plot showing a comparison of EMG activity from sternocleidomastoid (SCM), diaphragm (DIA), external intercostal (EIC), and latissimus dorsi (LAT) muscles between standing and lateral decubitus positions, in each breathing group, during normal quiet breathing (above), speaking the word "Mississippi" (middle), and forced deep breathing (below) (*p<0.05, **p<0.01; Wilcoxon rank-sum test).

Figure 1 shows the effect of body position on EMG activity in both breathing groups in all muscles studied.

EMG activity of DIA and EIC muscles was significantly higher during standing than in the lateral decubitus position in both breathing groups during all tasks (*p<0.05), except activity of DIA muscle in subjects with costodiaphragmatic breathing during task 2 (speaking) (p>0.05).

EMG activity of SCM muscle was the lowest of all muscles studied and did not change with body position or breathing type (p>0.05).

EMG activity of LAT muscle was higher in the standing than in the lateral decubitus position in both breathing groups, only during task 3 (forced deep breathing) (*p<0.05).

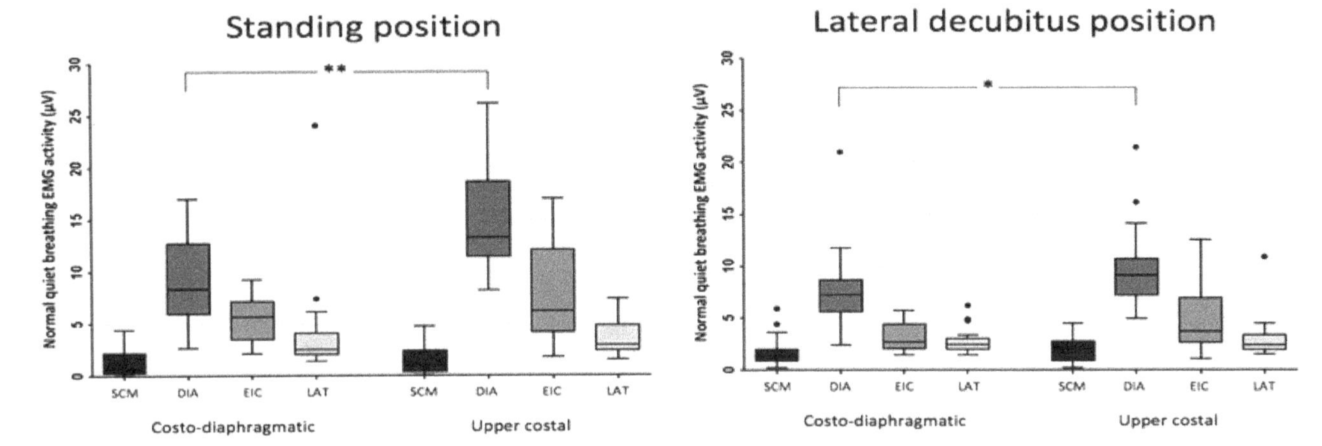

Figure 2: Box plot showing a comparison of EMG activity from sternocleidomastoid (SCM), diaphragm (DIA), external intercostal (EIC), and latissimus dorsi (LAT) muscles between subjects with costo-diaphragmatic and with upper costal breathing, during normal quiet breathing, at standing position (upper panel) and at lateral decubitus position (lower panel), (*p<0.05, **p<0.01; Mann-Whitney U-test).

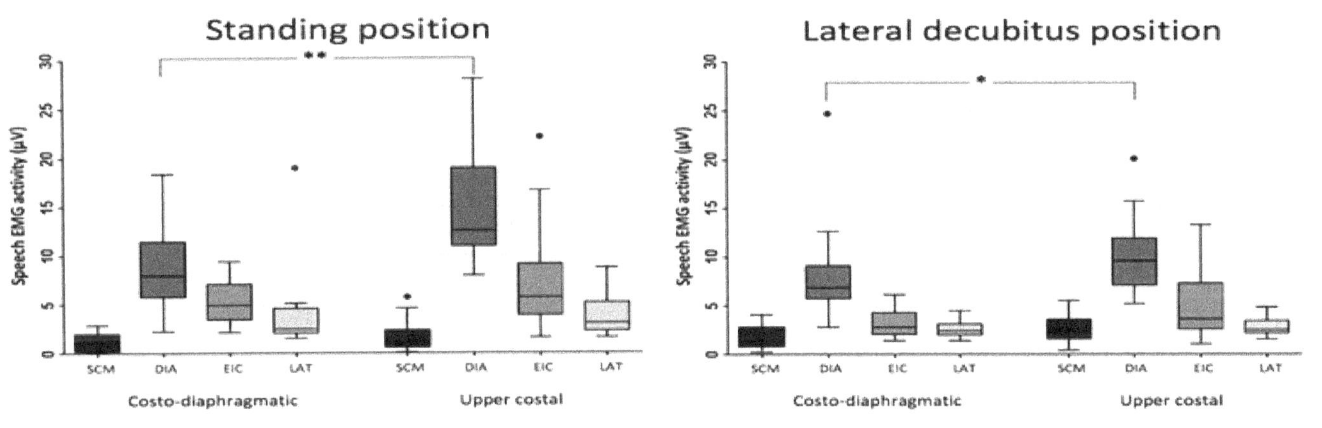

Figure 3: Box plot showing a comparison of EMG activity from sternocleidomastoid (SCM), diaphragm (DIA), external intercostal (EIC), and latissimus dorsi (LAT) muscles between subjects with costo-diaphragmatic and with upper costal breathing, speaking the word "Mississippi", at standing position (upper panel) and at lateral decubitus position (lower panel), (*p<0.05, **p<0.01; Mann-Whitney U-test).

Figures 2 and 3 show that EMG activity of DIA muscle was significantly higher during task 1 and 2, respectively, in subjects with upper costal than with costo-diaphragmatic breathing, in the standing position (**p<0.01; upper panel) and in the lateral decubitus position (*p<0.05; lower panel), whereas EMG activity of SCM, EIC and LAT muscles did not differ between both breathing types in the studied body positions (p>0.05).

Figure 4 shows that EMG activity of DIA muscle in the standing position (upper panel) was significantly higher during tasks 3 (forced deep breathing) in subjects with upper costal than in subjects with costo-diaphragmatic breathing type (*p<0.05); whereas EMG activity of SCM, EIC and LAT muscles did not differ between both breathing groups (p>0.05). EMG activity of all muscles was similar during task 3 in the lateral decubitus position (lower panel) between both breathing types (p>0.05).

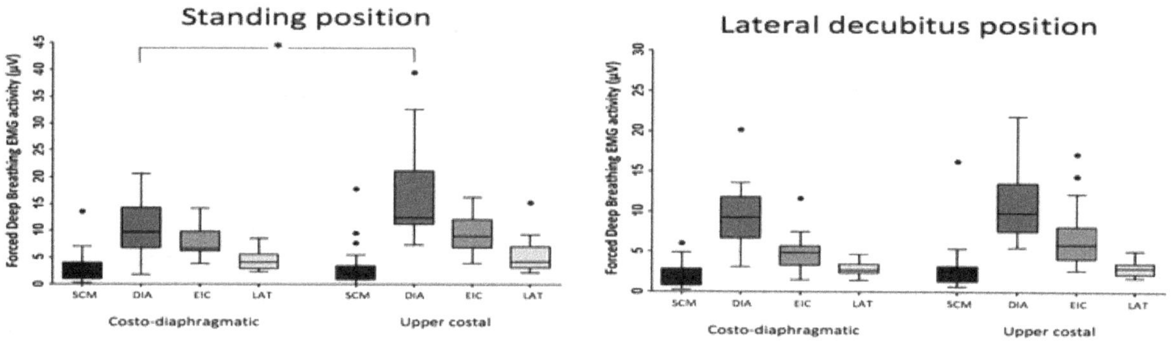

Figure 4: Box plot showing a comparison of EMG activity from sternocleidomastoid (SCM), diaphragm (DIA), external intercostal (EIC), and latissimus dorsi (LAT) muscles between subjects with costo-diaphragmatic and with upper costal breathing, during forced deep breathing, at standing position (upper panel) and at lateral decubitus position (lower panel), (*p<0.05; Mann-Whitney U-test).

Discussion

In the present study, the subjects were asked to perform all tasks voluntarily, in accordance to previous instructions. This is important, since it is well known that premotor drive from multiple descending pathways, i.e., from the motor cortex for voluntary respiratory tasks, are integrated at the spinal cord [16,17]. They may arise directly from oligosynaptic pathways from the motor cortex to the diaphragm and intercostal motoneurons [18] or from local spinal reflexes. At the spinal level, all inputs acting on motoneurons and interneurons, including spinal reflexes, are coordinated to produce the appropriate motor output [17].

The significantly higher EMG activity observed during standing than in the lateral decubitus position is important because it suggests differences in the respiratory effort depending on the body position. This finding can be explained by the fact that, in the standing position, intrapleural pressure is lower at the apex than in the base of the lungs [19]. This results in more expanded alveoli in the apex than the base, leading to lower alveolar ventilation in the apex, which is independent of the breathing type. In the right lateral decubitus position, the intrapleural pressure gradient goes from the left to the right lung, therefore, alveolar ventilation is higher in the right than in the left lung. Since the right lung is bigger than the left, respiratory effort is lower in the right lateral decubitus than in the standing position, thus explaining the lower EMG activity recorded in the former position.

The higher activity recorded in the standing position may also be due to a differential modulation of the motor neuron pools of respiratory muscles arising from different types of receptors, such as: plantar mechano-receptors, leg muscular proprioceptors, knee articular proprioceptors, vestibular and visual receptors. It is reasonable to assume that afferences stemming from these receptors are different in the standing than in the lateral decubitus positions. In addition, in our work, it is very important to consider the change in visual inputs, since in the standing position the subjects kept his eyes open and looked straight ahead, while in the lateral decubitus position, room light was turned off and the subjects kept his eyes closed.

The significantly higher EMG activity observed in DIA muscle of subjects with upper costal breathing, during standing at all tasks (Figures 2-4, upper panels), agrees with the result observed in previous works [13,14]. The higher activity of DIA muscle is contrary to that expected, since in the presence of a predominant superior thoracic expansion, a lower EMG activity would be expected in this muscle. Subjects that preferentially expand the superior part of the thorax (upper costal breathing), however, require higher respiratory effort to produce a normal alveolar ventilation, since, as mentioned above, respiratory effort is higher in the standing than in the right lateral decubitus position. Therefore, the higher EMG activity recorded in DIA muscle would result from the higher respiratory effort, depending on the breathing type which could reduce the adaptive capability of these subjects.

The higher EMG activity observed in DIA muscle of subjects with upper costal breathing in the right lateral decubitus position during tasks 1 and 2 (Figures 2 and 3, lower panels) is important because normal quiet breathing is frequent while resting in a bed and is also an habitual sleeping position and to speak is frequent during awake hours, respectively.

This higher EMG activity recorded in DIA muscle of subjects with upper costal breathing in the right lateral decubitus position, however, cannot be attributed to a higher respiratory effort, since alveoli expansion in the apex and in the base of the lung are similar in both breathing types. We do not know if subjects with upper costal breathing (diagnosed in the standing position) maintain their breathing type in the lateral decubitus position, therefore, in a future study this should be assessed.

Similar EMG activity of SCM muscles in the standing position, in both breathing groups, is in agreement with previous studies [5,13,14]. This same EMG activity pattern was observed in the lateral decubitus position in the present study. This behavior of SCM muscle could be explained by a predominant effect of vestibular and/or visual afferents than other influences on its pool of motoneurons, depending on the body position, due to its role as postural rather than respiratory muscle.

Similar EMG activity of LAT muscle in both breathing groups, during all studied tasks in the standing position, agrees with previous studies [13,14]. This same EMG activity pattern was observed in the lateral decubitus position in the present study, suggesting that activity of this muscle is more relevant during longer disturbances and/or critical conditions [10,11].

The present study has at least four limitations. First, subjects studied were only male which limits the ability to extrapolate these findings to the general population. Second, we do not have data regarding the difference or similarity in the smoking habit in both groups. Third, we only studied young subjects and it is possible that elderly subjects with lung or cardiac disease could present differences in the EMG pattern. Fourth, surface electrodes on the chest could capture electrocardiogram and/or pick up activity from neighboring muscles. In addition, EMG activity recorded in the left EIC muscle during right lateral decubitus position could be more influenced by cardiac activity than right EIC activity recorded in the left lateral decubitus position. This could be important and deserves to be assessed in a future study. In spite of these limitations, this is the first study that shows significant higher diaphragm EMG activity in the lateral decubitus position, in young adult subjects with upper costal breathing than in subjects with costo-diaphragmatic breathing during low effort (normal quiet breathing and speech).

Conclusion

- Higher EMG activity in the diaphragm and external intercostal muscles observed in both breathing types in the standing than in the lateral decubitus position, suggests differences in the respiratory effort depending on the body position.
- Higher EMG activity in the diaphragm observed in subjects with upper costal than in subjects with costo-diaphragmatic breathing, during normal quiet breathing and speaking the word "Mississippi", suggests a higher respiratory effort depending on the breathing type that could reduce their adaptive capability.

References

1. Rogers RR (2012) Past, present, and future use of oral appliance therapies in sleep-related breathing disorders. J Calif Dent Assoc 40: 151-157.
2. Cole AM (2014) The role of dentistry in the field of sleep medicine are we respecting the physiology? Cranio 32: 9-10.
3. Feldman JL, Del Negro CA (2006) Looking for inspiration: new perspectives on respiratory rhythm. Nat Rev Neurosci 7: 232-242.
4. Costa D, Vitti M, de Olivera Tossello D, Costa R (1994) Participation of the sternocleidomastoid muscle on deep inspiration in man. An electromyographic study. Electromyogr Clin Neurophysiol 34: 315-320.
5. De Mayo T, Miralles R, Barrero D, Bulboa A, Carvajal D, et al. (2005) Breathing type and body position effects on sternocleidomastoid and suprahyoid EMG activity. J Oral Rehabil 32: 487-494.
6. Cagnie B, Danneels L, Cools A, Dickx N, Cambier D (2008) The influence of breathing type, expiration and cervical posture on the performance of the cranio-cervical flexion test in healthy subjects. Man Ther 13: 232-238.
7. Tokizane T, Kawamata K, Tokizane H (1952) Electromyographic studies on the human respiratory muscles; studies on the activity pattern of neuromuscular units. Jpn J Physiol 2: 232-247.
8. Ratnovsky A, Elad D, Halpern P (2008) Mechanics of respiratory muscles. Respir Physiol Neurobiol 163: 82-89.
9. Hudson AL, Gandevia SC, Butler JE (2011) Control of human inspiratory motoneurones during voluntary and involuntary contractions. Respir Physiol Neurobiol 179: 23-33.
10. Gronbaek P, Skouby AP (1960) The activity of the diaphragm and some muscles of the neck and trunk in chronic asthmatics and normal controls. Acta Med Scand 168: 413-425.
11. Cala SJ, Edyvean J, Rynn M, Engel LA (1992) O2 cost of breathing: Ventilatory vs. pressure loads. J Appl Physiol 73: 1720-1727.
12. Orozco-Levi M, Gea J, Monells J, Aran X, Aguar M, et al. (1995) Activity of latissimus dorsi muscle during inspiratory threshold loads. Eur Respir J 8: 441-445.
13. Gutierrez MF, Valenzuela S, Miralles R, Portus C, Santander H, et al. (2014) Does breathing type influence electromyographic activity of obligatory and accessory respiratory muscles? J Oral Rehabil 41: 801-808.
14. Celhay I, Cordova R, Miralles R, Meza F, Erices P, et al. (2015) Effect of upper costal and costo-diaphragmatic breathing types on electromyographic activity of respiratory muscles. Cranio 33: 100-106.
15. McNeill CH (1997) Science and practice of occlusion. Quintessence Publishing Co, Illinois.
16. Aminoff MJ, Sears TA (1971) Spinal integration of segmental, cortical and breathing inputs to thoracic respiratory motoneurons. The Journal of Physiology 215: 557-575.
17. Bellingham MC (1999) Synaptic inhibition of cat phrenic motoneurons by internal intercostal nerve stimulation. Journal of Neurophysiology 82: 1224-1232.
18. Gandevia SC, Plassman BL (1988) Responses in human intercostal and truncal muscles to motor cortical and spinal stimulation. Respiration Physiology 73: 325-337.
19. West JB (2012) Respiratory Physiology: The Essentials. (9thedn) Lippincott Williams & Wilkins, Baltimore, USA: 95-124.

12

Evaluating of Sleep Quality in Shift-Work Nurses

Valiollah Akbari[1] **, Abbas Hajian**[2,*] **and Mahbubeh Sadat Mirhashemi**[3]

[1]*Medical Doctor, Assistant Professor of Psychiatry, Department of Psychology, University of Medical Sciences, Qom, Iran*

[2]*Medical Doctor,General Practitioner, University of Medical Sciences, Qom, Iran*

[3]*Medical Doctor, General Practitioner, University of Medical Sciences, Qom, Iran*

[*]**Corresponding author:** Abbas Hajian, Medical Doctor, General Practitioner, University of Medical Sciences, Qom, Iran, E-mail: abbashajian@ymail.com

Abstract

Sleep quality directly influences mental and physical acts of human. Shift workers, such as nurses are at extreme risk for poor sleep. In this article we have attempt to evaluate how the beliefs of nurses about their sleep quality were. The paper is a cross sectional study among 370 nurses and correlates to demographics. Totally 151 (41%) men and 219 (59%) women participated. All of them had nursing education degree and had work experience. We found the prevalence of sleep disturbances as high as 86% and total mean score of the Persian version of Pittsburg's Sleep Questionnaire Index (PSQI-P) calculated 7.13 ± 2.5 in the study. The most common complaint of shift-work nurses was delay in sleeping initiation. We did not find any significant relation between sleep disorders and gender, age, years of nursing and hospital department of service. Although, inadequate sleep quality is a worldwide problem, but the wide difference between subjective findings of nurses and those of the general population is very significant.

Keywords: Sleep quality; Shift-work nurses; PSQI-P

Introduction

Sleep is the complex bio-physiologic circadian vital process which directly and indirectly relates to many daily physical and mental functions of human. The most known hormonal mechanism of sleeping is the melatonin effect, the substance periodically secrets by pineal gland in brain [1]. The pineal secretion affects also cardiovascular, reproductive and neuroendocrine systems [1].

It may be a clue that while this small gland becomes calcified, mentioned systems and also sleeping features will negatively affect synchronously. Because of that darkness stimulates the pineal body, there is a rhythmic secreting pattern during every 24-hour. Since the serum level of melatonin –sleep hormone- maximizes at night [1], makes the desire of getting asleep. As shift-work staffs including nurses have to be awaked weather partial or total of some of their nights, they face to challenge with the hormone effects and this eventually makes them more susceptible to expose to sleep disorders. As nurses' work quality directly affects patient health status, it is very important to have regular observation programs and if needed, solve their sleep problems.

Insomnia or disturbed sleep as one of the most common sleep disorders has a wide range of definition including difficulty in sleep initiation or maintenance, early morning awakening and non-restorative sleep which may discover firstly by fatigue, irritability, malaise and decreasing in memory or concentration [1]. For instance about 32-54% of night workers have symptoms of insomnia or daytime sleepiness compared with 18% of day workers who claim of above symptoms [2].

The importance of paying more attention to sleep problems will be more bright when reports tell that about 1.3 million patient injuries and over 100,000 deaths occur annually due to hospital related errors or preventable adverse events [2,3]. These measures magnify as doubled when nurses worked over 12 consecutive hours [3]. In this study we have attempt to find the prevalence of shift-worked nurses' sleep problems and its possible relation to some other considered features.

Method and Material

This cross-sectional study was done among nursing staff who worked in hospitals of a Persian city in autumn 2014, Iran. Totally 370 nurses including 151 (40.8%) males and 219 (59.2%) females were selected over an automatic randomized sampling method among who had -at least cumulatively 24 hours per week - night shift in last four weeks. We considered just awaked time in each night shift that each nurse subjectively estimated for him/herself. For instance it was possible that a nurse had had four night shifts in shift-plan and the other had two, but based on subjective estimation both had at least 24 hours or more of awaking time along with all night shifts per each week.

In other word, the study criterion for considering shift working was the hours each nurse was awake in the work setting during the nights and not only having night shifts whether being awaked or not. All participants were 21 to 47 years old, married and had nursing education degree. Health status of them was subjectively near normal and they were under no regular prescription for sleep related or any other chronic disease. They did not drink or smoke. Females were not pregnant while study performed. All had work experience in range of one to 25 years. In order to measure the sleep quality, we used the Persian version of Pittsburg's Sleep Questionnaire Index (PSQI-P).

The PSQI-P is consisted of eighteen questions in a self-rating Likert answering system. The reliability of the alpha coefficient of Cronbach for this questionnaire was reported 0.77 [4]. This tool is well potent to distinguish sleep disorders such as primary insomnia, major depression and daytime over sleepiness from normal sleep [5,6]. The PSQI-P is constructed of seven parts based on international classification of sleep disorders to find sufferers in a period of last four weeks [5-7].

The parts are including of subjective sleep quality, sleep latency, sleep duration, sleep efficiency, and sleep disturbances, daytime dysfunction and hypnotic medications use. Each category scores from zero to 3. Thus a fully filled questionnaire has a score range of zero up to 21 [5,6]. There is also another classification for the PSQI-P, which breaks the contents into three bigger factors [6]. In both platforms, everybody scores ≥5 marked as a low sleep quality person and who makes the points <5 considered as a good sleeper without significant sleep disturbance [5].

Authors promised all participants to save their personal privacy and made oral satisfaction. We measured shift-work nurses' sleep quality and its probable relation to gender, age, level of education, place of work -servicing patients in internal, surgical, emergency and other hospital departments- and also years of work experience. We estimated statistic indexes including minimum, maximum, means and standard deviations by using the SPSS version 18.

To evaluate study hypothesis regarding that shift work nurses more suffer by sleep disturbances than general population, we applied the T-test and also used the Chi-square test in order to find any relation between study variables and the constant of sleep quality. We also used the One-way ANOVA test to calculate the means of answers of each seven part and other details of the PSQI-P between groups of poor and good sleepers. We considered value of significant p as less than 0.05.

Results

The observational study was performed by collecting 370 fully filled questionnaires of totally 151 (40.8%) males and 219 (59.2%) females as shift-work nurse. The mean age was 30.8 ± 5.3 with minimum age of 21 and maximum of 47 years. Females were 29.7 ± 4.8 and males were 32.3 ± 5.6 years old (p=0.05).

All respondents were in subjectively acceptable health status and did not use any prescribed medication or therapy for any health condition during last year of study performance.

They also did not drink or smoke regularly. All of them had nursing license degree (360 had license and 10 had higher degrees). Nurses were distributed in below hospital stations: internal medicine (102 persons, 27.6%), surgery (127, 34.3%), cardiac care unit (75, 20.3%) and other minor sections (66, 17.8%).

Based on study findings, there were 317 persons (85.7%) with sleep disturbances; it means they were bad sleepers and had PSQI-P score ≥5, and only 53 nurses (14.3%) were good sleepers and had PSQI-P score <5. Table 1 shows findings over the seven parts of the PSQI-P among nurses.

Symptom Severity					
Factor	Normal	Mild Dysfunction	Moderate Dysfunction	Severe Dysfunction	p
Subjective Sleep Quality	Very good	Fairly good	Fairly bad	Very bad	0.649
	41 (11%)	215 (58.1%)	86 (23.2%)	28 (7.5%)	
Sleep Latency	≤15 minutes	16-30 minutes	31-60 minutes	>60 minutes	0.143
	49 (13.2%)	105 (28.3%)	108 (29.1%)	108 (29.1%)	
Sleep Duration	>7 hours	6-7 hours	5-6 hours	<5 hours	0.714
	233 (62.9%)	84 (22.7%)	35 (9.4%)	18 (4.8%)	
Sleep Efficency*	>85%	75-84%	65-74%	<65%	0.383
	75 (20.2%)	148 (40%)	98 (26.4%)	49 (13.2%)	
Sleep Disturbances	Never	Once or twice	Once or twice each week	Three or more times each week	0.652
	3 (0.0%)	173 (46.7%)	181 (48.9%)	13 (3.5%)	
Daytime Dysfunction	0	1-2	3-4	5-6	0.114
	202 (54.5%)	93 (25.1%)	55 (14.8%)	20 (5.4%)	
Hypnotic Medication Use	Not during the past month	Less than once a week	Once or twice a week	Three or more times a week	0.318
	279 (75.4%)	47 (12.7%)	29 (7.8%)	15 (4%)	
*(Number of hours slept/Number of hours slept in bed) x 100					

Table 1: Prevalence of the PSQI-P parts in shift-work nurses. N=370.

The total score of each questionnaire was measured. The mean and the standard deviation of all total scores calculated 7.13 ± 2.5. Table 2 shows the questionnaire findings in detail. Data showed that the most common complaint among shift-work nurses was delay in sleeping initiation (29.2%) and duration of 30 ± 31 minutes.

Snoring (3%) placed in the bottom of the list of nurse complaints. The results showed no significant relation between sleep disturbances and other considered study features.

	Times of Experience				
Factor	**Not during the past month**	**Less than once a week**	**Once or twice a week**	**Three or more times a week**	**p**
Cannot go to sleep within 30 minutes	49 (13.2%)	105 (28.3%)	108 (29.1%)	108 (29.1%)	0.502
Wake up in the middle of the night or early morning	50 (13.5%)	131 (35.4%)	119 (32.1%)	70 (18.9%)	0.131
Have to get up to use the bathroom	209 (56.4%)	82 (22.1%)	66 (17.8%)	13 (3.5%)	0.102
Cough or snore loudly	242 (65.4%)	78 (21%)	39 (10.5%)	11 (2.9%)	0.086
Feel too cold	140 (37.8%)	108 (29.1%)	94 (25.4%)	28 (7.5%)	0.244
Feel too hot	111 (30%)	102 (27.5%)	108 (29.1%)	49 (13.2%)	0.502
Have bad dreams	172 (46.4%)	118 (31.8%)	52 (14%)	28 (7.5%)	0.173
Have pain	194 (52.4%)	107 (28.9%)	52 (14%)	17 (4.5%)	0.401
Concentration disturbances	75 (20.2%)	148 (40%)	98 (26.4%)	49 (13.2%)	0.077
Having problem to be awake while driving	202 (54.5%)	93 (25.1%)	55 (14.8%)	20 (5.4%)	0.387
Hypnotic medication use	279 (75.4%)	47 (12.7%)	29 (7.8%)	15 (4%)	0.056
Other problem	274 (74%)	27 (7.2%)	44 (11.8%)	25 (6.7%)	0.069

Table 2: Prevalence of detailed features of the PSQI-P contents. N=370.

Data showed that the mean years of nursing experience was 8 ± 5.3 with range of at least one year up to maximum 25 years. Suffering from low sleep quality had no relation with gender (p=0.7), as poor sleepers involved of 85.8% of men and 85.4% of women. There was same finding over the age (p=0.7). Data showed that the means for age of good and poor sleepers were 30.5 ± 5.8 and 30.8 ± 5.2 respectively. The number of years of the nursing experience did not influenced sleep quality (p=0.6), while the means for years of nursing experience were 7.7 ± 6.2 and 8 ± 5.8 among poor and good sleeper respectively. Contrary to expectations, working in different hospital sections also did not significantly affect the sleep quality (p=0.3). Therefore, working in more intensive parts such as CCU or emergency department in comparison with the other non-intensive one had same results and made problems up to 88.3% and 84.6% among intensive and non-intensive unit nurses, respectively. We also did not find any significant relation between poor sleep quality and the level of education (p=0.1). The prevalence of complaints among licensed and who had higher degrees was 86.1% and 70% respectively.

Discussion

This study was performed among shift-work nurses in order to detect how their sleep quality levels were. To achieve this goal we used the PSQI-P as a well-known scientific subjective self-answering questionnaire. Of all 370 participants who had subjectively acceptable health status the mean of the PSQI-P score was 7.13 ± 2.5 which was reported 6.8 ± 3.8 in another study [8]. The prevalence of poor sleep quality was as high as 86% in our study, while it was subjectively reported about 57-76% among nurses and 26-39% among general population by a Taiwanese study performed in 2013 [2]. The other authors described this prevalence as 73.3% [8], 71.4% [9] and 57% [10] in earlier studies. Our finding showed the highest percent of involvement and it also determined that sleep disturbances have increased specifically among nurses. The convergence of findings over the issue of inadequate sleep quality implies on a worldwide problem which may not greatly relate to divergence of ethical origins, cultures, climate of living region, economy and genetic differences among nations. We found no relation between degree of education and the level of sleep quality as found in another study [9]. Although, reports of other study showed nurses with high school or lower degree of education had much higher as doubled risk ratio to have sleep disorders compared with those with higher degrees [2]. This difference may due to sample characteristics or regional culture and national instructions to register graduated persons for work. We found delay in sleep initiation was the most common complaint among participants. This was different in other studies which reported decreased total sleep duration time [11], digestive disorders [12,13], mental or psychological problems [14], musculoskeletal complaints [15] and improper daily sleeping [16,17] as their most common symptom followed by low sleep quality. This may due to personal, professional, social, cultural and life style differences among respondents. Our findings were compatible with those studies evaluating probable relationship between sleep discomfort and age, gender, work experience, department of nursing and further marriage status or number of children that the latter was not considered in ours [2,18-20]. We did not find any major correlation between above variables and sleep quality, as the other authors did [2,8-10,18-20]. This compatible findings and considering that sleep complaints have increased during last decade, implies on having wider look to find causes of sleep problems is necessary, especially among nurses whose work outcomes directly influence patient health and prognosis. As mentioned above, over 2 million patient injuries occur annually due to preventable hospitalization errors if nurses have more working hour load and not enough restoration time [3]. Some Japanese studies revealed a great correlation between nursing errors and shifting work (odds ratio=1.1) [21], because of daily sleepiness and sleep latency [22]. Also in one Iranian study brightly stated poor sleepers suffered chiefly by disturbed sleep latency and this event induced in 2.58 time more daily sleepiness [23]. Eventually, considering this study and others' findings seems paying more attention to the issue of sleep problems and following adverse effects is a serious need for both general population and who has risky profession.

Limitation

Consideration of samples including shift-work staff without having synchronous data of non-shift work nurses - although it is almost always impossible to have statistically valuable samples of nurses whose shifts are only along with days - and general population prevented us to have wider comparison. Making objective examination of sleep will help to have more reliable results. Considering at least other demographic features for instance body mass index would help to estimate effects of fatness - known as a hormone related event - on the study objectives. However, we claim that there is a long list of variables exist that may affect sleep quality but have ignored since now.

Conclusion

This study showed that shift-work nurses are highly suffered by poor sleep quality. Gender, age, years of work experience and department of nursing have no significant effect on this issue. It seems planning new studies with deeper and more pervasive look to find what makes this highly poor sleep quality among nursing staff is a great need.

Acknowledgement

We kindly thank the department of psychology and nursing unit of University of Medical Sciences, Qom, Iran, observing the study steps by all.

Conflict of Interests

The team of authors promised that they had not any conflict of interests for making this paper.

References

1. Haghighi Kh, Aminian O, Pouryaghoub Gh, Yazdi Z (2008) Efficacy and Hypnotic Effects of Melatonin in Shift-Work Nurses: Double-Blind, Placebo-Controlled Crossover Trial. Journal of Circadian Rhythms 6:10.
2. Chien PL, Su HF, Hsieh PC, Siao RY, Ling PY, et al. (2013) Sleep Quality among Female Hospital Staff Nurses. Hindawi Publishing Corporation Sleep Disorders 283490.
3. Scott LD, Rogers AE, Hwang WT, Zhang Y (2006) Effects of Critical Care Nurses' Work Hours on Vigilance and Patients' Safety. American Journal of Critical Care 15:130-137.
4. Farrahi MJ, Nakhaee N, Sheibani V, Garrusi B, Amirkafi A (2012) Reliability and validity of the Persian version of the Pittsburgh Sleep Quality Index (PSQI-P). Sleep Breath 16: 79-82.
5. Akbari V, Hajian A, Hosseini SM (2015) Validity and Reliability of Persian Version of the Occupational Impact of Sleep Questionnaire (OISQ-P). Journal of Sleep Disorders and Therapy 4: 186.
6. Buysse DJ, Reynolds CF, Monk TH, Berman SR and Kupfer DJ (1989) The Pittsburgh Sleep Quality Index: A new instrument for psychiatric practice and research. Journal of Psychiatric Research 28: 193-213.
7. Akbari V, Hajian A, Damirchi P (2014) Prevalence of Emotional Disorders Among Students of University of Medical Sciences; Iran. The Open Psychology Journal 7: 29-32.
8. Rocha MCP, De Martino MMF (2010) Stress and Sleep Quality of Nurses Working Different Hospital Shifts. Rev Esc Enferm USP 44: 279-85.
9. Moradi S, Farahnaki Z, Akbarzadeh A, Gharagozlou F, Karchani M, et al. (2014) The Relationship between Shift Work and Job Satisfaction among Nurses: a Cross-sectional Study. International Journal of Hospital Research 3(2): 63-68.
10. Shao MF, Chou YC, Yeh MY, Tzeng WC (2010) Sleep Quality and Quality of Life in Female Shift-Working Nurses. J Adv Nurs 66: 1565-72.
11. Zverev YP, Misiri HE (2009) Perceived Effects of Rotating Shift Work on Nurses' Sleep Quality and Duration. Malawi Medical Journal 21: 19-21.
12. Ruggiero JS (2003) Correlates of Fatigue in Critical Care Nurses. Research in Nursing and health. Pubmed 26: 434–44.
13. Lee S, Colditz GA, Berkman LF, Kawachi I (2004) Prospective Study of Job Insecurity and Coronary Heart Disease in US Women. Ann Epidemiol 14: 24–30.
14. McVicar A (2003) Workplace Stress in Nursing: A Literature Review. J Adv Nurs 44: 633–42.
15. Fouman Golshani M (2010) Sociology of Education. Davaran publication. Third edition, Ninth publication.
16. Wetterberg L (1978) Melatonin in humans' physiological and clinical studies. J NeuralTransm Suppl 13: 289-310.
17. Fischer FM, Paraguay AIBB, Bruni AC, Moreno CRC, Berwerth A, et al. (1998) Working conditions, work organization and consequences on health of Brazilian petrochemical workers. Int J Ind Ergonom 21: 209-19.
18. Berenholtz SM, Dorman T, Pronovost PJ (2003) Improving Quality and Safety in the ICU. ontemp Crit Care 1: 1-8.
19. Baldwin DC, Daugherty SR, Tsai R, Scotti M (2003) A National Survey of Residents' Self-Reported Work Hours: Thinking Beyond Specialty. Acad Med 78: 1154-1164.
20. Landrigan CP, Rothschild JM, Cronin JW, et al. (2004) Effect of Reducing Interns' Work Hours on Serious Medical Errors in Intensive Care Units. N Engl J Med 351: 1838-1848
21. Arimura M, Imai M, Okawa M, Fujimura T, Yamada N (2010) Sleep, Mental Health Status, and Medical Errors among Hospital Nurses in Japan. Industrial Health 48: 811–7.
22. Suzuki K, Ohida T, Kaneita Y, Yokohama E, Uchiyama M (2005) Daytime Sleepiness, Sleep Habits and Occupational Accidents among Hospital Nurses. Journal of Advanced Nursing 52(4): 445–53.
23. Forouzi MAZ, Tirgari B, Iranmanesh S, Razban F, Sistani R (2014) Sleep Quality and Sleepiness in South East Iranian Nurses. Journal of Research & Health 4: 649-56.

13

Evaluation of Denture Wear on Upper Airway Dimensions and Oxygen Saturation in Completely Edentulous Patients

Gowda M[1*], Sahoo NK[1], Guruprasada[1], Naveen KS[2] and Verma K[3]

[1]*Command Military Dental Centre (WC), Chandimandir, Haryana, India*

[2]*Army Dental Centre (R and R), Delhi, India*

[3]*Military Dental Centre (BEG), East Kirkee, Pune, India*

[*]**Corresponding author:** Gowda M, Command Military Dental Centre (WC), Chandimandir, Haryana, India, E-mail: kamalverma_in@yahoo.com

Abstract

Background: Majority of the elderly people complain of difficulty in sleeping. Although the causes for the sleep disturbances may be multifactorial in nature, the sleep disordered breathing (SDB) is one of the primary disorder. The study was undertaken to study the effect of complete denture rehabilitation which could have profound impact on rehabilitation protocol on complete edentulous patients.

Aim: The aim of this study is to cephalometrically evaluate the effect of complete denture rehabilitation on upper airway dimensions and position of hyoid bone and also to examine if complete denture rehabilitation influences oxygen saturation and degree of sleepiness by overcoming upper airway collapsibility.

Material and Method: Of 30 edentulous patients who complained of snoring during sleep were selected for the study. The baseline lateral cephalogram of all the patients were taken by asking the patient to attain the natural head position. MAS (Minimal Airway Space), PAS (Posterior Airway Space), SAS (Superior Airway Space), MP-H (Perpendicular distance from hyoid bone to mandibular plane) were also recorded. The patients were also subjected to pulse oximetry test to assess the oxygen saturation and ESS (Epworth Sleepiness Scale) to assess the day time sleepiness. All these subjects were rehabilitated using conventional complete denture fabricated using standard prosthodontic protocol and after 6 weeks to 8 weeks they were subjected to same tests again with dentures *in situ*.

Results: The results of this study showed no statistically significant difference on minimal airway space (MAS), posterior airway space (PAS), superior airway space (SAS), perpendicular distance from hyoid bone to mandibular plane (MP-H), epworth sleepiness scale (ESS) and oxygen saturation.

Conclusion: Wearing the complete denture during night does not improve the airway space, oxygen saturation and day time sleepiness significantly among edentulous patients.

Keywords: Sleep disordered breathing; Obstructive sleep apnea; Epworth sleepiness scale

Introduction

Disturbed sleep is a common source of disgruntlement among elderly people. It is estimated that up to 50% of elderly adults complain of difficulty in sleeping, further aggravating the risks of morbidity in the ageing population [1]. It has been described that 43% of those over the age of 65 have difficulty in the onset and maintenance of sleep, while 25% report daily drowsiness [2].

Many authors in 1970 delineated the causes of upper airway sleep disorders and in 1980 they described the oral appliances as pivotal treatment modality. Drowsiness and symptoms of sleep disturbance have been associated with declining cognitive capacity, depression, falls and mortalities. Sleep disturbances are multifactorial in nature and could be impacted by alterations of the circadian rhythm, neuropsychological impairment, use of medications and some medical conditions.

In most of the cases disturbed sleep is constantly associated with sleep-disordered breathing (SDB) which can range from the cessation of respiration lasting for at least 10 seconds (apneas) and or partial or reduced respiration (hypopneas) during sleep [3].

One of the exacerbating factors that were recommended to worsen SDB is edentulism. Complete tooth loss sequels in anatomical changes that may sway upper airway dimensions and pass out by influencing the postural rest position of the mandible, muscle tone and tongue posture during sleep. A decrease in retropharyngeal space and or the hypotonicity of the pharyngeal musculature in edentulous people have been recommended to increase the collapsibility of airways [4].

Using supine lateral cephalometric studies in complete denture wearers, they substantiated decrease in retropharyngeal space and anteroposterior oropharyngeal distance in the absence of dentures. They found that there may be perpetuation of obstructive sleep apnea (OSA) and lower arterial hemoglobin oxygen saturation in patients following the removal of dentures. Thus, they collectively assign edentulism as a reason for exacerbation of OSA [5].

There are very few studies to analyze the role of complete denture rehabilitation on the upper air way dimension and its influence on oxygen saturation to analyze and assess whether edentulism favors the occurrence or alleviating of OSA which would have intense effect on rehabilitation protocol in complete edentulous patients with SDB.

Materials and Methods

A repeated design measure study was undertaken. The samples were selected from the completely edentulous patients visiting our institution seeking complete dentures. All patients were informed of the modalities and purpose of the study before obtaining consent to participate.

The inclusion criteria for the study were first time complete edentulous patients with well-formed residual ridges in class I relation, presence of snoring or known case of obstructive sleep apnea, age group of between 50 years to 70 years, clinically stable with no systemic involvement especially respiratory disease and infections. The exclusion criteria included any metabolic or craniofacial syndrome, BMI>3, nasal obstruction, pharyngeal tumours, history of tongue, palate or upper airway surgery, skeletal class III relationship, grossly resorbed residual alveolar ridges and musculoskeletal disorders.

All complete dentures were made and assessed by the same clinician at all stages and were fabricated by the same technician in accordance with the standard prosthodontic treatment and laboratory protocol.

The sample consisted of 30 edentulous patients who complained of snoring. Out of which 14 were males and 16 were females with mean age of 63 years. Baseline lateral cephalograms were recorded at the end expiration, palate not involved in deglutition and jaws in physiologic rest position by asking the patients to attain natural head position (NHP) (Figures 1 and 2).

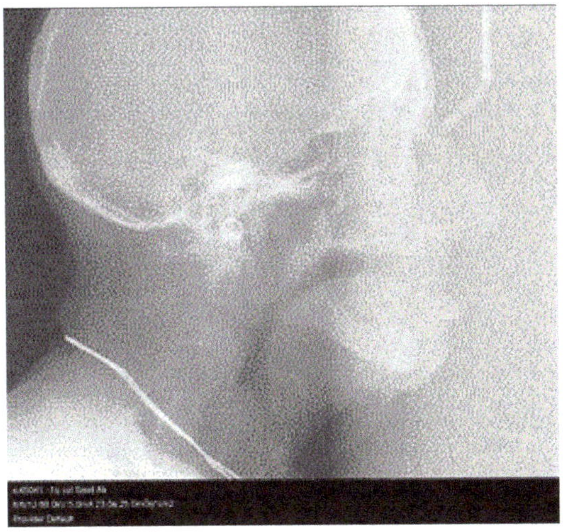

Figure 1: Pre-insertion cephalogram.

To attain NHP, patients were made to stand without head fixation in cephalostat, after moving head forward and backward 3 times, swallowing and lips at rest. Exposure time and other parameters were kept constant and radiographs were made with a film object distance of 180 cm and film to median plane distance of 10 cm which was constant for both pre and post cephalometric radiographs.

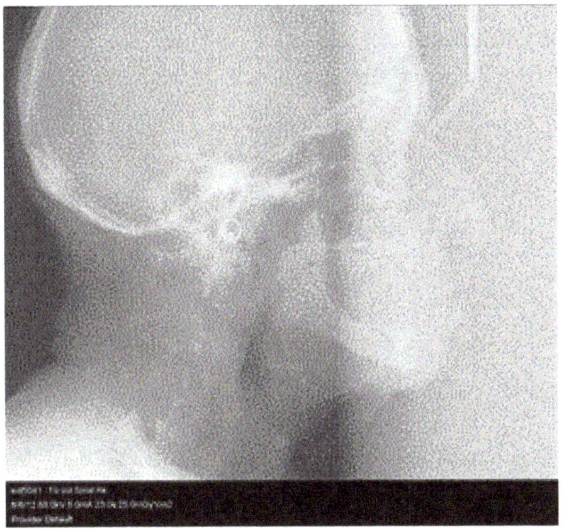

Figure 2: Post-insertion cephalogram.

All the patients were also subjected to overnight pulse oximetry test to assess oxygen saturation and epworth sleepiness scale (ESS) to assess day time sleepiness (Figures 3 and 4).

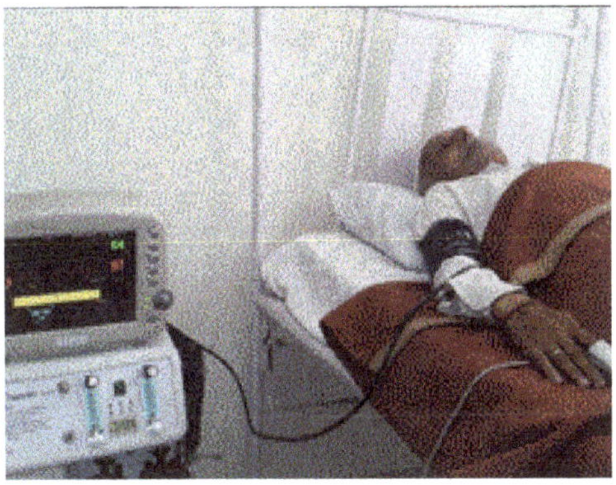

Figure 3: Sleep study being carried out.

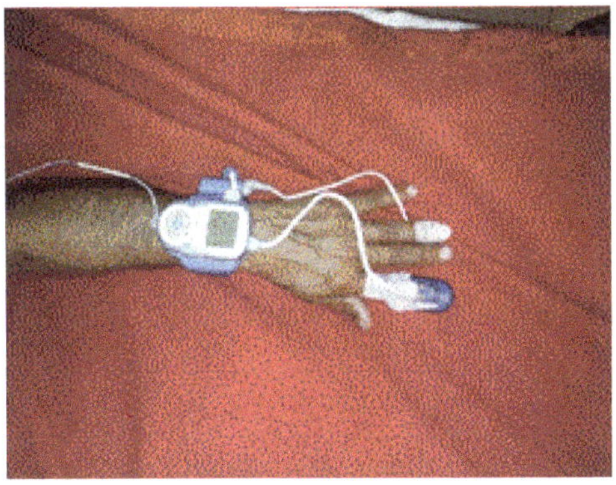

Figure 4: Electrodes attached while doing sleep study.

All the 30 study subjects were rehabilitated with conventional polymethyl methacrylate complete dentures (CD) using standard prosthodontic fabrication protocols.

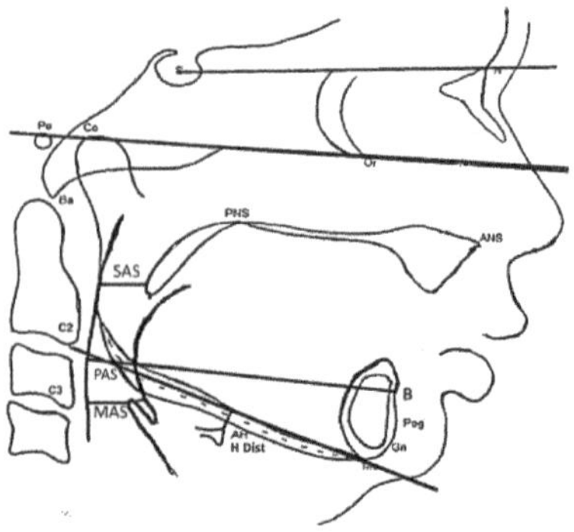

Figure 5: Cephalometric landmarks and measurements.

After 6 weeks to 8 weeks, following the use of CD and having observed the compliance of use, they were subjected to lateral cephalograms with CD *in situ* as per standardised protocol followed during pre-treatment cephalometry using the same cephalometric machine.

All the rehabilitated study subjects were also subjected to overnight pulse oximetry with wearing CD to assess oxygen saturation and ESS scores were evaluated.

The data recordings of sleep duration lasting for more than 4 h were considered as acceptable for the purpose of our study.

Based on the outer border of the radiograph, vertical and horizontal lines were traced perpendicular to each other.

These two lines acted as references to calculate the angles between the head and neck on the cephalograms and the measurements for posterior airway space (PAS), minimal airway space (MAS), superior airway space (SAS) and perpendicular distance from hyoid bone to mandibular plane (M-PH) (Figure 5 and Table 1).

Results

The mean SAS without dentures was 8.96 mm (± 1.84) and with denture wear was 8.90 mm (± 1.79) with difference in mean of 0.06 (± 0.52). The comparison of means was done using paired t-test, wherein p-value was of 0.48 indicating no statistically significant difference in SAS, between with and without denture wearers (Table 2).

The mean MAS without dentures was 7.00 mm (± 1.59) and with denture wear was 7.30 mm (± 1.46) with difference in mean of 0.30 (± 0.53).

The p-value was of 0.005 indicates statistically significant difference in MAS, between with and without denture wearers (Table 3).

The mean PAS without dentures was 11.76 mm (± 1.83) and with denture wear was 11.93 mm (± 2.08) with difference in mean of 0.16 (± 0.53). The p-value of 0.096 indicates no statistically significant difference in PAS, between with and without denture wearers (Table 4). The mean H-distance without denture was 11.73 mm (± 1.7) and with denture wear was 11.7 mm (± 2.08) with difference in mean was 0.03 (± 0.85). The p-value of 0.83 indicates no statistically significant difference in H-distance to the mandibular plane, between with and without denture wearers (Table 5).

S.No.	Cephalometric variables	Definition
1)	Superior airway space (SAS)	A horizontal distance from the tip of the soft palate to pharyngeal wall.
2)	Posterior airway space (PAS)	Horizontal distance from the posterior margin of the tongue to pharyngeal wall measured on the B-Go line.
3)	Minimum airway space (MAS)	Minimum horizontal distance between the anterior and posterior wall of pharynx in the oropharyngeal region (or) horizontal distance between the anterior and posterior wall at the narrowest part of oropharynx.
4)	Hyoid distance (H- MP)	A perpendicular distance between the superior most point on the body of hyoid bone and the mandibular plane.

Table 1: Definitions of various cephalometric measurements.

Variable	Pretreatment		Post treatment		Mean of diff	p-value
	Mean	SD	Mean	SD		
SAS	8.96	1.84	8.9	1.79	0.066	0.489

Table 2: Effect of wearing complete denture on SAS.

Variable	Pre treatment		Post treatment		Mean of diff	p-value
	Mean	SD	Mean	SD		
MAS	7	1.59	7.3	1.46	0.3	0.005

Table 3: Effect of wearing complete denture on MAS.

Variable	Pre treatment		Post treatment		Mean of diff	p-value
	Mean	SD	Mean	SD		
PAS	11.76	1.83	11.93	2.08	0.16	0.096

Table 4: Effect of wearing complete denture on PAS.

The ESS score without denture was 8.83 (± 1.64) and with denture wear was 8.83 (± 1.81) with difference in mean of 0.00 (± 0.74). The p-value of 1.00 indicating no statistically significant difference in ESS between with and without denture wearers (Table 6). The oxygen saturation percentage score without dentures was 93.30 (± 1.74) and with denture wear was 93.20 (± 1.58) with difference in mean of 0.10 (± 0.88). The p-value of 0.54 indicates no statistically significant difference in oxygen saturation percentage between with and without denture wearers (Table 7).

Variable	Pre treatment		Post treatment		Mean of diff	p-value
	Mean	SD	Mean	SD		
H - Distance	11.73	1.7	11.7	2.08	0.03	0.831

Table 5: Effect of wearing complete denture on H-distance.

Variable	Pre treatment		Post treatment		Mean of diff	p-value
	Mean	SD	Mean	SD		
ESS	8.83	1.64	8.83	1.81	0	1

Table 6: Effect of wearing complete denture on ESS.

Variable	Pre treatment		Post treatment		Mean of diff	p-value
	Mean	SD	Mean	SD		
Oxy Sat	93.3	1.74	93.2	1.58	0.1	0.541

Table 7: Effect of wearing complete denture on oxygen saturation.

Discussion

From a methodical viewpoint, sleep is defined on the basis of both the behavior of the person while asleep and related physiological changes that occur to the alert brain's electrical rhythms in sleep [6]. The behavioral criteria consist of a complete lack of mobility or slight mobility, sluggish eye movements, peculiar sleeping posture, decreased response to external stimulation, increased reaction time and arousal threshold, an impaired cognitive function and a reversible unconscious state. The physiological parameters are based on the findings of EEG, electro-oculography (EOG) and electromyography (EMG).

Sleep apnea, based on the denotation, should have at least five apneas or hypopneas per hour of sleep accompanied by excessive daytime sleepiness (EDS). The manifestations of OSAS can be divided into two groups; those occurring during sleep and those occurring during awake. Nocturnal symptoms includes choking during sleep. Habitual loud snoring and halting of breathing and abnormal motor activities during sleep, severe sleep disruption, heartburn as a result of gastro esophageal reflux, nocturnal enuresis which is seen mostly in children and profuse sweating at night. The daytime symptoms includes sleep attacks lasting 0.5 h to 2 h and occurring mostly when the patient is relaxing i.e. sitting down or watching television.

Increased pharyngeal collapsibility is a frequent cause of obstructive sleep apnea (OSA) [5] which results from the combination of anatomical abnormalities of the upper airway with changes in neural activation mechanisms. Innumerable structural changes in facial morphology have been associated with OSA pathogenesis like retrognathic mandibles, posteriorly placed pharyngeal walls, large tongues and soft palate. Missing teeth produces prominent anatomical changes that may influence upper airway size and function, such as decreased vertical dimension of occlusion, reduction of the lower third facial height and mandible rotation correlating its role in the pathogenisis of OSA [7].

Bucca et al. [5] and Gupta et al. [8] confirmed that removal of dentures significantly decreases the retropharyngeal space and sleeping without dentures is associated with significant decrease in apnea-hypopnea index (AHI) and decrease in mean arterial hemoglobin saturation. The authors stressed the fact of wearing complete dentures during night will negate the effects of OSA. Their results were in contrast to our study results, wherein there was no significant difference in cephalometric findings in superior airway space (SAS) (Table 2) and posterior airway space (PAS) (Table 4) whereas there was a significant difference in minimal airway space (MAS) (Table 3) between patients with and without complete dentures. This could be because our study sample was of non-confirmed cases of OSA with only snoring as an inclusion criteria.

Carossa et al. [9] described the effect of removal of dentures and modifications of prosthesis on pharyngeal collapse and showed statistically significant reduction in PAS. They concluded that wearing denture induces modifications in the position of tongue, the jaw and the pharyngeal air way space which was not in accordance with our study. This may be because of the selection of sample size of 27 subjects with reduced vertical dimension compared to our study sample of ideal jaw relations.

Gupta et al. [4] evaluated completely edentulous patients cephalometrically with increasing vertical jaw relation using an acrylic jig of 2 mm to 3 mm and revealed that there was a statistically significant correlation between PAS and retropharyngeal space between edentulous and patients with complete dentures and they concluded that increasing vertical dimension of occlusion within acceptable limits is beneficial to patients with OSA.

Ariska et al. [10] and Bucca et al. [11] had evaluated the risk for OSA in completely edentulous patients with and without complete dentures respectively and concluded that the episode of AHI increases along with reduction in oxygen saturation and retropharyngeal space without dentures indicating worsening of the OSA among subjects. But although there was a definite improvement of AHI among all denture wearers, the oxygen saturation level was recorded at 95.4 ± 2.4 without dentures and 95.6 ± 1.6 with dentures indicating no statistically significant difference. This result is in concurrence to our study wherein the oxygen saturation level was recorded at 93.30 ± 1.74 without dentures and 93.20 ± 1.58 reveling no statistically significant difference.

In a study by Tsuda et al. [12], they demonstrated that edentulism favors upper airway obstruction during sleep. In fact, both AHI and mean SaO_2 were significantly worse in the patients who slept without dentures than in the patients slept with dentures. Almeida analysed completely edentulous patients with OSA and contrary to other study findings concluded that dentures substantially increases AHI especially in supine position. They had the mean oxygen saturation percentage value of 94.2 ± 1.57, almost similar to our study findings 93.25 ± 1.31 (Table 7), which is almost nearer to the proved normal basal oxygen saturation of 95.5%. The findings may be attributed due to the recordings taken only during sleep and supine position and not compared with patients when awake. This can be attributed due to interruption of elevator muscles due to the denture wear during sleep leading to the more collapsibility of the airway thus leading to reduced oxygen saturation. The day time sleepiness measured using Epworth Sleepiness Scale score was 10.2 ± 4.4 compared to our results of 8.83 ±

1.72 (Table 6), indicating there was no EDS compared between patients with or without complete dentures. The variation between the results may be attributed to the selection of subjects with non-confirmed OSA subjects selected by us.

Our study results showed no correlation between oxygen saturation and hyoid bone distance to mandibular plane. The anteroposterior measurement of retro pharyngeal space on cephalograms at three areas of SAS, PAS and MAS, revealed only MAS significant when compared between completely edentulous patients wearing with and without complete denture.

Conclusion

Within the limitation of the study it is concluded that denture wearing at night in healthy completely edentulous patients will not significantly improve quality and quantity of sleep as determined by oxygen saturation levels and ESS scoring. There is no significant increase in airway space and oxygen saturation levels are not affected with the use of complete dentures during sleep. It is recommended that further studies involving large sample size with OSAS may be required to be studied to conclusively prove the hypothesis of wearing denture at night improves the air way space and reduces the symptoms of OSAS. Further studies with confirmed OSA patients and varying the prosthesis vertical dimension of occlusion and MRI study with 3D measurements may give definite insight on understanding their effect on sleep parameters and on airway changes.

References

1. Foley DJ, Monjan A, Simonsick EM, Wallace RB, Blazer DG (1999) Incidence and remission of insomnia among elderly adults: an epidemiologic study of 6,800 persons over three years. Sleep 22: S366-S372.
2. Fragoso CAV, Gill TM (2007) Sleep complaints in community- living older persons: a multifactorial geriatric syndrome. J Am Geriatr Soc 5: 1853-1866.
3. Ivanhoe JR, Cibirka RM, Lefebvre CA, Parr GR (1999) Dental considerations in upper airway sleep disorders: A review of the literature. J Prosthet Dent 82: 685-698.
4. Gupta P, Thombare R, Pakhan AJ, Singhal S (2011) Cephalometric evaluation of the effect of complete dentures on retropharyngeal space and its effect on spirometric values in altered vertical dimension. ISRN Dent 51: 69.
5. Bucca C, Carossa S, Pivetti S, Gai V, Rolla G, et al. (1999) Edentulism and worsening of obstructive sleep apnoea. Lancet 353: 121-122.
6. Chokroverty S (2009) An overview of normal sleep. Sleep disorders medicine: Basic science, technicalconsiderations and clinical aspects. (3rd edn), Elsevier Publications, Philadelphia, USA.
7. Morelli DL, Jackson N, Gislason T, Arnardottir ES (2011) The effect ofedentulismon ahi, odi, and tongue morphology in iceland sleep apnea cohort (ISAC). Am J Respir Crit Care Med 183: 3676.
8. Gupta P, Thombare R, Singhal S, Pakhan AJ (2010) Obstructive sleep apnea and edentulism-role of complete dentures/oral appliance from prosthodontic respective: a review. Indian J Sleep Med 5: 116-119. Bucca C, Cicolin A, Brussino L, Arienti A, Graziano A, et al. (2006) Tooth loss and obstructive sleep apnoea. Respir Res 7: 8.
9. Carossa S, Bucca C, de Lillo A, Corsalini M, Rizzatti A, et al. (2000) Correlation between edentulism, sleep disorders and arterial hypertension. Preliminary research. Minerva Stomatol 49: 399-404.
10. Arisaka H, Sakuraba S, Tamaki K, Watanabe T, Takeda J, et al. (2009) Effects of wearing complete dentures during sleep on the apnea-hypopnea index. Int J Prosthodont 22: 173-177.
11. Bucca C, Cicolin A, Brussino L, Arienti A, Graziano A, et al. (2006) Tooth loss and obstructive sleep apnoea. Respir Res 7: 8.
12. Tsuda H, Almeida FR, Walton JN, Lowe AA (2010) Questionnaire-based study on sleep-disordered breathing among edentulous subjects in a university oral health center. Int J Prosthodont 23: 503-506.

Hypothesizing that Putative Dopaminergic, Melatonin, Benzodiazepine Reward Circuitry Receptor(s) Activator Provides Sleep Induction Benefits

Kenneth Blum[1,3*], Marlene-Oscar-Berman[2], William Downs B[3], Eric R Braverman[1,4], Florian Kreuk[4], Kristina Dushaj[4], Courtney Truesdell[4], Mona Li[4], John Giordano[5], Joan Borsten[6], Thomas Simpatico[7], Debmayla Barh[8], Margaret A Madigan[3,4,9], Scott Jones[5] and Stephen Schoenthaler[5,10]

[1]*Department of Psychiatry, University of Florida, McKnight Brain Institute, USA*

[2]*Departments of Psychiatry and Anatomy & Neurobiology, Boston University School of Medicine, and Boston VA Healthcare System, Boston, USA*

[3]*Impact genomics, Inc., Lederoch, Pennsylvania, USA*

[4]*Department of Clinical Neurology, Path Research Foundation, USA*

[5]*Department of Holistic Medicine, National Institute for Holistic Addiction Studies, USA*

[6]*Department of Addiction Research & Therapy, Malibu Beach Recovery Center, USA*

[7]*Human Integrated Services Unit University of Vermont Center for Clinical & Translational Science, College of Medicine, USA*

[8]*Institute of Integrative Omics & Applied Biotechnology, India*

[9]*Department of Personalized Genomics, IGENE LLC., USA*

[10]*Department of Sociology, California State University, USA*

Abstract

The issue of insomnia is a global phenomenon which requires additional in-depth research. Insomnia especially in alcohol-dependent patients, for example, may lead to suicide. It is noteworthy that childhood sleep problems predict the onset of drinking in boys. We now know that while there are multi-faceted reasons for sleep problems and disturbances (e.g. sleep drive homeostasis, circadian rhythm physiology, and genetic influences), the scientific community has not been able to deliver an appropriate solution. Some benefit has been noted with cognitive behavioral therapy, but it has minimal effects in patients relapsing from drugs especially alcohol, cocaine and opiates. While there are a number of pharmaceutical drugs developed to treat insomnia, most have associated side effects and even addiction liability. We do know that benzodiazepines hijack the midbrain dopamine system leading to addiction. Finally, it has been proposed that dopamine D2 receptors are involved in rapid eye movement sleep, suggesting as proposed herein that dopaminergic activation is a worthwhile mechanism to explore in the future. The concepts presented herein on potential nutrigenomic therapy warrants further in-depth analysis. In this regard we hypothesize based on both literature review and empirical data that a putative dopaminergic, melatonin, benzodiazepine reward circuitry receptor(s) activator provides sleep induction benefits.

Keywords: Insomnia; Reward circuitry; Reward Deficiency Syndrome (RDS); Melatonin; Benzodiazepines, Nutrigenomics; Rapid-eye movement; Sleep

Introduction

Considering the benefits provided by typical hypnotic and non-hypnotic medication for the treatment of chronic insomnia such as barbiturates, benzodiazepines, as well as Zolpidem, versus the risk of both abuse liability and toxicity is a challenging calculation. The calculation is confounded by the paucity of evidence-based data on the hypnotic efficacy of sleep inducing pharmacological and non pharmacological treatments for chronic insomnia. While inducing sleep, many hypnotic-type medications may also induce potential abuse liability for the patient and other side effects. For example, benzodiazepines, prescription drugs remedying anxiety and insomnia, are recreationally abused; the number of individuals abusing the benzodiazepines is on the rise [1]. Importantly, the mechanism of benzodiazepine activation of midbrain dopamine neurons is well-known, with the mesocorticolimbic reward system affected by benzodiazepine [1].

Others have suggested that non-pharmacological approaches can facilitate sleep and reduce sleep disruption without the specter of side effects and may be a satisfactory regimen in the potential of regaining restorative sleep patterns. In this hypothesis paper, we attempt to show certain neurological mechanisms involved in normal sleep patterns may provide a blueprint to the development of a non-pharmacological treatment for chronic insomnia.

Insomnia Definition and Prevalence

Sleep disorders affect one fifth of Americans [2] and manifest in impaired function or excessive sleepiness due to reduced sleep quality [3]. For persons with sleep disorders, quality of life is greatly affected, for example, attention is reduced, concentration limited, memory negatively affected, reasoning and problem solving skills decreased, and reaction time to emotional and physical pain worsened in persons with insomnia compared to matched controls [4]. Classified by the International Classification of Sleep Disorders (ICSD) as a dyssomnia [5], insomnia is the chief sleep disorder [6].

A condition which negatively affects the ability of an individual to fall asleep or maintain desirable sleep duration or quality, insomnia has

***Corresponding author:** Kenneth Blum, Department of Psychiatry, University of Florida, McKnight Brain Institute, Gainesville, Florida, USA,
E-mail: drd2gene@gmail.com

several risk factors. Age and gender have been implicated as risk factors for insomnia, with the elderly more likely to experience insomnia and women more likely to experience difficulties sleeping than men [7]. Older individuals have trouble maintaining sleep, while falling asleep is the primary sleep issue in younger individuals [8]. 95% of adults had experienced insomnia in 1979, according to a Gallup poll survey, indicating that most people are vulnerable to some instances of sleep disorder [8].

The range of adults with chronic insomnia, ~10% to 15%, and the range of adults with transient insomnia, 25% to 35%, can be explained by the variable diagnostic measures and differing definitions in the study of sleep disorders [7]. Recent changes in the definitions of insomnia now reflect perceptions of sleep problems in patients and include the effect poor quality sleep has on daily function [8]. The constantly evolving definitions in the study of sleep disorders limit the potential for determining the scope of the problem. However, comprehensive surveys in large cohorts provide opportunities to measure this scope-one third of all people experiencing sleep issues annually, half of which seek medical advice for the issue, with only 15% of people actually reported as having sleep disorders [8]. To effectively treat a sleep disorder, the differences between sleep disorders must be understood fully and undoubtedly, such that diagnosis is accurate and treatment is pointed and geared specifically to each respective condition.

According to a 1995 report from the National Sleep Foundation, in a primary care population study, only 6% of insomniacs had gone to their physician specifically for this complaint. Additionally, insomnia in psychiatric patients is under-recognized [9]. While insomnia has been investigated in depth, insomnia is still not completely understood, the study hindered by inconsistent diagnostic criteria and variable definitions.

Insomnia and Sleep Disorder Comorbidities

Primary sleep disorders, not accompanied by other conditions, occur in some cases; however, many sleep disorders occur concomitantly with other medical and/or psychiatric conditions [10]. Latest sleep surveys indicate that of the general adult population, insomnia affects 10% to 17%, and increased rates of insomnia occur in patients with psychiatric conditions [11]. In example, Okuji et al. [11] determined that 69% of patients with mood disorder spectrum, 63% of patients with anxiety disorder, and 50% of patients with an ICD-10 schizophrenia spectrum complained of insomnia.

It is well known that insomnia commonly occurs concomitantly with depression, and it is generally thought of as a symptom in mood disorder [12]. Some studies, however, have claimed that depression and insomnia are disorders distinct in etiology and of genetic influences [13]. Utilizing a 15,000 subject European cohort and longitudinal study, in 40% of cases insomnia occurred before depression and in 56% of cases insomnia occurred before recurrent depression [13]. Insomnia has been implicated as a risk factor for depression. Individuals with a history of insomnia have four times the risk for depression as those that do not [14]. Moreover, the Breslau et al. [14] study also found that prior insomnia history significantly correlated with substance use disorder (S.U.D.), smoking, and risk for anxiety. Finally, following successful treatment for depressive symptoms, as measured with the Hamilton Rating Scale for Depression (HAM-D) scores, patients still reported sleeping difficulties [14].

Many of the symptoms that occur in insomniacs also occur in other sleep disorders; furthermore, sleep disorders, in general, are associated with a myriad of additional co morbidities. For example, the relationship of sleep and suicide has been investigated. A 1997 study conducted by Ağargün determined that persons with the worst quality of sleep, as measured through the Pittsburgh Sleep Quality Index (PSQI), consequently scored the highest suicide subscale scores, indicating an inverse relationship between suicide and sleep quality [15].

In regards to stress, numerous anxiety disorder patients report problems falling and staying asleep; in support, polysomnographic tests of panic disorder patients indicate a reduced efficiency in sleep patterns when compared to normal controls-with increased time awake and increased time before falling asleep [16]. Interestingly, REM sleep measures do not differ significantly nor does sleep architecture for panic disorder patients and normal subjects [16]. For patients with generalized anxiety disorder, 60% to 70% complain that they have issues sleeping; polysomnographs of these patients showed an increase in the time it took to fall asleep as well as a reduction in ability to maintain sleep [16]. Similarly, the REM sleep measures and sleep architecture were not significantly different from controls. Obsessive-compulsive disorder (OCD) patients, though reporting poor sleep, did not show significant difference from controls; patients with social phobias have not been shown to differ in sleep parameters from controls [16].

More recently, utilizing a cohort of 375,653 US adults (≥ 18 years of age) in a 2013 study, Liu et al. [17] investigated the relationship between chronic disease and insufficient sleep. Controlling for various demographics and adjusting for covariates, a significant positive relationship ($p<0.0001$) was observed between six chronic diseases and insufficient sleep [17]. These relationships were modestly explained by frequent mental distress; the relationships between both high blood pressure and diabetes and insufficient sleep were modestly explained by obesity [17]. While the relationship between insufficient sleep and chronic diseases has been investigated, the comprehensive cause-and-effect relationship is impossible to infer from such studies; thus, relationships between these conditions remains unclear [7].

Post-traumatic Stress disorder (PTSD) has also been associated with degradation in sleep quality, 70% to 91% of patients with PTSD have reported issues falling to and maintaining sleep, and 19% to 71% of patients report nightmares, dependent on PTSD severity and physical aggression exposure [18]. The studies relating sleep patterns of PTSD patients and controls are presently inconclusive; however, for PTSD patients the system of REM sleep control seems to be dysregulated [18]. Interestingly, PTSD patients are more predisposed to sleep disordered breathing (SDB) and disorders involving movement during sleep; these comorbidities have been implicated as playing roles in the sleep deficiencies of PTSD patients [18].

Other conditions associated with insomnia are Chronic Obstructive Pulmonary Diseases, Obstructive Sleep Apnea, and Restless Leg Syndrome (RLS).

Insomnia and Sleep Disorder Management

Sleep disorders are presently managed with pointed and treat-to-target techniques depending on condition, with the type and etiology of the condition influencing ideal management [19]. The initial treatment regimen for sleep disorders involves improving sleep hygiene; this is completed by utilizing routine strategies to promote a healthy and silent sleep situation, reducing caffeine or alcohol consumption prior to bed, adhering to a non-disruptive exercise schedule, limiting exposure to stimulates, and employing wind-down sessions prior to sleep [20].

Determined through a comprehensive 59 trial meta-analysis, sleep induction and sleep maintenance have both been improved by non-pharmacological treatments for insomnia [21]. In these studies, sleep restriction therapy and stimulus control therapy were associated with the strongest evidence [21]. Moreover it was found that an average of 5 hours of intervention was shown to reduce time of onset latency and time awake after sleep onset [21].

Furthermore, cognitive behavioral therapy is utilized to treat insomnia and nightmares in PTSD patients by utilizing specialized strategies such as the imagery rehearsal therapy (IRT), a technique in which alternate positive endings are imagined and discussed for nightmares of the patient between a therapist and the patient [18]. While there have been only a few studies on the matter, significant reductions in insomnia and nightmares have been demonstrated through IRT therapy in PTSD patients [18]. Some uncontrolled experiments implicate continuous positive airway pressure as also improving sleep quality, with reduction in nightmare incidence, insomnia and other PTSD symptoms [18]. Continued research is necessary to determine the value of behavioral therapies for sleep disorders.

Additional sleep disorder treatment techniques include behavioral therapy such as biofeedback, as well as light therapy, chronotherapy, and pharmacotherapy, using sedatives and/or hypnotics [19,22-24]. Relaxation therapy, stimulus control therapy [25], sleep restriction therapy [26], and cognitive behavioral therapy (CBT) [27] are other interesting non-pharmacological techniques utilized to treat sleep disorders.

Pharmacotherapeutic Intervention

In the search for a drug which induces sleep without the usual hypnotic–abuse liability and toxicity has been a real challenge for the pharmaceutical industry. Griffiths et al. [28] evaluated 19 hypnotic drugs for both abuse liability and toxicity and found that Phenobarbital has the highest abuse liability and toxicity and Trazodone (a non-approved anti-insomniac drug) while having no abuse liability potential does have significant toxicity [28]. However, one drug, ramelteon, was found not to have any abuse liability or toxicity. This is quite interesting considering that this substance does not bind to the typical GABA receptor. Unlike all other hypnotic drugs used to treat insomnia, ramelteon is amelatonin receptor agonist acting at MT1 MT2 receptors located at/in the superachiasmatic nucleus, which affects the circadian sleep-wake cycle. The MT1 receptor seems to be associated with direct promotion of sleep. This receptor is believed to play a role in helping to quiet down arousal and allow sleepiness to take over. The MT2 receptor seems to be acting primarily with respect to the reinforcement of the whole 24-hour cycle. Ramelteon has negligible affinity for the MT3 receptors, which are widely distributed throughout the body, or for other major neurotransmitter receptors such as GABA, histamine, opioid, dopamine, or acetylcholine. A recent PubMed search revealed a total of 1,138 papers regarding pharmacological and non-pharmacological treatment of chronic insomnia of which 755 were pharmacological.

Hypothesis

It is hypothesized that measurement of various genetic mutations through gene expression, single nucleotide polymorphisms, as well as additional phenotypic and genetic diagnostics, with the interest of changing the makeup and creation of nutritional supplements, will shift the diagnostic, stratification, prognostic, and treatment paradigm for sleep in humans. Furthermore, mesolimbic neurochemical reward circuitry manipulation inducing dopamine release at the Nucleus accumbens will offer benefits in stress and pain relief, both major factors in sleep processes [29]. Specifically, the present theoretical notion includes proprietary algorithms that combine genetic mutations into index values, referred to as Genoscores, to represent specific pre-defined formulations. We hereby propose that a number of experiments be performed to further our scientific credibility. The experiments will include both genetic and non-genetic subjects and the formulations will include both "one-size-fits all" as well as DNA-based customized formulations to induce sleep. The trials will also include comparisons with known FDA approved sleep medications. The protocol will consist of a double-blind randomized placebo-controlled cross-over study. The measurement scales will include one of the following instruments: Fatigue Severity Scale (FSS); Stanford Sleepiness Scale (SSS); Epworth Sleepiness Scale (ESS) and/or Chalder Fatigue Scale (CFS) or Empirical Sleepiness & Fatigue Scales developed by Bailes and associates.

EZ-Sleep™

EZ-sleep™ is a unique formula and method to safely and naturally induce effective sleep. This novel technology contrasts with existing tactics to manipulate three important pathways in sleep induction. Moreover we are hypothesizing that EZ-Sleep™, a putative dopaminergic, melatonin, benzodiazepine reward circuitry receptor(s) activator, may become an important front-line non-pharmacological treatment for chronic insomnia. We further hypothesize that utilization of this nutraceutical may result in significant reduction of hypnotic medication abuse and toxicity liability thereby increasing benefit over risk.

Rationale

This novel approach utilizes synergistic nutraceutical components to exploit symbiotic mechanisms stimulating metabolism and healthy sleep through:

1. Pleasure mechanisms that effect stress

2. The metabolic and immunological mechanisms that effect sleep induction.

3. The neuroendocrine system that affects circadian rhythm

Importantly, these three systems are homeostatic and compensatory, intimately interactive and interdependent in ensuring optimal sleep and metabolic function. This novel nutraceutical technology optimizes sleep mechanisms especially those tied to stress. Table 1 lists the ingredients in EZ-Sleep™. A careful review of the existing literature reveals that the ingredients in EZ-Sleep™ should lead to enhance sleep function. In the arsenal of nutrients, EZ-Sleep™ primarily contains sleep inducing ingredients.

Ingredients & Scientific Explanation

EZ-Sleep™ complex: stress reduction components

Manipulation of pleasure mechanisms that effect stress is exploited by some of the ingredients of EZ-Sleep™, especially through promotion of dopamine release at the Nucleus accumbens, stimulating stress reduction and pain reduction.

In humans, an imaging study by Hilker and associates (2006) found that marked striatal dopamine depletion was demonstrated in patients with REM sleep behavior disorder utilizing functional MRI [30]. Dopamine is also involved in other sleep disorders including Restless Leg syndrome (RLS). A neurological disorder affecting 1-10% of the population, RLS induces urges to move ones extremities in an effort to address paraesthetic sensations [31]. RLS symptoms are heightened when going to sleep in the evening and interrupt/delay desired sleeping

Supplement Facts
Serving Size: 1 Tablet, 45 minutes before bedtime without food
Serving per container: 60
Amount per Serving
Vitamin B6 (as Pyridoxine HCL, Pyridoxal-5-Phosphate)
Calcium (as hydroxycitrate)
Magnesium (as magnesium citrate and oxide) (aspartate is better!)
Manganese (ascorbate)
Potassium (as hydroxycitrate)
Synaptamine Proprietary Complex
Chromium picolinate
DL-phenylalanine (D-PhenEze™)
L-Glutamine
Rhodiola rosea Extract (3%)‡ (RhodiGen™
Grifonia simplicifolia Extract (5-HTP)
**EZ Sleep™ Proprietary Calming blend
Passiflora incarnata L. Extract Δ (EM103 Passiflora incarnata)
Protykin (50% trans-resveratrol)
Melatonin
* Daily Value not established.
**Chamomile, Valerian, and Hops Flower (33 mg each)
TOTAL MGs

Table 1: Ingredients of EZ-Sleep™: the putative dopaminergic, melatonin, benzodiazepine reward circuitry receptor(s) activators that enable sleep induction benefits.

and waking times. While the etiopathogenesis of RLS remains unknown, a dopaminergic system is hypothesized to play an important role in RLS manifestation-the use of dopamine agonists in treatment, such as 2005 FDA approved ropinirole, offer valuable therapeutic solutions to RLS [31].

Dopaminergic involvement of sleep and wakefulness is very complex, and exact mechanisms are still unclear. The various receptors of dopamine (D1-D5) all have very distinct properties and may interact at different sleep processes. While dopamine agonists seem to induce sleep interaction of dopamine at various dopamine receptor sites, there may be differential sleep induction and wakefulness depending on the dopamine receptor targeted. For example, recent hypotheses implicate D3 receptor involvement in pramipexole stimulated sleep increase and locomotor activity reduction [32]. Furthermore, high dose pramipexole stimulated postsynaptic D2 receptor activation has been hypothesized to increase motor behavior and wakefulness [32]. REM latency has been increased in rats that were administered a dopamine D4 receptor antagonist (L-741,741), and these results suggest a role for D4 receptors in the regulation of wake and sleep [33].

Lima et al. [34] following animal experimentation, proposed that blockage of dopaminergic D2 receptors produce a decrease of REM but not of slow wave sleep in rodents after REM sleep deprivation [34]. This work suggests that in regards to sleep and wake state maintenance and regulation, dopamine acts as a key substance [34].

While there is sufficient evidence for serotonergic involvement in stress induced insomnia and SSRI's may work in certain instances, long term treatment of insomnia with these agents have been somewhat disappointing, in spite of significant animal work suggestive of serotonin involvement in sleep disorders.

The serotonergic synthesis inhibitor para-chlorophenylalanine, p-CPA, pretreatment has been studied in a murine model, utilizing young male Charles Foster rats subjected to acute immobilization stress, to investigate their resultant sleep-wake patterns [35]. Three groups of rats, subjected to (i) acute immobilization stress, (ii) p-CPA pretreatment and acute immobilization stress, and (iii) neither p-CPA pretreatment nor acute immobilization stress, were monitored in their sleep quality and resultant wakefulness [35]. As a result, p-CPA pretreatment successfully reversed the detrimental effects following acute immobilization stress, including changes in total sleep time and total time of REM sleep [35]. Other work from the laboratory of Geller and Blum initially showed that p-CPA caused an enhancement of stress related conflict in rats [36].

The following ingredients promote stress manipulation through synergistic and symbiotic mechanisms.

Passiflora incarnate: Passionflower is the name of several plants stemming from the Passiflora genus [37]. The origin of Passiflora is in the tropical and subtropical regions of the western hemisphere, and there are over 40 different species in the genus. First transported by Spanish conquerors from Mexico to Europe in the sixteenth century, Passionflower has been utilized as a calming tea remedying menstrual pain, conjunctivitis, hemorrhoids, diarrhea, colic, dysentery, skin eruptions, and muscle spasms and is now a worldwide medical herb. The inclusion of Passionflower in sleep inducing formulas exploits its effect on the central nervous system (CNS) and its stress reduction effects [38]. When in a comfortable sleep environment a reduction in stress should be associated with sleepiness.

A problem with Passionflower is its identity since a number of alkaloids have been sold under its name; however, *Passiflora incarnate* (P. incarnata) stands out as the most important, being the most consistently effective. The total alkaloid content of P. incarnate, as listed on the U.S. Agricultural Research Service's ethno botanical database, is 100 to 900 ppm, and it has a 1.2% to 3.9% total flavonoid content. In P. incarnata, there are twenty flavonoids, amongst them gynocardine and cyanogenic glycoside, as well as six alkaloids, and some researchers have attributed the sedative effects from *P. incarnatato* the alkaloids: Harmane and relatives, harmol and harmaline. In contrast, other researchers have attributed CNS bioactivity to flavonoids such as luteolin, apigenin, or their glycosides, stating that the alkaloid content of P. incarnatais not high enough to cause CNS effects.

Most recently, a highly anxiolytic, tri substituted benzoflavone moiety has been isolated from a P. incarnata extract. P. incarnata extract has effectively restored the libido of older male rats [39]; restored fertility and libido previously compromised by tetra hydro cannabinol, nicotine and alcohol addiction [40]; and compared to oxazepam, double-blind randomized studies have indicated that Passiflora extract has been proven to be a fairly effective means for managing generalized anxiety [39]. Interestingly, other double-blind randomized controlled trials have suggested the potential for Passiflora extract as a valuable adjuvant for managing opiate withdrawal [41]. In a mice model, Passiflora has been shown to decrease benzodiazepine dependence. Moreover, the sedative effects of P. incarnata have been verified in numerous pharmacological investigations. EZ-Sleep™ was formulated with information from Euro med (source of dried aerial EM103 P. incarnata parts, cut or fragmented). Separated leaves have been demonstrated as affording the highest possible CNS results, and excluding the flowers, the usage of all aerial parts may prove to be the best method for maximizing bioactive EM103 P. incarnata plant parts. Passiflora preparation standardization has been studied actively, in special regard to its relation on anxiolytic activity.

It was suggested in the early 1970's, by one of us (KB), that serotonin was a biological substrate of stress. Through injections of p-CPA, a serotonin chemical synthesis depletor in rodents, the initiation of stress in rodents was attenuated. Other researchers have also recognized and shown serotonin and dopamine involvement in the production of stress in humans and other animals. By comparing skin conductance levels in a double-blind randomized controlled human trial, stress levels have been shown to be reduced by amino acid and enkephalinase inhibition therapy. These results support Passiflora extract use for anxiety disorder treatments, especially for serotonin mediated disorders. Interestingly, this is homologous to a Passiflora extract phyto constituentindole.

The genus Passiflora comprises about 500 species [37]. The substance Passiflora incarnata and its benzoflavone isolate binds to the benzodiazepine receptor [42]. As such, it has many biological effects including promotion of sleep, anxiolytic activity [43], anti-alcohol and opiate craving activity [40], promotion of sexual appetite [39], and hypnotic activity [44].

11.1.2 DL-Phenylalanine (validated via FTIR verified reference standard D-PhenEze™): DL-phenylaline (DLPA) inhibits the breakdown of the opioid peptides and has been shown to reduce stress in a double blind placebo controlled study. DLPA has been found to reduce stress by anti-craving reward mechanism.

D-phenylalanine inhibits the enzyme enkephalinase, which metabo¬lizes or breaks down enkephalins, thereby increasing enkephalins availability and, most likely, increasing dopamine availability at reward sites (under stressful conditions especially) [45-47].

Furthermore, L-phenylalanine is utilized to stimulate dopamine production and/or increase brain reward neither area nor epinephrine levels. A significant problem with L-phenylalanine is potential competition with other amino-acids, i.e. blood born L-tyrosine and L-tryptophan at the large neutral amino-acid brain carrier system. However, for the first time, other data has demonstrated synthesis and release responses to several dopaminergic agents may be stemming from synaptosomal dopamine, a product of the hydroxylation of phenylalanine. Dopamine created from 14C-phenylalanine in the Caudate nucleus of a rat through synaptosomal preparation was increased and concomitantly stimulated by Cogentin and Amphetamine. A net increase in dopamine also occurs due to amfoelic acid. In this regard, synaptosomal particles are potential components that can synthesize dopamine from L-phenylalanine; synthesis from L-phenylalanine potentially under regulatory control by synaptosomal particles.

L-Tyrosine: L-tyrosine is utilized to increase dopamine levels in the brain as an amino-acid synthesis promoter, direct precursor. L-tyrosine is used for repletion of metabolized neurotransmitters (i.e. dopamine).

EZ Sleep™ Proprietary Calming Blend: The following ingredients constitute the calming blend to promote sleep: Chamomilia flower, hops flower, valerian root extract, Jamaican dogwood extract, valanic acid, and kava kava. Chamomile extract leads to a significant decrease in sleep latency in rats [48]. Kava Kava reduced generalized anxiety disorder in humans [49,50]. A combination of Valerian-Hops is used as a sleep aid [51]. Binding affinities were observed for this combination of serotonin receptor subtypes including 5-HT7 that promotes sleep. Valerian and valanic acid are partial agonists of the 5-HT5A receptor, a substrate involved in insomnia. Valanic acid enhances the sedative effects of Valarian. Trends toward increase in slow-wave sleep and lack of effect on REM sleep were observed in 1994. There have been studies on Hops that show a sedative effect [52].

Pyridoxal-5-phosphate: Pyridoxal-5-phosphate is the active ingredient of vitamin B_6, important as a co-factor in neurotransmitter production and gastrointestinal amino acid absorption improvement.

Calcium: Calcium promotes release of neurotransmitters. Many metabolic events require calcium, and calcium nutrient inclusion is therefore proposed by the authors to promote sleep. Calcium in a number of species induces a sleep-like state [53,54].

EZ-Sleep™ complex: sleep induction enhancement components

While stress-reduction plays an important role in enabling sleep induction, other components of EZ-Sleep™ directly promote sleep induction through various other mechanisms. Most of the hypnotic drugs on the market are central nervous depressants acting at the gamma- aminobutyric acid $(GABA)_A$ receptor. In this regard, wisdom dictates that only a few hypnotic-like drugs have been approved to treat insomnia, but not beyond short term therapy because of the abuse liability. The benzodiazepine hypnotics are only approved for short term use, as are zolpidem immediate-release (Ambien) and zaleplon (Sonata) the non-benzodiazepine agents that act at the same benzodiazepine-activated $GABA_A$ receptor complex. The following ingredients make use of the GABA complex and serotonergic mechanisms to aid sleep induction.

L-Glutamine: L-glutamine, a precursor amino-acid for GABA, is utilized to increase GABA levels in the brain at anxiety associated receptors. L-glutamine maintains balance in case of D-phenylalanine over-inhibition. The inhibitory action of GABA on brain function is tied to integrated sleep processes [55]. GABA shuts off the neurotransmitters that induce wakefulness. Chronic excess of GABA in the brain induces increased slow-wave sleep [56]. Studies have shown that Adenosine A2A receptor agonist induced sleep by inhibiting the histaminergic system through increasing GABA release in the tuberomammillary nucleus [57]. GABA is linked to the benzodiazepine receptor. The sedative hypnotic benzodiazepine-GABA receptor agonist (BzRas) Zaleplon induces a long-term anti-insomnia effect in older patients [58]. The $GABA_A$ receptor is the target for most widely prescribed sleep medications [59]. The stimulation of the benzodiazepin-GABA site induces sedation, hypnosis, and anxiolytic activity.

Grifoniasimplicifolia Extract, 5-HTP (optional): 5-HTP is an amino acid precursor to brain serotonin. Serotonin levels rise during sleep stages. Sleep is a problem with age and many old people complain about insomnia. It is known that age induces a decrease in serotonergic receptors. The serotonin precursor 5-HTP causes a reversal of insomnia by para-chlorophenylalanine induced serotonin brain depletion [60]. While Serotonin-2A and 2C receptor gene polymorphisms may associate with sleep problems in Japanese patients, these polymorphisms did not associate with apnea [61]. However, both age and BMI did associate. Sleep apnea syndrome is associated with serotonin transporter gene polymorphism [62]. While the 5-HT2A receptor may be involved in insomnia (whereby antagonists may be helpful), 5-HT7 promotes REM sleep [63,64]. Injection of a 5-HT1A -receptor agonist directly into the dorsal midbrain promotes sleep.

Utilizing brain micro dialysis, lateral hypothalamus serotonin release was examined following systemic administration of 5-hydroxy-1-tryptophan in an in vivo rat model [65]. A long lasting, dose-dependent and immediate increase in dialysates 5-HT is observed with the administration of 5-HTP. The 5-HTP- induced response of 5-HT was significantly attenuated and levels of basal 5-HT decreased significantly, when calcium was not included in the perfusion medium, thereby limiting exocytosis.

Chromium Salts (Nicotinate and Picolinate): Chromium is a tryptophan enhancing substance, which increases the brain content of serotonin. Serotonin is involved in the natural sleep process [66]. Brain serotonin production has been shown to be promoted by an oxygen-coordinated chromium nicotinate. Picolinate, another chromium salt, effects the production of serotonin. Since brain serotonin is important as a sleep neurotransmitter, the EZ-sleep™ formula will contain this salt [67].

Rhodiola rosea Extract (3%) (validated via FTIR verified reference standard RhodiGen™): As demonstrated in several clinical trials with double-blind placebo controls, Rhodiola rosea (R. rosea) positively enhances mood, reduces stress and has no detectable toxicity levels. R. rosea extract positively influences the higher nervous system, improving memory and attention span. Where lower dopamine and serotonin brain levels are observed, it is hypothesized that R. rosea can potentially act as a COMT inhibitor. COMT activity has been decreased by 60% and neurotransmitter levels by 30% by R. rosea. This phenomenon will assist in sleep induction. Moreover, the plant adaptogen R. rosea promotes positive effects on sleep [68]. R. rosea has a positive effect on paradoxical sleep deprivation [69]. R. rosea improves endurance exercise in healthy young adults [70]. R. rosea reduces stress and improves sleep [71]. R. rosea improves mental capacity in a double-blind study [72]. R. rosea was effective in improving sleep quality in young men living in high altitudes [73].

Manganese (ascorbate) (ManganEze™): Manganese is found in a large variety of minerals, sea and fresh water, marine and land plants, and animals [74]. Manganese is an essential trace element, human requirements being estimated at between 3 and 9 mg per day. 15 studies have described the adverse mood effects of Manganese (Mn) overexposure, specifically in six dimensions of mood: (i) irritability, nervousness and anxiety; (ii) emotional disturbance; (iii) psychotic experiences; (iv) sleep disturbance, lack of vigor and fatigue; (v) aggression hostility; (vi) compulsive and/or impulsive behavior [75]. 1:15 studies utilized standardized measures of mood. When the Brief Symptom Inventory (BSI) and Profile of Moods State (POMS) standardized mood scales were used to evaluate low Mn levels of exposure and its consequence on mood, results indicated that older men with higher Mn levels showed significant disturbances on four of the six mood dimensions relative to men with lower MN levels, including irritability, nervousness and anxiety; aggression hostility; and emotional disturbance [75]. The POMS and BSI are useful standardized mood scales for the assessment of Mn/mood effects [75]. However, optimal doses produce health benefits. Mn has hypnotic-like effects and as such, enhances alcohol-induced sleeping time in mice. There are no human studies directly involving the effects of Mn on sleep performance, but it has been considered as a sedative inducing nutrient for years.

EZ-Sleep™complex: neuroendocrine circadian rhythm manipulation components

Circadian rhythm, created by molecular mechanisms, is considered a biological property universal to the majority of living things on earth; in which, the regulation of clock genes through a transcription feedback loop is vital to all studied species [76]. The clock genes observed in insects and mammals have been remarkably alike, indicating genetic level, evolutionary circadian rhythm conservation [76]. Homeostasis and circadian rhythms work concomitantly to regulate arousal and sleep in mammals; however, the underlying genetic pathway through which sleep is regulated is not readily understood. Similarities in the molecular arousal regulation pathways between insects and mammals have been discovered; in example, dopamine has been implicated as a key player in the regulation of arousal and sleep-like behavior in ants [76].

Interestingly there is strong evidence for the interaction of melatonin and dopamine D2 receptor. Both the melatonin and dopaminergic systems regulate the light/dark cycles in the animal as well as in the human [77].

Acknowledged to play a role in numerous mammalian brain regions such as the retina, hypothalamus, and nigrostriatal system, the presence of a dopamine-melatonin association is of particular interest. For example, in C57BL/6 mice nigrostriatal damage is caused by the effect of melatonin on 1 methyl-4-phenyl-1, 2, 3, 6-tetrahydropyridine [78]. In C57BL/6 mice, however, the interaction between striatal dopamine and melatonin rhythmic production is not readily understood [77].

Work utilizing the C57BL/6 mice model has investigated circadian rhythm variations in striatal dopamine levels and pineal production of melatonin [78]. This work has indicated the possibility for a series of significant dopamine and melatonin interactions. In mice controls, melatonin has a narrow circadian rhythm peak at midnight, striatal dopamine reaches a low-point at midnight, and 3,4-dihydroxyphenylacetic acid (DOPAC) levels, a primary dopamine metabolite, increase shortly after a decrease in striatal dopamine levels [78]. Following pineal gland removal, the cyclic changes in dopamine and DOPAC levels were less pronounced; however, administration of melatonin over a 6 day period to pinealectomized mice dose-dependently repaired this rhythm [78]. This suggests a potential murine linkage between pineal melatonin secretion and dopamine circadian rhythm [78].

Ramelteon, approved by the Food and Drug Administration (FDA) in 2005, is presently the only medication utilized for long-term insomnia treatment and works by exploiting the soporific property of melatonin; it works as a melatonin receptor agonist [79]. The efficacy of ramelteon is not presently known, although findings have been promising; the efficacy will rely on the results of additional placebo-controlled trials [79]. The effectiveness of melatonin and ramelteon in treating insomnia requires further attention, as present data on the topic is based on studies with several limitations, and there have been only three control trials for ramelteon [79]. It is important to note that sleep maintenance has not been shown to improve with zolipidem controlled-release or eszopiciline, a GABAA agonist. In fact, according to Johnson and Griffiths (2005) subjective comparisons have characterized the hypnotic effect of ramelteon relative to the benzodiazepine and non-benzodiazepine $GABA_A$ active agents as "more subtle" and "less prominent" [28]. Furthermore, post -sleep questionnaires have indicated that ramelteon's hypnotic effect may be experienced as less robust than could be expected from polysomnography data [80].

The following EZ-Sleep™ ingredients affect circadian rhythms, promoting improved sleep quality and improved duration.

Melatonin: Existing as a hormone, endogenous melatonin is secreted by the pineal gland and linked to circadian rhythm [81]. A study of melatonin in the 1970's and 1980's revealed sedative/hypnotic effects of this compound [82,83]. In a recent meta-analysis of 16 studies by Buscemi et al. [84]. It has been concluded that while melatonin may not be effective in primary sleep disorder treatment, it is potentially useful in short term DSPS treatment [84]. The use of melatonin for a short period, 3 months or less, has been implicated as safe.

The pineal gland hormone melatonin improves sleep quality [85]. A recent meta-analysis reveals melatonin treatment significantly reduced sleep onset latency and increased total sleep duration [86]. Melatonin secretion helps regulate sleep and circadian rhythms [87]. Beta-Methyl-6 chloromelatonin significantly decreases sleep latency in insomnia

[88]. Melatonin improves sleep behavior in children with epilepsy [89]. While one study was negative with respect to the effectiveness in melatonin versus placebo with regard to sleep deprivation of winter depression, other studies are positive in terms hypnotic actions [90]. It seems that the effects of melatonin on sleep works best in patients that have abnormal sleep patterns compared to health individuals [91, 92].

Magnesium (ligand? aspartate?) (MagNezyum™?): Chronic stress reduces intracellular magnesium [93]. Aging effects sleep and magnesium reverses these age-related effects and promotes sleep [94]. EEG blood magnesium levels are under strong genetic control, whereas brain magnesium levels are not [95]. Optimal levels of magnesium are required for normal sleep regulation [96].

INGREDIENT	DOSE	FINDING
Pyridoxine HCL Pyridoxal 5-Phosphate	20 mg (20% PHCL; 80% P-5-P	Catalyst for synthesis of neurotransmitters
Chromium[a,b]	400 mcg	Chromium is a tryptophan enhancing substance, which increases the brain content of serotonin. Serotonin is involved in the natural sleep process [66].
DL-phenylalanine[c,d,e,f]	2000 mg	DLPA inhibits the breakdown of the opioid peptides and has been shown to reduce stress in a double blind placebo controlled study. DLPA has been found to reduce stress by anti-craving reward mechanism.
L-Glutamine[g,h,i,j,k]	150 mg	L-Glutamine is the precursor amino-acid for GABA. The inhibitory action of GABA on brain function is tied to integrated sleep processes [55]. GABA shuts off the neurotransmitters that induce wakefulness. Chronic excess of GABA in the brain induces increased slow–wave sleep [56]. Studies have shown that Adenosine A2A receptor agonist induced sleep by inhibiting the histaminergic system through increasing GABA release in the tuberomammillary nucleus [57]. GABA is linked to the benzodiazepine receptor. The sedative hypnotic benzodiazepine–GABA receptor agonist (BzRas) Zaleplon induces a long-term anti-insomnia effect in older patients [58]. The GABAA receptor is the target for most widely prescribed sleep medications [59]. The stimulation of the benzodiazepin –GABA site induces sedation, hypnosis, and anxiolytic activity.
Grifoniasimplicifolia Extract (5-HTP)[l,m,n,o,p,q,r,s,t,u]	100 mg	5-HTP is an amino acid precursor to brain serotonin. Serotonin levels rise during sleep stages. Sleep is a problem with age and many old people complain about insomnia. It is known that age induces a decrease in serotonergic receptors. The serotonin precursor 5-HTP causes a reversal of insomnia by para-chlorophenylalanine induced serotonin brain depletion [60]. While Serotonin-2A and 2C receptor gene polymorphisms may associate with sleep problems in Japanese patients, these polymorphisms did not associate with apnea [61]. However, both age and BMI did associate. Sleep apnea syndrome is associated with serotonin transporter gene polymorphism [62]. While the 5-HT2A receptor may be involved in insomnia (whereby antagonists may be helpful), 5-HT7 promotes REM sleep [63,64]. Injection of a 5-HT1A –receptor agonist directlyinto the dorsal midbrain promotes sleep.
Melatonin	10 mg	The pineal gland hormone melatonin improves sleep quality [85]. A recent meta-analysis reveals melatonin treatment significantly reduced sleep onset latency and increased total sleep duration [86]. Melatonin secretion helps regulate sleep and circadian rhythms [87]. Beta-Methyl-6 chloromelatonin significantly decreases sleep latency in insomnia [88]. Melatonin improves sleep behavior in children with epilepsy [89]. While one study was negative with respect to the effectiveness in melatonin versus placebo with regard to sleep deprivation of winter depression, other studies are positive in terms hypnotic actions [90]. It seems that the effects of melatonin on sleep works best in patients that have abnormal sleep patterns compared to health individuals [91,92].
Rhodiola rosea	100 mg	The plant adaptogen rhodiola rosea promotes positive effects on sleep [68]. Rhodiola rosea has a positive effect on paradoxical sleep deprivation [69]. Rhodiola rosea improves endurance exercise in healthy young adults [70]. Rhodiola rosea reduces stress and improves sleep [71]. Rhodiola rosea improves mental capacity in a double-blind study [72]. Rhodiola was effective in improving sleep quality in young men living in high altitudes [73].
Passion Flower	300 mg	The genus Passiflora comprises about 500 species [37]. The substance Passifloraincarnita and its benzoflavobe isolate binds to the benzodiazepine receptor [42]. As such, it has many biological effects including promotion of sleep, anxiolytic activity [43], anti-alcohol and opiate craving activity [40], promotion of sexual appetite [39], and hypnotic activity [44].
Calming Blend		
(The following ingredients constitute the calming blend to promote sleep: Chamomilia flower, hops flower, valerian root extract, Jamaican dogwood extract, valanic acid, and kava kava)	200 mg	Chamomiles extract lead to a significant decrease in sleep latency in rats [48]. Kava Kava reduced generalized anxiety disorder in humans [49,50]. A combination of Valarian–Hops is used as a sleep aid [51]. Binding affinities were observed for this combination of serotonin receptor subtypes including 5-HT7 that promotes sleep. Valarian and Valanic acid are partial agonists of the 5-HT5A receptor a substrate involved in insomnia. Valanic acid enhances the sedative effects of Valarian. Trends toward increase in slow-wave sleep and lack of effect on rapis eye movement (REM) sleep were observed in 1994. There have been studies on Hops that show a sedative effect [52].
Magnesium	270 mg	Chronic stress reduces intracellular magnesium [93]. Aging effects sleep and magnesium reverses these age-related effects and promotes sleep [94]. EEG blood magnesium levels are under strong genetic control, whereas brain magnesium levels are not [95]. Optimal levels of magnesium are required for normal sleep regulation [96].
Calcium	555 mg	Calcium in a number of species induces a sleep-like state [53, 54].
Manganese ascorbate	13.25 mg	Manganese is found in a large variety of minerals, sea and fresh water, marine and land plants, and animals [74]. Manganese is an essential trace element, human requirements being estimated at between 3 and 9 mg per day. 15 studies have described the adverse mood effects of Manganese (Mn) overexposure, specifically in six dimensions of mood: (i) irritability, nervousness and anxiety; (ii) emotional disturbance; (iii) psychotic experiences; (iv) sleep disturbance, lack of vigor and fatigue; (v) aggression hostility; (vi) compulsive and/or impulsive behavior [75]. 1:15 studies utilized standardized measures of mood. When the Brief Symptom Inventory (BSI) and Profile of Moods State (POMS) standardized mood scales were used to evaluate low Mn levels of exposure and its consequence on mood, results indicated that older men with higher Mn levels showed significant disturbances on four of the six mood dimensions relative to men with lower MN levels, including irritability, nervousness and anxiety; aggression hostility; and emotional disturbance [75]. The POMS and BSI are useful standardized mood scales for the assessment of Mn/mood effects [75]. However, optimal doses produce health benefits. Mn has hypnotic-like effects and as such, enhances alcohol sleeping time in mice. There are no human studies directly involving the effects of Mn on sleep performance, but it has been considered as a sedative inducing nutrient for years.

Table 2: Clinical support for ingredients of EZ-Sleep™: the relative dosage and scientific findings in clinical support of various ingredients to be utilized in the EZ-Sleep™ formula.

EZ-Sleep™ complex: additional components

The final components of EZ-Sleep™ are supplements and proprietary complexes involved in antioxidant support and sleep mechanism facilitation.

Protykin (50%): Protykin is an extract of Polygonumcuspidatum which supplies antioxidant and hormone support.

Potassium

Synaptamine Proprietary Complex: Table 2 lists the relative dosages and summarizes the clinical support for the ingredients of EZ-Sleep™.

Conclusion

The issue of insomnia is a global phenomenon which requires additional in-depth research. Insomnia especially in alcohol-dependent patients, for example, may lead to suicide. It is noteworthy that childhood sleep problems predict the onset of drinking in boys [97]. We now know that while there are multifaceted reasons for sleep problems and disturbances (e.g. sleep drive homeostasis, circadian rhythm physiology and genetic influences), the scientific community has not been able to deliver and appropriate solution. Some benefit has been noted with cognitive behavioral therapy, but it has minimal effects in patients relapsing from drugs especially alcohol, cocaine and opiates. While there are a number of pharmaceutical drugs developed to treat insomnia, most have associated side effects and even addiction liability. We do know that benzodiazepines hijack the midbrain dopamine system leading to addiction. Finally, Lima et al. [34] proposed that dopamine D2 receptors are involved rapid eye movement sleep, suggesting as we have proposed herein that dopaminergic activation is one mechanism worthwhile exploring in the future [34]. The concepts presented herein on potential nutrigenomics therapy warrants further in-depth analysis [98-105].

Acknowledgement

The writing of this paper was supported in part by funds from the National Institutes of Health, NIAAA (RO1-AA07112 and K05-AA00219) and the Medical Research Service of the US Department of Veterans Affairs (MOB). TS is partially support by SAHMSA grants as well. The writing of this paper was funded in-part by a grant awarded to Kenneth Blum and Eric R. Braverman from Life Extension Foundation, Ft. Lauderdale, Florida to PATH Foundation NY.

Conflicts of Interest

Kenneth Blum, PhD, holds US and foreign patents on nutraceutical complex. Kenneth Blum, Bernard W. Downs, Margaret Madigan are owners and employees of IGENE and Impact Genomics. There are no other conflicts.

References

1. Lalive AL, Rudolph U, Lüscher C, Tan KR (2011) Is there a way to curb benzodiazepine addiction? Swiss Med Wkly 141: w13277.
2. National Institute of Health (2003) National Sleep Disorders Research Plan.
3. Roller L (2002) Treating sleep disorders. Australian Journal of Pharmacy 83: 443-447.
4. Zammit GK, Weiner J, Damato N, Sillup GP, McMillan CA (1999) Quality of life in people with insomnia. Sleep 22 Suppl 2: S379-385.
5. Cartwright R (2000) Sleep-related violence: does the polysomnogram help establish the diagnosis? Sleep Med 1: 331-335.
6. Grunstein R (2002) Insomnia. Diagnosis and management. Aust Fam Physician 31: 995-1000.
7. Doghramji K (2006) The epidemiology and diagnosis of insomnia. Am J Manag Care 12: S214-220.
8. Rosekind MR (1992) The epidemiology and occurrence of insomnia. J Clin Psychiatry 53 Suppl: 4-6.
9. Berlin RM, Litovitz GL, Diaz MA, Ahmed SW (1984) Sleep disorders on a psychiatric consultation service. Am J Psychiatry 141: 582-584.
10. American Psychiatric Association (1994) American Psychiatric Task Force on DSM-IV Diagnostic and Statistical Manual of Mental Disorders: DSM IV (4thedn), American Psychiatric Association, Washington, DC.
11. Okuji Y, Matsuura M, Kawasaki N, Kometani S, Shimoyama T, et al. (2002) Prevalence of insomnia in various psychiatric diagnostic categories. Psychiatry Clin Neurosci 56: 239-240.
12. Jindal RD, Thase ME (2004) Treatment of insomnia associated with clinical depression. Sleep Med Rev 8: 19-30.
13. Ohayon MM, Roth T (2003) Place of chronic insomnia in the course of depressive and anxiety disorders. J Psychiatr Res 37: 9-15.
14. Breslau N, Roth T, Rosenthal L, Andreski P (1996) Sleep disturbance and psychiatric disorders: a longitudinal epidemiological study of young adults. Biol Psychiatry 39: 411-418.
15. AÄŸargÃ¼n MY, Kara H, Solmaz M (1997) Subjective sleep quality and suicidality in patients with major depression. J Psychiatr Res 31: 377-381.
16. Papadimitriou GN, Linkowski P (2005) Sleep disturbance in anxiety disorders. Int Rev Psychiatry 17: 229-236.
17. Liu Y, Croft JB, Wheaton AG, Perry GS, Chapman DP, et al. (2013) Association between perceived insufficient sleep, frequent mental distress, obesity and chronic diseases among US adults, 2009 behavioral risk factor surveillance system. BMC Public Health 13: 84.
18. Maher MJ, Rego SA, Asnis GM (2006) Sleep disturbances in patients with post-traumatic stress disorder: epidemiology, impact and approaches to management. CNS Drugs 20: 567-590.
19. Reite M, Ruddy J, Nagel K (2002) Evaluation and Management of Sleep Disorders (3rdedn), American Psychiatric Publishing Inc., Washington, DC.
20. Neubauer DN (2003) Pharmacologic approaches for the treatment of chronic insomnia. Clin Cornerstone 5: 16-27.
21. Morin CM, Culbert JP, Schwartz SM (1994) Nonpharmacological interventions for insomnia: a meta-analysis of treatment efficacy. Am J Psychiatry 151: 1172-1180.
22. Wagner DR (1999) Circadian Rhythm Sleep Disorders. Curr Treat Options Neurol 1: 299-308.
23. Czeisler CA, Kronauer RE, Allan JS, Duffy JF, Jewett ME, et al. (1989) Bright light induction of strong (type 0) resetting of the human circadian pacemaker. Science 244: 1328-1333.
24. Reiter RJ (2003) Melatonin: clinical relevance. Best Pract Res Clin Endocrinol Metab 17: 273-285.
25. Bootzin RR, Perlis ML (1992) Nonpharmacologic treatments of insomnia. J Clin Psychiatry 53: 37-41.
26. Spielman AJ, Saskin P, Thorpy MJ (1987) Treatment of chronic insomnia by restriction of time in bed. Sleep 10: 45-56.
27. Smith MT, Neubauer DN (2003) Cognitive behavior therapy for chronic insomnia. Clin Cornerstone 5: 28-40.
28. Griffiths RR, Johnson MW (2005) Relative abuse liability of hypnotic drugs: a conceptual framework and algorithm for differentiating among compounds. J Clin Psychiatry 66 Suppl 9: 31-41.
29. Brown RJ, Blum K, Trachtenberg MC (1990) Neurodynamics of relapse prevention: a neuronutrient approach to outpatient DUI offenders. J Psychoactive Drugs 22: 173-187.
30. Hilker R, Burghaus L, Razai N, Jacobs AH, Szelies B, et al. (2006) Functional brain imaging in combined motor and sleep disorders. J Neurol Sci 248: 223-226.

31. Fulda S, Wetter TC (2005) Dopamine agonists for the treatment of restless legs syndrome. Expert Opin Pharmacother 6: 2655-2666.

32. Lagos P, Scorza C, Monti JM, Jantos H, Reyes-Parada M, et al. (1998) Effects of the D3 preferring dopamine agonist pramipexole on sleep and waking, locomotor activity and striatal dopamine release in rats. Eur Neuropsychopharmacol 8: 113-120.

33. Canvas M, Navarro JF (2006) Effects of selective dopamine D4 receptor antagonists, L-741,741, on sleep and wakefulness in rats. Prog Neuropsychopharmacol Biol Psychiatry 30: 668-678.

34. Lima MM, Andersen ML, Reksidler AB, Silva A, Zager A, et al. (2008) Blockage of dopaminergic D(2) receptors produces decrease of REM but not of slow wave sleep in rats after REM sleep deprivation. Behav Brain Res 188: 406-411.

35. Sinha RK (2006) P-CPA pretreatment reverses the changes in sleep and behavior following acute immobilization stress rats. J Physiol Sci 56: 123-129.

36. Geller I, Blum K (1970) The effects of 5-HTP on para-Chlorophenylalanine (p-CPA) attenuation of "conflict" behavior. Eur J Pharmacol 9: 319-324.

37. Dhawan K, Dhawan S, Sharma A (2004) Passiflora: a review update. J Ethnopharmacol 94: 1-23.

38. Dhawan K, Kumar S, Sharma A (2001) Anti-anxiety studies on extracts of Passiflora incarnata Linneaus. J Ethnopharmacol 78: 165-170.

39. Dhawan K, Sharma A (2003) Restoration of chronic-Delta 9-THC-induced decline in sexuality in male rats by a novel benzoflavone moiety from Passiflora incarnata Linn. Br J Pharmacol 138: 117-120.

40. Dhawan K, Kumar S, Sharma A (2002) Suppression of alcohol-cessation-oriented hype-anxiety by the benzoflavone moiety Passiflora incarnate Linneaus in mice. J Etnopharmacology 81: 239-244.

41. Akhondzadeh S, Kashani L, Mobaseri M, Hosseini SH, Nikzad S, et al. (2001) Passionflower in the treatment of opiates withdrawal: a double-blind randomized controlled trial. J Clin Pharm Ther 26: 369-373.

42. Dhawan K, Dhawan S, Chhabra S (2003) Attenuation of benzodiazepine dependence in mice by a tri substituted benzoflavone moiety of Passiflora incarnate Linneasus: a non-habit forming anxiolytic. J Pharm Pharm Sci 6: 215-222.

43. Dhawan K, Kumar S, Sharma A (2001) Anxiolytic activity of aerial and underground parts of Passiflora incarnata. Fitoterapia 72: 922-926.

44. Krenn L (2002) [Passion Flower (Passiflora incarnata L.)--a reliable herbal sedative]. Wien Med Wochenschr 152: 404-406.

45. Blum K, Briggs AH, Trachtenberg MC, Delallo L, Wallace JE (1987) Enkephalinase inhibition: regulation of ethanol intake in genetically predisposed mice. Alcohol 4: 449-456.

46. Blum K, Trachtenberg MC, Ramsay JC (1988) Improvement of inpatient treatment of the alcoholic as a function of neurotransmitter restoration: a pilot study. Int J Addict 23: 991-998.

47. Blum K, Trachtenberg MC, Elliot CE, Dingler ML, Sexton RL, et al. (1988) Enkephalinase inhibition and precursor amino acid loading improves inpatient treatment of alcohol and polydrug abusers: Double-blind placebo-controlled study of the nutritional adjunct SAAVE. Alcohol 5: 481-493.

48. Shinomiya K, Inoue T, Utsu Y, Tokunaga S, Masuoka T, et al. (2005) Hypnotic activities of chamomile and passiflora extracts in sleep-disturbed rats. Biol Pharm Bull 28: 808-810.

49. Cauffi JS, Forbes HJ (1999) Dietary supplements used in the treatment of depression, anxiety, and sleep disorders. Lippincotts Prim Care Pract 3: 290-304.

50. Boerner RJ, Sommer H, Berger W, Kuhn U, Schmidt U, et al. (2003) Kava-Kava extract LI 150 is as effective as Opipramol and Buspirone in Generalized anxiety Disorder--an 8 week randomized, double –blind multicentre clinical trial in 129 out patients. Phytomedicine 4: 38-49.

51. Fernández S, Wasowski C, Paladini AC, Marder M (2004) Sedative and sleep- enhancing properties of linarin, a flavonoid-isolated from Valeriana officinalis. Pharmacol Biochem Behav 77: 399-404.

52. Abourashed EA, Koetter U, Brattström A (2004) In vitro binding experiments with a Valerian, hops and their fixed combination extract (Ze91019) to selected central nervous system receptors. Phytomedicine 11: 633-638.

53. Veale WL, Myers RD (1971) Emotional behavior, arousal and sleep produced by sodium and calcium ions perfused within the hypothalamus of the cat. Physiol Behav 7: 601-607.

54. Erickson CK, Tyler TD, Beck LK, Duensing KL (1980) Calcium enhancement of alcohol and drug-induced sleeping time in mice and rats. Pharmacol Biochem Behav 12: 651-656.

55. Gottesmann C (2004) Brain inhibitory mechanisms involved in basic and higher integrated sleep processes. Brain Res Brain Res Rev 45: 230-249.

56. Arnulf I, Konofal E, Gibson KM, Rabier D, Beauvais P, et al. (2005) Effect of genetically caused excess of brain gamma-hydroxybutyric acid and GABA on sleep. Sleep 28: 418-424.

57. Hong ZY, Huang ZL, Qu WM, Eguchi N, Urade Y, et al. (2005) An adenosine A receptor agonist induces sleep by increasing GABA release in the tuberomammillary nucleus to inhibit histaminergic systems in rats. J Neurochem 92: 1542-1549.

58. Ancoli-Israel S, Richardson GS, Mangano RM, Jenkins L, Hall P, et al. (2005) Long-term use of sedative hypnotics in older patients with insomnia. Sleep Med 6: 107-113.

59. Bateson AN (2004) The benzodiazepine site of the GABAA receptor: an old target with new potential? Sleep Med 5 Suppl 1: S9-15.

60. Petitjean F, Buda C, Janin M, Sallanon M, Jouvet M (1985) [Insomnia caused by administration of para-chlorophenylalanine: reversibility by peripheral or central injection of 5-hydroxytryptophan and serotonin]. Sleep 8: 56-67.

61. Sakai K, Takada T, Nakayama H, Kubota Y, Nakamata M, et al. (2005) Serotonin-2A and 2C receptor gene polymorphisms in Japanese patients with obstructive sleep apnea. Intern Med 44: 928-933.

62. Ylmaz M, Bayazit YA, Ciftci TU, Erdal ME, Urhan M, et al. (2005) Association of serotonin transporter gene polymorphism with obstructive sleep apnea syndrome. Laryngoscope 115: 832-836.

63. Fish LR, Gilligan MT, Humphries AC, Ivarsson M, Ladduwahetty T, et al. (2005) 4-Fluorosulfonylpiperidines: selective 5-HT2A ligands for the treatment of insomnia. Bioorg Med Chem Lett 15: 3665-3669.

64. Hedlund PB, Sutcliffe JG (2004) Functional, molecular and pharmacological advances in 5-HT7 receptor research. Trends Pharmacol Sci 25: 481-486.

65. Levkovitz Y, Richter-Levin G, Segal M (1994) Effect of 5-hydroxytryptophane on behavior and hippocampal physiology in young and old rats. Neurobiol Aging 15: 635-641.

66. Evans GW (1993) Chromium picolinate is an efficacious and safe supplement. Int J Sport Nutr 3: 117-122.

67. Jha SK, Ross RJ, Morrison AR (2005) Sleep-related neurons in the central nucleus of the amygdala of rats and their modulation by the dorsal raphe nucleus. Physiol Behav 86: 415-426.

68. Panossian A, Wagner H (2005) Stimulating effect of adaptogens: an overview with particular reference to their efficacy following single dose administration. Phytother Res 19: 819-838.

69. Provalova NV, Skurikhin EG, Pershina OV, Suslov NI, Minakova MY, et al. (2002) Mechanisms underling the effects of adaptogens on erythropoiesis during paradoxical sleep deprivation. Bull Exp Biol Med 133: 428-432.

70. De Bock K, Eijnde BO, Ramaekers M, Hespel P (2004) Acute Rhodiola rosea intake can improve endurance exercise performance. Int J Sport Nutr Exerc Metab 14: 298-307.

71. Earnest CP, Morss GM, Wyatt F, Jordan AN, Colson S, et al. (2004) Effects of a commercial herbal-based formula on exercise performance in cyclists. Med Sci Sports Exerc 36: 504-509.

72. Shevtsov VA, Zholus BI, Shervarly VI, Vol'skij VB, Korovin YP, et al. (2003) A randomized trial of two different doses of a SHR-5 Rhodiola rosea extract

versus placebo and control of capacity for mental work. Phytomedicine 10: 95-105.

73. Ha Z, Zhu Y, Zhang X, Cui J, Zhang S, et al. (2002) [The effect of rhodiola and acetazolamide on the sleep architecture and blood oxygen saturation in men living at high altitude]. Zhonghua Jie He He Hu Xi Za Zhi 25: 527-530.

74. Hine CH, Pasi A (1975) Manganese intoxication. West J Med 123: 101-107.

75. Bowler RM, Mergler D, Sassine MP, Larribe F, Hudnell K (1999) Neuropsychiatric effects of manganese on mood. Neurotoxicology 20: 367-378.

76. Kume K (2006) [Molecular biology of biological clock--genetic regulation of circadian rhythm and sleep]. No To Hattatsu 38: 247-252.

77. Sumaya IC, Byers DM, Irwin LN, Del Val S, Moss DE (2004) Circadian-dependent effect of melatonin on dopaminergic D2 antagonist-induced hypokinesia and agonist-induced stereotypies in rats. Pharmacol Biochem Behav 78: 727-733.

78. Khaldy H, León J, Escames G, Bikjdaouene L, García JJ, et al. (2002) Circadian rhythms of dopamine and dihydroxyphenyl acetic acid in the mouse striatum: effects of pinealectomy and of melatonin treatment. Neuroendocrinology 75: 201-208.

79. Bellon A (2006) Searching for new options for treating insomnia: are melatonin and ramelteon beneficial? J Psychiatr Pract 12: 229-243.

80. Roth T, Stubbs C, Walsh JK (2005) Ramelteon (TAK-375), a selective MT1/MT2-receptor agonist, reduces latency to persistent sleep in a model of transient insomnia related to a novel sleep environment. Sleep 28: 303-307.

81. Reiter RJ (2003) Melatonin: clinical relevance. Best Pract Res Clin Endocrinol Metab 17: 273-285.

82. Cramer H, Rudolph J, Consbruch U, Kendel K (1974) On the effects of melatonin on sleep and behavior in man. Adv Biochem Psychopharmacol 11: 187-191.

83. Arendt J, Borbely AA, Franey C, Wright J (1984) The effects of chronic, small doses of melatonin given in the late afternoon on fatigue in man: a preliminary study. Neurosci Lett 45: 317-321.

84. Buscemi N, Vandermeer B, Hooton N, Pandya R, Tjosvold L, et al. (2005) The efficacy and safety of exogenous melatonin for primary sleep disorders. A meta-analysis. J Gen Intern Med 20: 1151-1158.

85. España RA, Scammell TE (2004) Sleep neurobiology for the clinician. Sleep 27: 811-820.

86. Brzezinski A, Vangel MG, Wurtman RJ, Norrie G, Zhdanova I, et al. (2005) Effects of exogenous melatonin on sleep: a meta-analysis. Sleep Med Rev 9: 41-50.

87. Burch JB, Yost MG, Johnson W, Allen E (2005) Melatonin, sleep, and shift work adaptation. J Occup Environ Med 47: 893-901.

88. Zemlan FP, Muchahey JJ, Scharf MB, Mayleben DW, Rosenberg R, et al. (2005) The efficiency and safety of the melatonin against beta-methyl-6 chloromelatonin in primary insomnia: a randomized, placebo-controlled, crossover clinical trial. J Clin Psychiatry 66: 384-90.

89. Gupta M, Aneja S, Kohli K (2005) Add-on melatonin improves sleep behavior in children with epilepsy: randomized, double-blind, placebo-controlled trial. J Child Neurol 20: 112-115.

90. Danilenko KV, Putilov AA (2005) Melatonin treatment of winter depression following total sleep deprivation: waking EEG and mood correlates. Neuropsychopharmacology 30: 1345-1352.

91. Zhdanova I (2005) Reply to the comment on Melatonin as a hypnotic: Pro. J smrv 9: 69-70.

92. Dolberg OT, Hirschmann S, Grunhaus L (1998) Melatonin for the treatment of sleep disturbances in major depressive disorder. Am J Psychiatry 155: 1119-1121.

93. Tanabe K, Osada N, Suzuki N, Nakayama M, Yokoyama Y, et al. (1997) Erythrocyte magnesium and prostaglandin dynamics in chronic sleep deprivation. Clin Cardiol 20: 265-268.

94. Chollet D, Franken P, Raffin Y, Henrotte JG, Widmer J, et al. (2001) Magnesium involvement in sleep: genetic and nutritional models. Behav Genet 31: 413-425.

95. Held K, Antonijevic IA, Künzel H, Uhr M, Wetter TC, et al. (2002) Oral Mg(2+) supplementation reverses age-related neuroendocrine and sleep EEG changes in humans. Pharmacopsychiatry 35: 135-143.

96. Takase B, Akima T, Uehata A, Ohsuzu F, Kurita A (2004) Effect of chronic stress and sleep deprivation on both flow-mediated dilation in the brachial artery and the intracellular magnesium level in humans. Clin Cardiol 27: 223-227.

97. Brower KJ (2013) Treating Insomnia in alcohol-dependent patients. Presented at Omics 2nd International Conference on addiction research & Therapy, July 22-24, Las Vegas, NV, USA

98. Wyatt JK (2004) Delayed sleep phase syndrome: pathophysiology and treatment options. Sleep 27: 1195-1203.

99. Dulcis D, Jamshidi P, Leutgeb S, Spitzer NC (2013) Neurotransmitter switching in the adult brain regulates behavior. Science 340: 449-453.

100. Comings DE, Muhleman D, Gysin R (1996) Dopamine D2 receptor (DRD2) gene and susceptibility to posttraumatic stress disorder: a study and replication. Biol Psychiatry 40: 368-372.

101. Anderson RA (1998) Recent advances in the clinical and biochemical manifestation of chromium deficiency in human and animal nutrition. Journal of Trace Elements in Experimental Medicine 11: 2-3.

102. Petijean F, Buda C, Janin M, Touret M, Salvert D, et al.(1978) Sleep and monoamines: differential radioautography of central neurons after systematic injection of tritiated 5-hydroxytryptophane (5 hTP 3H) or of dihydroxyphenylalanine (DOPA 3H). C R Acad Sci Hebd Seances Acad Sci D 287: 1135-1139.

103. Capasso A, Sorrentino L (2005) Pharmacological studies on the sedative and hypnotic effect of Kava kava and Passiflora extracts combination. Phytomedicine 12: 39-45.

104. Akhondzadeh S, Naghavi HR, Vazirian M, Shayeganpour A, Rashidi H, et al. (2001) Passionflower in the treatment of generalized anxiety: a pilot double-blind randomized controlled trial with oxazepam. J Clin Pharm Ther 26: 363-367.

105. Lechin F, Pardey-Maldonado B, van der Dijs B, Benaim M, Baez S, et al. (2004) Circulating neurotransmitters during the different wake-sleep stages in normal subjects. Psychoneuroendocrinology 29: 669-685.

15

Family History of Successful CPAP Treatment is Associated with Improved CPAP Compliance

Jeffrey J Stanley*

Department of Otolaryngology, Head and Neck Surgery and Neurology, University of Michigan, USA

***Corresponding author:** Jeffrey J Stanley, Departments of Otolaryngology, Head and Neck Surgery and Neurology, University of Michigan, USA

Abstract

Background: Non-compliance with continuous positive airway pressure (CPAP) is a significant problem in the treatment of obstructive sleep apnea (OSA). When compliance is defined as an average CPAP use >4 hours/night, 46%-83% of patients are non-compliant. Poor compliance leaves undertreated patients at increased risk for cardiovascular and neurocognitive sequelae of OSA. Factors known to affect CPAP compliance include disease severity, perceived symptomatic benefit, and intensive and early support through the sleep clinic.

Objectives: The objective of this study was to assess the effect of a family history of successful CPAP treatment on CPAP compliance.

Methods: An anonymous survey of 410 adult patients attending CPAP follow-up clinic at a tertiary medical center was conducted between March 2010 and February 2011. Patterns of CPAP use were assessed. Compliance was defined as an average CPAP use >4 hours/night. Subjects were also surveyed regarding the presence of first degree relatives with a diagnosis of OSA, their use of CPAP, whether they described their CPAP as "helpful" and whether or not they "liked" using their CPAP.

Results: Thirty-eight percent of the patients surveyed (n=157) had a family member who also had a diagnosis of OSA and used CPAP. Of those with a family history of CPAP use, 92% of compliant patients had a family member who described their CPAP as "helpful" *vs.* 71% of non-compliant patients (p=0.002). Logistic regression analysis to predict compliance *vs.* non-compliance, controlling for age, gender, ethnicity, and a diagnosis of co-morbid hypertension or diabetes showed that having a family member who found CPAP "helpful" was associated with an odds ratio for compliance of 4.70 (95% CI 1.99-11.07, p value <0.001). In addition, 72% of compliant *vs.* 60% of non-compliant patients had a family history of CPAP use with a family member who "liked" their CPAP (p=0.3).

Conclusion: CPAP non-compliance is a complex multifactorial clinical problem. This study shows that familial social support, in the form of modeling CPAP use and self-described helpfulness of CPAP therapy, is associated with CPAP compliance.

Keywords: CPAP treatment; CPAP compliance; Memory; Neurocognitive

Introduction

Obstructive sleep apnea is characterized by recurrent episodes of partial or complete upper airway obstruction. The prevalence of OSA in the general adult population varies between 2 and 4%. During episodes of upper airway obstruction, a subsequent increase in sympathetic nerve activity and transient decrease in oxygen saturation are believed to be account for an increase in cardiovascular risk. This includes an increased risk of hypertension, cerebrovascular accident and myocardial infarction. OSA is also associated with neurocognitive symptoms such as excessive daytime sleepiness, poor concentration and memory impairment [1].

Continuous positive airway pressure (CPAP) is the most effective treatment for OSA. CPAP establishes a pneumatic splint and prevents collapse of the upper airway associated with muscular relaxation during sleep. The effectiveness of CPAP therapy is dependent on its frequency and duration of use. CPAP compliance is frequently defined as use of the device for greater than 4 hours per night. Using this definition, 46%-83% of patients are non-compliant. Patients with adequate CPAP compliance are observed to have improvement in disease specific quality of life measures, including daytime sleepiness, as well as a decrease in new-onset hypertension and cardiovascular events. Factors known to affect CPAP compliance include disease severity, perceived symptomatic benefit, associated co-morbidities and early support through the sleep clinic. However, compliance is likely effected by additional factors as well. Identification of compliance predictors could help in the planning of early interventions to improve CPAP use. CPAP compliance depends to a great extent not only on the subject (severity of disease, symptomatology, etc.), but also on education and professional medical support with therapy and additional factors in the home environment. This includes the influence of marital status and other close personal relationships/ support structure outside of the hospital setting [2,3].

Methods

An anonymous survey of 410 adult patients attending CPAP follow-up clinics at the University of Michigan was conducted between March 2010 and February 2011. Patterns of CPAP use were assessed. Compliance was defined as an average CPAP use >4 hours/night. Demographic factors including age, gender, ethnicity and a diagnosis of co-morbid hypertension and diabetes were recorded. Subjects were also surveyed regarding the presence of first degree relatives with a diagnosis of OSA, their use of CPAP, whether they described their CPAP as "helpful" and whether or not they "liked" using their CPAP.

Logistic regression analysis was utilized to predict compliance *vs.* non-compliance for patients with a family member also diagnosed with OSA and using CPAP, controlling for age, gender, ethnicity, diagnosed hypertension and diagnosed diabetes. Age was treated as a categorical variable using the following categories: 18-20, 21-40, 41-60, 61-80 and >81 years of age. A p value <0.05 was considered to be significant [4-9].

Results

The majority of patients were male, Caucasian and of middle age. Less than fifty percent had a diagnosis of co-morbid hypertension or diabetes. Thirty-eight percent of the patients surveyed (n=157) had a family member who also used CPAP.

Of those with a family history of CPAP use, 92% of compliant patients had a family member who described their CPAP as "helpful" *vs.* 71% of non-compliant patients (p=0.002).

Regression analysis to predict compliance *vs.* non-compliance, controlling for age, gender, ethnicity, diagnosed hypertension and diagnosed diabetes showed that having a family member who found CPAP "helpful" was associated with an odds ratio for compliance of 4.70 (95% CI 1.99-11.07, p value <0.001). In addition, 72% of compliant *vs.* 60% of noncompliant patients had a family history of CPAP use with a family member who "liked" their CPAP (p=0.3) [10].

Discussion

The current study provides insight into additional social factors that may have an effect on CPAP compliance. Previous studies which explored predictors of long-term CPAP compliance showed that perceived symptomatic benefit and intensive and early support through the sleep clinic played an important role. Other studies have shown that disease severity, age, gender and associated co-morbidities, such as hypertension, are also associated with adherence to CPAP therapy. This study is the first to examine the role of familial experience with CPAP treatment as a potential factor influencing CPAP use in other affected family members. Social influences, especially those of close relatives, have been previously shown to play a significant role in health behaviors of other family members ranging from dietary habits to smoking to seat belt use. Over ninety percent of patients in this study with a family member also diagnosed with OSA who described their CPAP as "helpful" were CPAP compliant. This compliance rate was significantly higher than those with a family member who did not describe their CPAP use as particularly "helpful" [11-13].

CPAP compliance is critical to improving the quality of life and cardiovascular outcomes of patients diagnosed with OSA. However, many potential predictors of adherence to this therapy remain unevaluated. Personalized therapeutic decision-making tools may be helpful in the management of sleep apnea and improvement in rates of CPAP compliance. Interestingly, our study suggests that one of the predictors of adequate CPAP compliance is a family history of successful use.

During the past decade, there has been an increasing focus on personalized medicine. One of the goals of personalized medicine is to identify specific factors among individuals with a particular disease to more precisely target therapy and improve treatment outcomes. Patients with OSA have different clinical presentations as well as different social support structures. By identifying these patient variables, providers may be better able to develop a personalized treatment program for each patient including early and frequent intervention for those at highest risk of poor compliance with therapy. Patients with a negative family experience with CPAP use may benefit from early intervention and support [14-16].

There are certain limitations of the current study. First, this study evaluated primarily male, Caucasian and middle aged subjects. Second, this study only surveyed CPAP compliance in patients who were using or still attempting to use CPAP. Therefore, the results of this study may not be generalizable to patients of other demographic backgrounds or who were diagnosed with OSA but no longer using CPAP. Finally, this study did not account for all potential confounding factors that may ultimately influence CPAP compliance, including disease severity [17,18].

Conclusion

CPAP non-compliance is a complex multifactorial clinical problem. This study shows that familial social support, in the form of modeling CPAP use and self-described helpfulness of CPAP therapy, is associated with CPAP compliance.

References

1. Al Lawati NM, Patel S, Ayas NT (2009) Epidemiology, risk factors, and consequences of obstructive sleep apnea and short sleep duration. Prog Cardiovasc Dis 51: 285-293.
2. Aloia MS, Arnedt J, Riggs RL, Hecht J, Borrelli B (2004) Clinical management of poor adherence to CPAP: Motivational enhancement. Behav Sleep Med 2: 205-222.
3. Aloia MS, Arnedt JT, Millman RP, Stanchina M, Carlisle C, et al. (2007) Brief behavioral therapies reduce early positive airway pressure discontinuation rates in sleep apnea syndrome: Preliminary findings. Behav Sleep Med 5: 89-104.
4. Aloia MS, Arnedt JT, Stepnowsky C, Hecht J, Borrelli B (2005) Predicting treatment adherence in obstructive sleep apnea using principles of behavior change. J Clin Sleep Med 1: 346-353.
5. Sleep-related breathing disorders in adults (1999) Recommendations for syndrome definition and measurement techniques in clinical research. The report of an American academy of sleep medicine task force. Sleep 22: 667-689.
6. Chervin RD, Theut S, Bassetti C, Aldrich MS (1997) Compliance with nasal CPAP can be improved by simple interventions. Sleep 20: 284-289.
7. Engleman HM, Martin SE, Douglas NJ (1994) Compliance with CPAP therapy in patients with the sleep apnoea/hypopnoea syndrome. Thorax 49: 263-266.
8. Engleman HM, Wild M (2003) Improving CPAP use by patients with the sleep apnoea/hypopnoea syndrome (SAHS). Sleep Medicine Reviews 7: 81-99.
9. Hoy CJ, Vennelle M, Kingshott RN, Engleman HM, Douglas NJ (1999) Can intensive support improve continuous positive airway pressure use in

patients with the sleep apnea/hypopnea syndrome? Am J Respir Crit Care Med 159: 1096-1100.

10. Kribbs NB, Pack AI, Kline LR, Smith PL, Schwartz AR, et al. (1993) Objective measurement of patterns of nasal CPAP use by patients with obstructive sleep apnea. Am Rev Respir Dis 147: 887-895.
11. Krieger J (1992) Long-term compliance with nasal continuous positive airway pressure (CPAP) in obstructive sleep apnea patients and nonapneic snorers. Sleep 15: S42-S46.
12. Lewis K, Seale L, Bartle IE, Watkins AJ, Ebden P (2004) Early predictors of CPAP use for the treatment of obstructive sleep apnea. Sleep 27:134-138.
13. Nieto F, Young T, Lind B, Shahar E, Samet J, et al. (2000) Association of sleep-disordered breathing, sleep apnea, and hypertension in a large community-based study. JAMA 283: 1829-1836.
14. Peppard P, Young T, Palta M, Skatrud J (2000) Prospective study of the association between sleep-disordered breathing and hypertension. N Engl J Med 342: 1378-1384.
15. Sin D, Mayers I, Man G, Pawluk L (2002) Long-term compliance rates to continuous positive airway pressure in obstructive sleep apnea: A population-based study. Chest 121: 430-435.
16. Stepnowsky C, Marler MR, Ancoli-Israel S (2002) Determinants of nasal CPAP compliance. Sleep Med 3: 239-247.
17. Weaver TE, Grunstein RR (2008) Adherence to continuous positive airway pressure therapy: The challenges to effective treatment. Proc Am Thorac Soc 5: 173-178.
18. Weaver TE, Maislin G, Dinges DF, Bloxham T, George CFP, et al. (2007) Relationship between hours of CPAP use and achieving normal levels of sleepiness and daily functioning. Sleep 30: 711-719.

Gender differences in Health among Unemployed Adults

Mohammad Ashraf Malik*

Department of Psychology, Government Degree College Sopore, Jammu and Kashmir, India

***Corresponding author:** Mohammad Ashraf Malik, Department of Psychology, Government Degree College Sopore, Jammu and Kashmir, India
E-mail: malikashraf43@gmail.com

Abstract

Background: Health simply means a psychological, physical and social wellbeing of an individual. In the present world human health is facing challenges especially among unemployed adults. It has been reported that there are a lot of differences in health between male and female adults.

Aim: The study sought to determine gender differences in health among unemployed adults.

Methods: The present paper consists of 300 unemployed adult, out of which 200 were male and 100 female. General Health Questionnaire (GHQ)-28 were used to collect data from the participants. For data analysis, t-test was used to determine the significance of difference between the means of the sample.

Results: The results revealed the Mean value (M=28.73) among females is higher compared to male unemployed adults (M=26.18).

Conclusion: The study revealed that unemployed females showed high mean score than male unemployed adults. This is an indication that females' health is poorer than male unemployed adults.

Keywords: Health; Gender; Unemployed; Adults

Introduction

Health is a state of wellbeing with physical, cultural, psychosocial, economic and spiritual attributes, not the absence of illness. WHO [1] defined health as 'a state of complete physical, social and spiritual wellbeing, not merely the absence of illness." Argele, Martin and Crossland [2] understood the health in terms of three components: positive affect (pleasant mood and emotions), absence of negative affect (unpleasant mood and emotions) and satisfaction with life as whole. According to Webster [3] Dictionary, health is defined as the "state of being hale sound or whole, in body, mind, or soul, especially the state of being free from physical disease or pain. Gender determines the sex of a person as male and female.

Unemployment is known as one of the prevailing social problems in the world. Unemployment is said to be a key player in deteriorating health of an individual. Various studies on unemployment and its consequences show a strong association between unemployment and ill health. Unemployment might be expected to increase anxiety and depression, lead to lower self-esteem, and produce adverse physical health consequences, particularly when efforts to locate work are met with failure over a long period of time.

Numerous literatures showed that unemployment has affected male and female adults differently. Leeflang, Klein-Hesselink, and Spruit (1992) compared life situation and health effects of short term and long term unemployed in 30-50 years old urban men and women. They concluded that present or anticipated financial problems were the mediating factors between unemployed status and reported health problems in both men and women.

Analysis of the Census Longitudinal Study for England and Wales showed that for younger unemployed men, mortality from injuries and poisoning including suicide was particularly high. Unemployed young women were found to have high mortality from coronary heart disease and from injuries and poisonings, including suicide [4]. It has also been revealed that the mental health consequences appear to be more apparent among middle aged people, rather than the younger or older unemployment, among men and single women, rather than married women, and among long term unemployed (i.e. over four months) rather than those that experience a short period of unemployment [5].

A study [6] shows that unemployment had more of an effect on the mental health of men than that of women. The study [6] further argued that gender differences in effects were related to family responsibilities and social class.

McKee-Ryan et al. [7] also found that unemployed women have worse mental health and Paul and Moser [8] find that men are more distressed by unemployment than women.

Strandh et al. [9] in a longitudinal showed that unemployment was more negatively related to mental health in men than among women in Ireland, while men and women were equally affected by unemployment in Sweden. The study [9] further revealed that factors related to the family and economic situation, as well as gender selection into the unemployment population, explains the differences in mental health between unemployed men and women in Ireland.

Aim of the study

Health is a main issue in this contemporary world as regards to gender and there are a lot of differences in health between men and women. It has been found that men have a low life expectancy and high mortality rate while women show greater morbidity rate. The main objective of the research is to determine the gender differences in health among male and female unemployed adults.

Methods

Study Participants

The present study consists of 300 unemployed adults, 200 of whom were males and 100 were female participants. Those participants who have completed at least first degree were recruited into the study. The participants were selected through random sampling method (Figure 1).

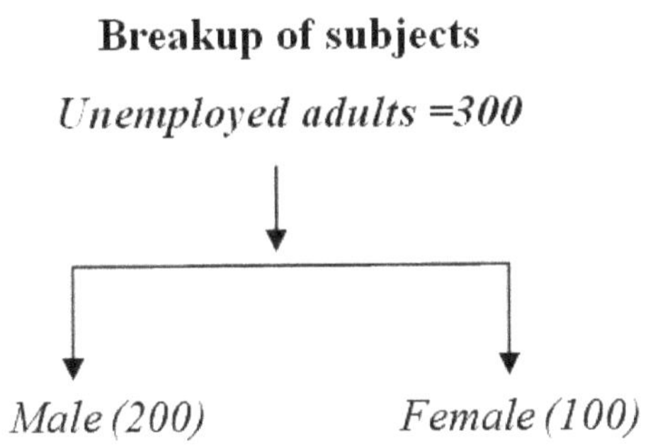

Figure 1: Participant's selection through random sampling method.

Data Collection Tools

The General Health Questionnaire-28(GHQ-28) developed by Goldberg in 1978 was devised in this study [10]. The instrument consists of items and each item is followed by four options that is "Not at all", "No more than usual", "Rather more than usual" and "Much More than usual". Through factor analysis, GHQ-28 was divided into four factors namely somatic (item 1-7), anxiety/insomnia (item 8-14), social dysfunctioning (item 15-21) and severe depression (item 22-28). The GHQ-28 can be scored from 0 to 3 for each response with total possible scores ranging from 0 to 84. The total score of 23-24 is the threshold for the presence of distress. For the purpose of reliability of present scale, Cronbach's alpha was applied on 300 unemployed adults. Further, the Cronbach's alpha of GHQ-28 was found to be 0.88 which is quite high and shows reliability of the said scale.

Recruitment Procedure

First of all, the investigator met with the participants personally, to explain the purpose of the study and solicit their support in completion of questionnaire. Thereafter, he reassured them of utmost confidentiality of data obtained from them in the course of the study. Having obtained their consent to participate, the General Health Questionaire-28 along with personal data sheet was administered to recruited unemployed educated adults individually.

Data analysis

The data was analyzed using Statistical Package for Social Science (SPSS) version 16.0 to determine the Mean and SD of the sample as well as t-test was computed to determine the significant difference in health among male and female unemployed adults.

Results

The present study sought to determine the gender difference in health among unemployed adults. The results of present study are given below. Table 1, shows that the Mean value among unemployed females (M=28.73) is higher than male unemployed adults (M=26.18).

Gender	N	Mean (M)	Stnd. Deviation (S.D.)
Male	200	26.18	12.43
Female	100	28.73	11.94

Table 1: Mean and S.D of male and female unemployed adults.

Gender	N	M	S.D.	M.D	S.ED	t	Sig.
Male	200	26.18	12.43	2.54	1.5	1.69	0.91
Female	100	28.73	11.94				

Table 2: Difference in health between male and female unemployed adults.

The results given in the Table 2, shows that the obtained t value (t=1.693>0.05) is not significant. It means that there is no significance of difference in health among male and female unemployed adults.

Discussion

The main aim of the present paper was to determine the gender difference in health among unemployed adults. The results showed that the Mean and S.D (M=28.73, S.D=13.94) in female unemployed adults was higher as compared to male unemployed adults (M=26.18, S.D. = 12.43). The result of the present study can be corroborated with the findings of O'Leary and Helgeson [11] which shows that financial barriers may prevent more women, more than men, from engaging in healthier lifestyles and desirable behavior change. While further comparing the both groups that is male and female unemployed adults, the results further indicate that no significance difference (t= 1.695 >.05) in health among unemployed male and female unemployed adults. It means that there is no or slight difference in health among unemployed adults.

Conclusion

The overall result of the study suggested that women showed worse health as compared to their male counterparts on the basis of mean score differences and no or slight significance differences were found in health among male and female unemployed adults. So, we can interpret that unemployed women are mostly affected as compared to male adults in respect of their health concerns. Due to the external demands and requirements of daily life and male partner could not manage it alone in this existing world. So, female also wants to share the burden of family expenses but due to limited jobs opportunities for females, they become more vulnerable to mental disorders like depression, stress and anxiety etc. In addition, sexual violence against women as compared to men also debars females to enter into the job market. Strandh, et al. [9] also argued that factors related to the family and economic situation, as well as gendered selection into the unemployment population, explains the difference in mental health between unemployed men and women in Ireland.

Recommendations

Unemployment is said to be great cause of mental disorders. So, application of psychological interventions for unemployed people would have positive effects on mental health.

More and more job opportunities should be generated by government and private entrepreneur and selection should be done on non-discriminative basis. So that each and every person can get his livelihood easily

Clinical counseling centers should be opened in those areas where a chance of unemployment rate is high. So that they can provide help whenever there is unemployment crisis.

Job oriented courses and placement cells as well should be open in colleges and universities and skills training programs should be provided so that unemployed people could also develop the idea of small businesses, probably receiving government funding.

Each state government should advance women through policy changes and provide more conducive working environment for women.

Women should be given equal respect as men and gender discrimination and gender discrimination and violence at work places should be looked into. Punishment should be instituted at workplace to deter perpetrators.

Sexual harassment at work places is commonly found. Lot of womens are not willing to work because of sexual violence. There should be a vigilant organization that will look upon all these crimes happened at workplaces.

Limitations

In this study, only gender was taken into consideration while other variables like age, socioeconomic status, residence etc. were not taken into with considered in the study.

Acknowledgement

I would like to thank Almighty Allah, who is most merciful and kind to all his creation. I also express my gratitude to all those participants who show their interest during the process of data collection, without their active participation this research work was incomplete and impossible. At last I would like express my thankfulness to all those who help me in one way or the other in carrying out this piece of research work.

References

1. W.H.O (1946) W.H.O, definition of health, preamble to the constitution of the world health organization's adopted by the international health conference, New York: WHO.
2. Argyle M, Martin M, Crossland J (1989) Happiness as a function of personality and social encounters. In: Forgas JP, Innes M (eds), Recent advances in social psychology: An international perspective. North Holland.
3. Webster Dictionary (1913) Definition of health. Retrieved from http://www.pnf.org/Definitions_of_Health _C.pdf.
4. Bethune A (1997) Unemployment and mortality. In: Drever F, Whitehead M (ed.). Health Inequalities: Decennial Supplement, Ds Series No. 15, London: The Stationery Office.
5. Bartley M (1994) Unemployment and ill health: understanding the relationship. J Epidemiol Community Health 48: 333-337.
6. Artazcoz L, Benach J, Borrell C, Cortès I (2004) Unemployment and mental health: understanding the interactions among gender, family roles, and social class. Am J Public Health 94: 82-88.
7. McKee-Ryan F, Song Z, Wanberg CR, Kinicki AJ (2005) Psychological and physical well-being during unemployment: a meta-analytic study. J Appl Psychol 90: 53-76.
8. Paul KI, Moser K (2009) Unemployment impairs mental health: Meta-analyses. Journal of Vocational Behavior 3: 264-282.
9. Strandh M, Hammarström A, Nilsson K, Nordenmark M, Russel H (2013) Unemployment, gender and mental health: the role of the gender regime. Sociol Health Illn 35: 649-665.
10. Goldberg D (1978) Manual of the general health questionnaire. Windsor: NFER-Nelson.
11. O'Leary A, Helgeson VS (1997) Psycho-social factors and women's health: Integrating mind, heart, and body. In S. J. Gallant, G. P. Keita, & R. Royak-Schaler (Eds.), Health care for women: Psychological, social, and behavioral influences (pp.25-40) Washington, D.C.: American Psychological Association.

17

Health Related Quality of Life in Adult Obstructive Sleep Apnea

Naveen Dutt[1,*], Kirti Chaudhry[2], Nishant Kumar Chauhan[1], Ashok Kuwal[1], Lokesh Kumar Saini[1], Swetabh Purohit[1] and Sunil Kumar[1]

[1]*Department of Pulmonary Medicine, All India Institute of Medical Sciences, Jodhpur, India*
[2]*Department of Dentistry, All India Institute of Medical Sciences, Jodhpur, India*

Abstract

Objective: To review the literature on Obstructive Sleep Apnea (OSA) and Health Related Quality of Life (HRQoL).

Method: We conducted systematic review of the literature on HRQoL and OSA.

Summary: Our review of published literature on quality of life in adult OSA suggest that there is significant impairment of HRQoL in obstructive sleep apnea but the magnitude of QoL impairment is not proportional to the severity of OSA as determined by AHI. There is paucity of data over effect of treatment on quality of life but the available data suggest that there is improvement in QoL with CPAP treatment at least in moderate and severe OSA patients. Effect of other treatment modalities is unclear yet.

Keywords: Health; Quality of life; Obstructive sleep apnea; Adult

Introduction

OSA is the most common form of sleep-disordered breathing (SDB) which is characterized by recurrent episodes of upper airway obstructions during sleep, resulting in reduction or cessation of airflow which leads to recurrent arousals, nocturnal desaturation and sleep fragmentation. When the obstructive sleep apnea is accompanied by daytime sleepiness it is referred to as obstructive sleep apnea syndrome (OSAS) [1]. Patients of OSA usually presents with excessive daytime sleepiness or insomnia, morning headache, nocturia, lethargerness, poor concentration and memory impairment.

Studies done across various ethnic groups and geographical regions shows high prevalence of OSA. Winconsin sleep cohort [2] is one of the extensive study on prevalence of OSA using in-laboratory polysomnography and found prevalence of OSA (AHI ≥ 5) 9% in females and 24% in males. OSA syndrome (AHI ≥ 5 and daytime sleepiness) was present in 2% in females and 4% in males. Diagnosis of OSA is made on night time polysomnography if number of apneas and hypoapneas per hour of sleep (called as Apnea Hypopnea Index or AHI) is more than 5.

There are several risk factors that have been implicated for OSA but amongst them, obesity is one of the strongest risk factor. Others are male gender, ageing, craniofacial abnormalities, genetic predisposition, alcohol, and ethnicity [3].

Significant clinical consequences of OSA cover a wide spectrum of conditions including daytime hypersomnolence, neurocognitive dysfunction, cardiovascular disease (Hypertension, Coronary artery disease, Heart failure, Stroke, Atrial fibrillation), metabolic dysfunction (Obesity, Type 2 Diabetes, Dyslipidemia), Respiratory failure and cor-pulmonale. Sleep apnea has also been linked to an increased risk of road traffic accidents [4].

Apart from these obvious clinical consequences, OSA has significant impact on QoL of the affected patients which cannot be explored in the sleep laboratory. Symptomatic measures and polysomnographic parameter like AHI and sleep fragmentation [5,6] have failed to adequately measure the rather broad impact of this disorder on human life. Symptoms are usually a subset of overall QoL of patients thus it is more important to measure the overall impact on QoL.

Materials and Methods

This study was a systematic review of literature from 1990 to 2015. We used pubmed database for our search. We used search terms "Obstructive Sleep Apnea" and "Quality of Life" and their commonly used synonyms and acronyms. We reviewed all the abstracts for inclusion in the study. We excluded the articles involving paediatric population.

Why do we need to measure QoL in OSA?

Generally AHI and other polysomnography indices are laboratory parameters which are used to gauge the severity and symptomatology of the patient. But there is lack of association between these polysomnography indices and real world clinical outcomes like QoL, patient perception of disease or survival [7].

Further the criteria used to define apneas, hypopneas and AHI threshold for severity are all arbitrary values without any objective physiological basis behind them [6]. Understandably the parameters derived from them may not be true representative of real effect of disease on the life of patient. Two recent large scale multi institutional studies on CPAP recognized these issues and used QoL measures and functional status as primary outcome for their assessment rather than AHI [8,9].

Concept of quality of life (QoL) and health related quality of life (HRQoL)

QoL has become a very important health outcome in clinical research. The concept of QoL represents the human desire to live a happy, productive, and meaningful and disease free life. When we

***Corresponding author:** Naveen Dutt, Assistant Professor, department of Pulmonary Medicine, All India Institute of Medical Sciences, Jodhpur, India, E-mail: drnaveendutt@yahoo.co.in

discuss QoL in relation to a disease, it represents desire not just to be free of symptoms of the disease but being free of any impact of disease or its treatment on happiness, productivity and meaningful life. It has become a frequently used tool to evaluate the burden of disease and to evaluate medical treatment. Only improvement in symptoms or increased life span is no longer sufficient for a successful treatment.

Although the term QoL was coined and defined much later but the concept and its importance has been duly addressed importance in the history of mankind. Renowned philosopher Aristotle (384-322 BC) not only described the importance of good life but talks about ultimate good being eudaimonia- a good life [10] In 1946 World Health Organisation (WHO) constitution declared health as "a state of complete physical, mental and social well-being and not merely the absence of disease or infirmity"[11]. After this WHO definition the importance of concept of QoL again came into prominence as it was totally in sync with the new definition of health.

The concept of QoL has different meaning for different individuals, populations and societies so it is very difficult to reach a consensus definition. World Health Organisation Quality of Life (WHOQOL) group defined QoL as "an individual's perception of their position in life, in context of the culture and values in which they live and in relation to their goals, expectations, standards and concerns" [12] QoL has several domains like functional competence, health related complaints, psychological and social functioning etc. HRQoL is an integral domain of QoL. When QoL is discussed in relation with health or diseases, it almost always means HRQoL unless specified otherwise. HRQoL is evaluated subjectively with the help of Questionnaires. These Questionnaires have multiple domains representing different aspects of life.

Quality of life instruments for obstructive sleep apnea (OSA)

There are two broad categories of QoL instruments which can be used to measure QoL in patients of OSA: Generic and OSA specific instruments. Generic instruments can be used to measure QoL in all kind of clinical conditions including OSA. Some of these generic QoL instruments have been widely used and validated in OSA. SF-36, a generic instrument is the most commonly used instrument in QoL studies in OSA, OSA Specific instruments are specifically designed for OSA and can be used to determine QoL in OSA patients only.

QoL instruments may also classified on the basis population they are used upon e.g. OSA-18 is an OSA specific QoL Instrument used in pediatric patients only.

Measuring tools

Details of OSA specific QoL instruments and frequently used generic instruments are listed in Table 1.

Which type of instrument should be used for measuring QoL

Generic and the OSA specific instruments have their own positives and negatives (Table 2). The structure of Generic instruments is more comprehensive as they cater to wide range of clinical conditions. They allow comparison to be made between studies, populations, or diseases but they may have some domains which are not related to OSA. Thus they may be lesser sensitive as compared to the disease specific instruments. In case person is suffering from more than one disease, Generic Instruments are more appropriate. Generic Instruments may have questions unrelated to the condition of the patient so may have less acceptability [27].

OSA specific instruments are specifically made for OSA patients so all their content is relevant to OSA. This makes them more sensitive to detect subtle changes in QoL for OSA. Their contents are related to patient's clinical condition so they tend to have higher acceptability and completion rates. This feature makes them more suitable for clinical use, due to their use being restricted to single disease, OSA specific instruments doesn't allow inter disease comparisons.

Thus, the choice of Instrument should be based on research question. If the researcher wants to compare QoL among two conditions then obviously only generic Instruments can be used. Otherwise the recent trend is towards use of OSA specific Instruments because of their better acceptability and completion rates (Table 2).

Assessment of QoL in OSA; role in clinical practice

Initially QoL (QoL) Instruments were developed as a research tool to study QoL impairment in OSA patients. They were not intended to be used in each and every patient for clinical assessment but as the researches showed that physiological parameters like Apnea-Hypoapnea Index (AHI), sleep fragmentation and other parameters recorded in sleep laboratory are inadequate to capture the complete spectrum of human suffering caused by OSA, importance of QoL assessment is increasingly being recognized and used in clinical care. It can be used to assess patient's health status before treatment; a significantly impaired QoL may itself be an indication to start CPAP therapy in mild OSA. They may also be used after treatment to evaluate the response of the treatment and if found inadequate, may help in modifying treatment decision.

OSA specific Instruments are more suitable for clinical use as inter-disease comparisons are not required. An ideal Instrument for use in clinical practise should be self- administered, easy to understand and short. Most of the present day instruments are too long to be used in clinical cases. SAQLI is long as well as interviewer administered so not suitable for clinical use. A short QoL Instrument may hasten the routine assessment of QoL in all OSA patients (Table 3).

Discussion

Our present review discusses various studies conducted on assessment of QoL in untreated and treated OSA patients. Our study also illustrates variety of HRQoL instruments used to measure QoL in OSA.

The choice of QoL instrument depends upon the purpose of its use and the setting in which they are being used. For clinical purpose, OSA specific instrument tend to perform better owing to their higher sensitivity, acceptability and completion rates. A short instrument which can be filled by the patient himself and doesn't take too long to answer is likely to be more acceptable for clinical use [14]. For research purpose choice of instrument depends on the research question being answered. If the researcher wants to do inter-disease comparison of QoL, only generic instrument can be used. For general purpose use of at least one generic and one OSA specific instrument is likely to be advantageous [27]. We feel that all the present instruments for measuring quality of life in OSA have one shortcoming or the other. A short questionnaire covering all important domains which can be answered in short time is still required.

A recent systematic review of measurement properties of patient reported outcome measures (PROM) used in OSA observed that most of the generic instruments with the exception of PGI (in which the patient himself write down and score the area of life which he feels is the most affected by the disease) have poor content validity for the

Instruments	Year	Domains	Items (No.)	Comments
Generic Instruments				
Short Form 36 (SF-36) [13]	1992	Physical functioning Role limitations because of physical health problems Bodily pain Social functioning General mental health Role limitations because of emotional problems Vitality General health perceptions	36	Poor content validity Mental health component and specifically it's vitality domain is probably best generic QoL instrument for OSA (14)
Nottingham Health Profile (NHP) [14]	1985	Paid employment Jobs around the house Social life Personal relationships Sex life Hobbies and interests Holidays	7	Allow only yes/No answers, so not likely to provide sensitive scores. Not frequently used, so less suitable to compare scores across diseases.
Sickness Impact Profile (SIP) [15] Functional Limitations Profile (FLP), 1981 [16] *FLP is the British version of SIP	1976	Ambulation, Body care and movement Mobility Household management Recreation and pastimes Social interaction Emotional behaviour Alertness behaviour Sleep and rest Eating Communication Work	136	Too large number of items Not frequently used, so less suitable to compare scores across diseases.
EuroQoL (EQ-5D) [17]	1990	Mobility Self-care Usual activities Pain/ discomfort Anxiety/depression + Global indication of health status	5 + 1	Studies suggest poor correlation with SF-36 and PGI(18)
Patient-generated index (PGI) [18]	1994	Patient select 5 affected areas in life	19	Good content validity as patient choose his own areas. Difficult to compare scores across diseases as no uniformity in ares chosen by patients.
Munich Life Quality Dimension List (MLQDL) [19]	1998	Physical condition Psyche Social life Everyday life	19	
MSE-P (Minor Symptom Evaluation- Profile) [20]	1999	Vitality (5 items) Contentment (7items) Sleep (3 items) Miscellaneous (9 items)	24	
Specific Instruments				
Functional Outcomes of Sleep Questionnaire (FOSQ) [21]	1997	Activity level Vigilance Intimate and sexual relationships General productivity Social outcome	30	Measures the impact of sleepiness on functional status.
Obstructive Sleep Apnea Patient-Oriented Severity Index (OSAPOSI) [22]	1998	Sleep problems Awake problems Medical problems Emotional and personal problems Occupational impact	32	Covered some domains not covered in other instruments (eg. Occupational impact like loss of job) Not publicly available (14)
Sleep Apnea Quality Of Life Index (SAQLI) [23]	1998	Daily functioning Social interactions Emotional functioning Symptoms + Treatment related symptoms	56 + 28 Treatment related symptoms	Good content validity Good pool of quality evidence Large number of items Interviewer administered
Quebec Sleep Questionnaire (QSQ) [24]	2004	Sleepiness Diurnal symptoms Nocturnal symptoms Emotions Social interactions	32	Original questionnaire in French Good content validity
Functional Outcomes Of Sleep Questionnaire-10 (FOSQ-10 -shorter version of the FOSQ) [25]	2009	Activity level Vigilance Intimate and sexual relationships General productivity Social outcome	10	Paucity of data
Maugeri Obstructive Sleep Apnea Syndrome (MOSAS) questionnaire [26]	2011	Sleep apnea psychological Impact Sleep apnea physical Impact Discomfort and nuisance caused by CPAP	16 + 7, CPAP related	Shorter Self-administered No questions on nocturnal symptoms (14)

Table 1: Details of OSA specific QoL instruments and frequently used generic instruments.

Generic QoL instruments	OSA Specific QoL instruments
Poor content validity. Some domains might be unrelated to OSA.	Good content validity, as they are more specific for OSA
Lower acceptability and completion rates.	Higher acceptability and completion rates
More comprehensive allow interdisease comparisons.	Doesn't allow interdisease comparisons.
More suitable for research studies	Better suitable for clinical use
Less sensitive	More sensitive to detect subtle changes in QoL

Table 2: Comparison of generic and OSA specific QoL instruments.

Study	Sample size	AHI	Instrument used	Setting	Observation
Gall et al. [28]	42 OSA patients (All Males)	RDI ≥ 20	SF-36	Untreated	Mild OSA patients had impairment in Social Functioning, Role limitations-Physical and Emotional, lowered mental health and well-being.
Fornas et al. [29]	103 OSA Patients and 40 healthy controls	38 ± 27	NHP	Untreated	SAHS patients showed a deterioration of general health status parameters in comparison with healthy subjects, these parameters do not correlate with the physiological disturbances of SAHS, expressed as the number of respiratory events per hour
Jenkinson et al. [30]	108 Patients of OSA		SF-36, FLP and EQ-5D (This study used 3 QoL measures)	Before and after 5 months of nasal CPAP therapy	SF-36 an FLP showed that there was significant baseline impairment of QoL in the patients and post CPAP QoL improved significantly. Surprisingly EuroQoL scores were higher at baseline indicating apparently good health and showed very little change. This study shows lack of correlation among the eneric questionnaire. nCPAP therapy returns patients to a QoL similar to the normal population.
Bolitschek et al. [19]	21 untreated OSA patients (QoL of 16 patients was evaluated) 67 patients with AHI > 20 and using CPAP more than 3 months 113 healthy controls	47.08/49.94 (Treated/Untreated)	MLQDL	Untreated verses treated	QoL was impaired in untreated patients there were no difference in QoL among nCPAP patients and healthy controls
Jenkinson et al. [31]	n = 89 for PGI and EuroQol, n= 86 for SF-36		PGI, EuroQoL SF-36	Before and after 3 months CPAP	It was done to compare the 3 QoL instruments. After CPAP, QoL was improved on PGI, normalized with SF-36 but there was no/little improvement on EuroQoL.
Piccrillo et al. [32]	119 OSA patients- 71 given CPAP, 48 underwent surgery	Mean= 40.0	SF-36, OSAPOSI	Before and after CPAP/Surgery	Scores on the role-physical, vitality, and emotional wellbeing subscales of the SF-36 increased significantly. OSAPOSI awake and sleep subscales and total instrument score increased
Flemons et al. [33]	SAQLI was tested in 24 OSA patients.	N.A.	SAQLI SF-36	Before starting and 4 week after CPAP	SAQLI had a high correlation with SF-36 among patients successfully completing CPAP
Bennett et al. [34]	51 OSA patients (46 M and 5 F)	Median apnea/ hypopnea index [AHI] 25, 90% central range: 1 to 98	SF-36	Before and after 4 week CPAP	In OSA patients SF-36 subscale scores for role-physical and vitality were impaired prior to CPAP as compared to normal population, which improved to normal levels after CPAP therapy.
D'Ambrosio et al. [35]	OSA patients (AHI > 15) = 29 (23 M, 6 F)	77 ± 9	SF-36	Before and after 8 weeks of CPAP therapy	All domains of SF were impaired as compared to control. Post treatment QoL improved significantly in vitality, social functioning and mental health domains
Engleman et al. [36]	34 OSA patients (AHI 5-15 + daytime sleepiness) Cross over trial- patients on 4 weeks of CPAP and 4 weeks of oral placebo therapy alternatively	NA	NHP, SF-36	Before and after 4 week CPAP or oral placebo	In OSA patients SF-36 scores were impaired on most subscales (except general health perceptions). After CPAP treatment, significant improvements were seen in most of the subscales as compared to placebo. There was no change in QoL after CPAP therapy on NHP for health and functional status.
Jokic et al. [37]	13 positional OSA patients (12 M, 1 F) cross over trial- patients on 2 weeks of CPAP and 2 weeks of Positional therapy	17 ± 8	NHP	Before and after each 2 week treatment limb	No significant difference in overall QoL between CPAP and positional therapy. (Energy level scores on the NHP were slightly better with CPAP).

Yang et al. [38]	Patients without OSA (AHI < 5)- 46 Mild OSA patients (AHI 5-15)- 16 Moderate to severe OSA (AHI > 15)- 21	NA	SF-36		
Stepnowsky et al. [39]	n = 69 (29 M, 40 F)	22 ± 19	MOS QWB	Untreated	OSA patients with AHI < 15 had significant impairment in general physical functioning and mental health functioning (not those with AHI > 15).
Walker-Engstrom et al. [20]	84 OSA patients- 41 in oral appliance group 43 in UPPP group (4 patients from oral appliances group stopped using appliances after 6 months and excluded from study)		MSE-P	Before and 1 year after UPPP or dental Device	The mean values for the three dimensions vitality, contentment and sleep improved significantly 1 year after intervention in the dental appliance and UPPP groups. One year after intervention the UPPP group showed significantly more contentment than the dental appliance group. In contrast, vitality and sleep dimensions did not differ between the two treatment groups. No significant correlations were observed between the QOL scores and somnographic values.
Baldwin et al. [40]	2398 OSA patients 5-14 AHI=1473, 15 + = 916	NA	SF-36	Untreated	Sleep disturbances are associated with worse physical and better mental HR-QOL than the U.S. norm.
Akashiba et al. [44]	60 OSAS patients (AHI > 20 + EDS) and arterial oxygen desaturation (SpO_2 < 80%), 34 healthy controls	51.6 ± 26.6	SF-36	Untreated	Six of eight domains and the total score on the SF-36 were significantly lower than those in the control subjects.
Lacasse [42]	OSA patients n=100 (82 male)	41 + 24	Self constructed 33 items questionnaire	Untreated	OSA significantly contributes to the impairment of all domains of what is usually referred to as "health-related QoL"
Parish and lyng [43]	54 patients and their bed partners	48.4 + 33.3	SF-36 and SAQLI	Before and 6 weeks after CPAP therapy	OSA results in impaired QOL in both the patients and their bed partners. Treatment with CPAP improves QOL of both the groups
Pichel et al. [44]	42 in 6 months CPAP group, 42 in 18 months CPAP group and 84 control	NA	SF-36	One group Treated with 6 month CPAP therapy and other with 18 months CPAP therapy	6 months group showed improvement in the vitality dimension while 18 months group showed improvement in four out of the eight SF-36 dimensions (physical function, role physical, vitality and general health perception). This study shows that QoL improves with long term use of CPAP
Mulgrew et al. [45]	68 Patients (35 in PSG group and 33 in ambulatory group)	(Median RDI) 31 in PSG group, 27 in ambulatory group	SAQLI	Before and after 3 months of CPAP therapy	This study was done to test utility of diagnostic algorithm with ambulatory CPAP titration without PSG. In ambulatory group no PSG was done before starting treatment. SAQLI score improved in all patients
Ye et al. [46]	176 OSA patients (152 male, 24 female)	63.9 ± 29.4	FOSQ	Before and after 3 months of CPAP treatment	women showed a greater improvement in the overall functional status compared to men
Weaver et al. [8]	239 OSA patients with AHI 5-30 were randomized to active CPAP (n=121) and sham CPAP (n=118, CPAP pressure < 1 cm H_2O)	12.8 + 6.4 and 12.5 + 6.5 in active CPAP and sham group respectively	SF-36, POMS and FOSQ	Before and after 8 weeks of CPAP treatment	There was greater improvement in QoL in active CPAP group as compare to sham CPAP group after 8 weeks of therapy
Dutt et al. [47]	69 OSA patients(57 M + 12 F) 41 healthy controls	26.39 ± 16.62	SAQLI	Untreated	QoL was impaired in OSA patients in all the four domains of Calgary SAQLI. QoL impairment not directly proportional to severity of OSA.
Quan el al. [48]	199 mild OSA (AHI 5-15) patients and 40 controls with no OSA	10.9 + 2.5	SAQLI	Untreated	It evaluated mild OSA patients only. No significant difference in QOL between patient having mild OSA and no OSA
Mohanty et al. [49]	18 OSA patients	47.7 + 10.7	FOSQ	Before and after 3 months of surgery	OSA patients were not compared with controls but there was improvement in QOL after laser assisted uvulopalatopharyngoplasty

Table 3: Studies exploring QoL in patients of OOSA [28-49].

disease. The study further observed that mental health component and in particular vitality domain of SF-36 is possibly the best generic QoL instrument for OSA. It is also observed that OSAPASI, SAQLI, QSQ and MOSAS questionnaires are the only QoL instruments with good content validity. SAQLI has the best quality evidences among them but it is relatively long and interviewer administered [14].

The First study that explored QoL in OSA patients was published by Gall et al in year 1993 which used SF-36 questionnaire to measure QoL [28]. The study was conducted among 42 males only and observed that QoL was significantly impaired in OSA patients. Interestingly in some severe OSA patients there was little impairment of QoL. After that, there have been many studies exploring QoL in patients of OSA which have been summarised in Table 3. The initial studies used only generic instruments to measure HRQoL in these patients. In 1997 Weaver et al developed FOSQ (Functional outcome of sleep questionnaire) an

OSA specific instruments to measure QoL in OSA patients [21]. After this other OSA specific Instruments like SAQLI (Sleep Anea QoL Questionnaire), OSAPOSI (OSA Patient Oriented Severity Index) and QSQ (Quebec Sleep Questionnaire) have also been used. Among the Generic Questionnaires SF-36 has been used most. Among the generic instruments studies have shown significant variability in QoL assessment even among same patients [31]. Jenkinson et al used SF-36, PGI and Euro QoL among same group of OSA patients and observed that while SF-36 and PGI showed significant life impairment in OSA, in contrast to the EuroQoL, which showed little QoL impairment [31].

Most of the studies suggest that there is significant impairment of QoL in OSA patients but interestingly the QoL impairment has not been found to be directly proportional to the severity of OSA as determined by AHI [29,35,38]. Even no other polysomnographic variable has been consistently found to be associated with QoL impairment. It has been suggested that HRQoL deteriorates only to a certain level with increasing RDI, but then plateaus [5].

The question of effect of treatment on QoL in OSA patients has not been answered convincingly. Different studies have shown divergent results. Some studies have shown that CPAP treatment improves QoL so much so that it reaches the level of healthy controls but some studies did not observed significant improvement in QoL. In many studies of the CPAP trials, the issue of compliance has not been addressed properly and proper adjustment to take compliance into account has not been done. A 2006 Cochrane review on Continuous positive airways pressure for obstructive sleep apnoea in adults concluded that CPAP improves QoL in people with moderate and severe OSA [50]. There is paucity of data regarding effect of other treatment modalities on QoL.

Conclusion

OSA has significant impact on most of the domains of human life. Different generic and OSA specific QoL instruments have been used to assess QoL in OSA. Choice of the instrument should be based on settings and the research question. The review of available literature suggests that there is considerable impairment of HRQoL in OSA. The impairment in QoL is not proportional to the disease severity measured by AHI and has not been consistently found to be associated with any other polysomnographic variable. The impact of various treatment modalities of OSA on QoL has not been explored adequately but the available data suggest that there is improvement in QoL with CPAP treatment at least in moderate and severe OSA patients.

Future Perspective

Most of the studies in this review evaluated HRQoL in patients treated only with CPAP but the effect of other treatment modalities like surgery, dental appliances and life style modification on QoL is yet to be explored. Although short term impact of treatment on QoL is promising but the long term impact of treatment on QoL needs further studies.

We believe that none of the questionnaires presently being used is close to perfect and still there is space for development of a small yet adequate questionnaire to measure QoL in OSA which can be used both in clinical and research setting. Only few of the present questionnaires having adequate backing literature so more studies including inter-instrument comparative studies are required.

Conflict of Interest

There is not conflict of interest in this research.

References

1. American Academy of Sleep Medicine (2005) International classifi- cation of sleep disorders. (2ndedn) Diagnostic and coding manual. Westchester, IL: American Academy of Sleep Medicine.
2. Young T, Palta M, Dempsey J, Skatrud J, Weber S, et al. (1993) The occurrence of sleep-disordered breathing among middle-aged adults. N Engl J Med 328: 1230-1235.
3. Lee W, Nagubadi S, Kryger MH, Mokhlesi B (2008) Epidemiology of Obstructive Sleep Apnea: a Population-based Perspective. Expert Rev Respir Med 2: 349- 364.
4. Patil SP, Schneider H, Schwartz AR, Smith PL (2007) Adult obstructive sleep apnea: pathophysiology and diagnosis. Chest 132: 325-337.
5. Moore P, Bardwell WA, Ancoli-Israel S, Dimsdale JE (2001) Association between polysomnographic sleep measures and health-related quality of life in obstructive sleep apnea. J Sleep Res 10: 303-308.
6. Tam S, Woodson BT, Rotenberg B (2014) Outcome measurements in obstructive sleep apnea: beyond the apnea-hypopnea index. Laryngoscope 124: 337-343.
7. Weaver EM, Woodson BT, Steward DL (2005) Polysomnography indexes are discordant with quality of life, symptoms, and reaction times in sleep apnea patients. Otolaryngol Head Neck Surg 132: 255-262.
8. Weaver TE, Mancini C, Maislin G, Cater J, Staley B, et al. (2012) Continuous positive airway pressure treatment of sleepy patients with milder obstructive sleep apnea: results of the CPAP Apnea Trial North American Program (CATNAP) randomized clinical trial. Am J Respir Crit Care Med 186: 677-683.
9. Kushida CA, Nichols DA, Holmes TH, Quan SF, Walsh JK, et al. (2012) Effects of continuous positive airway pressure on neurocognitive function in obstructive sleep apnea patients: The Apnea Positive Pressure Long-term Efficacy Study (APPLES). Sleep 35: 1593-602.
10. Macaro A (2012) Aristotle and the Good Life.
11. WHO (1947) World Health Organization: The constitution of the World Health Organization. WHO Chronicle 1: 6-24.
12. WHOQOL Group (1994) Development of the WHOQOL: Rationale and current status. Int J Mental Health 23: 24-56.
13. Ware JE, Sherbourne CD (1992) The MOS 36-item short-form health survey (SF-36). I. Conceptual framework and item selection. Med Care 30: 473-483.
14. Hunt SM, McEwen J, McKenna SP (1985) Measuring health status: a new tool for clinicians and epidemiologists. J R Coll Gen Pract 35: 185-188.
15. Bergner M, Bobbitt RA, Kressel S, Pollard WE, Gilson BS, et al. (1976) The sickness impact profile: conceptual formulation and methodology for the development of a health status measure. Int J Health Serv 6: 393-415.
16. Abma IL, van der Wees PJ, Veer V, Westert GP, Rovers M (2015) Measurement properties of patient-reported outcome measures (PROMs) in adults with obstructive sleep apnea (OSA): a systematic review, Sleep Medicine Reviews.
17. EuroQol Group (1990) EuroQol-a new facility for the measurement of health-related quality of life. Health Policy Amst Neth 16: 199-208.
18. Ruta DA, Garratt AM, Leng M, Russell IT, MacDonald LM (1994) A new approach to the measurement of quality of life. The Patient-Generated Index. Med Care 32: 1109-1126.
19. Bolitschek J, Schmeiser-Rieder A, Schobersberger R, Rosenberger A, Kunze M, et al. (1998) Impact of nasal continuous positive airway pressure treatment on quality of life in patients with obstructive sleep apnoea. Eur Respir J Off J Eur Soc Clin Respir Physiol 11: 890-894.
20. Walker-Engström ML, Wilhelmsson B, Tegelberg A, Dimenäs E, Ringqvist I (2000) Quality of life assessment of treatment with dental appliance or UPPP in patients with mild to moderate obstructive sleep apnoea. A prospective randomized 1-year follow-up study. J Sleep Res 9: 303-308.

21. Weaver TE, Laizner AM, Evans LK, Maislin G, Chugh DK, et al. (1997) An instrument to measure functional status outcomes for disorders of excessive sleepiness. Sleep 20: 835-843.
22. Piccirillo JF (2000) Outcomes research and obstructive sleep apnea. Laryngoscope 110: 16-20.
23. Flemons WW, Reimer MA (1998) Development of a disease-specific health-related quality of life questionnaire for sleep apnea. Am J Respir Crit Care Med 158: 494-503.
24. Lacasse Y, Bureau MP, Sériès F (2004) A new standardised and self-administered quality of life questionnaire specific to obstructive sleep apnoea. Thorax 59: 494-499.
25. Chasens ER, Ratcliffe SJ, Weaver TE (2009) Development of the FOSQ-10: a short version of the Functional Outcomes of Sleep Questionnaire. Sleep 32: 915-919.
26. Moroni L, Neri M, Lucioni AM, Filipponi L, Bertolotti G (2011) A new means of assessing the quality of life of patients with obstructive sleep apnea: the MOSAS questionnaire. Sleep Med 12: 959-965.
27. Moyer CA, Sonnad SS, Garetz SL, Helman JI, Chervin RD (2001) Quality of life in obstructive sleep apnea: a systematic review of the literature. Sleep Med 2: 477-491.
28. Gall R, Isaac L, Kryger M (1993) Quality of life in mild obstructive sleep apnea. Sleep 16: S59-61.
29. Fornas C, Ballester E, Arteta E, Ricou C, Diaz A, et al. (1995) Measurement of general health status in obstructive sleep apnea hypopnea patients. Sleep 18: 876-879.
30. Jenkinson C, Stradling J, Petersen S (1997) Comparison of three measures of quality of life outcome in the evaluation of continuous positive airways pressure therapy for sleep apnoea. J Sleep Res 6: 199-204.
31. Jenkinson C, Stradling J, Petersen S (1998) How should we evaluate health status? A comparison of three methods in patients presenting with obstructive sleep apnoea. Qual Life Res 7: 95-100.
32. Piccirillo JF, Gates GA, White DL, Schectman KB (1998) Obstructive sleep apnea treatment outcomes pilot study. Otolaryngol Head Neck Surg 118: 833-844.
33. Flemons WW, Reimer MA (2002) Measurement properties of the calgary sleep apnea quality of life index. Am J Respir Crit Care Med 165: 159-164.
34. Bennett LS, Barbour C, Langford B, Stradling JR, Davies RJ (1999) Health status in obstructive sleep apnea: relationship with sleep fragmentation and daytine sleepiness, and effects of continuous positive airway pressure treatment. Am J Respir Crit Care Med 159: 1884-1890.
35. D'Ambrosio C, Bowman T, Mohsenin V (1999) Quality of life in patients with obstructive sleep apnea: effect of nasal continuous positive airway pressure--a prospective study. Chest 115: 123-129.
36. Engleman HM, Kingshott RN, Wraith PK, Mackay TW, Deary IJ, et al. (1999) Randomized placebo-controlled crossover trial of continuous positive airway pressure for mild sleep Apnea/Hypopnea syndrome. Am J Respir Crit Care Med 159: 461-467.
37. Jokic R, Klimaszewski A, Crossley M, Sridhar G, Fitzpatrick MF (1999) Positional treatment vs continuous positive airway pressure in patients with positional obstructive sleep apnea syndrome. Chest 115: 771-781.
38. Yang EH, Hla KM, McHorney CA, Havighurst T, Badr MS, et al. (2000) Sleep apnea and quality of life. Sleep 23: 535-541.
39. Stepnowsky C, Johnson S, Dimsdale J, Ancoli-Israel S (2000) Sleep apnea and health-related quality of life in African-American elderly. Ann Behav Med Publ Soc Behav Med 22: 116-120.
40. Baldwin CM, Griffith KA, Nieto FJ, O'Connor GT, Walsleben JA, et al. (2001) The association of sleep-disordered breathing and sleep symptoms with quality of life in the Sleep Heart Health Study. Sleep 24: 96-105.
41. Akashiba T, Kawahara S, Akahoshi T, Omori C, Saito O, et al. (2002) Relationship between quality of life and mood or depression in patients with severe obstructive sleep apnea syndrome. Chest 122: 861-865.
42. Lacasse Y, Godbout C, Sériès F (2002) Health-related quality of life in obstructive sleep apnoea. Eur Respir J 19: 499-503.
43. Parish JM, Lyng PJ (2003) Quality of life in bed partners of patients with obstructive sleep apnea or hypopnea after treatment with continuous positive airway pressure. Chest 124: 942-947.
44. Pichel F, Zamarrón C, Magán F, del Campo F, Alvarez-Sala R, et al. (2004) Health-related quality of life in patients with obstructive sleep apnea: effects of long-term positive airway pressure treatment. Respir Med 98: 968-976.
45. Mulgrew AT, Fox N, Ayas NT, Ryan CF (2007) Diagnosis and initial management of obstructive sleep apnea without polysomnography: a randomized validation study. Ann Intern Med 146: 157-166.
46. Ye L, Pien GW, Ratcliffe SJ, Weaver TE (2009) Gender differences in obstructive sleep apnea and treatment response to continuous positive airway pressure. J Clin Sleep Med 5: 512-518.
47. Dutt N, Janmeja AK, Mohapatra PR, Singh AK (2013) Quality of life impairment in patients of obstructive sleep apnea and its relation with the severity of disease. Lung India 30: 289-294.
48. Quan SF, Budhiraja R, Batool-Anwar S, Gottlieb DJ, Eichling P, et al. (2014) Lack of Impact of Mild Obstructive Sleep Apnea on Sleepiness, Mood and Quality of Life. Southwest J Pulm Crit Care 9: 44-56.
49. Mohanty S, Gopinath M, Subramanian M, Sudhir A (2014) Quality of Life Measures Following Laser Assisted Uvulopalatopharyngoplasty (LAUP) in Obstructive Sleep Apnoea Syndrome (OSAS). Indian J Otolaryngol Head Neck Surg 66: 52-59.
50. Giles TL, Lasserson TJ, Smith BJ, White J, Wright J, et al. (2006) Continuous positive airways pressure for obstructive sleep apnoea in adults. Cochrane Database Syst Rev 1: CD001106.

18

Health-related Quality of Life in Patients with Sleep-Related Breathing Disorder

Philipp Hessmann[1,2*], **Jörg Heitmann**[3], **Sandra Apelt**[4], **Monika Balzer-Geldsetzer**[1], **Richard Dodel**[1] **and Geert Mayer**[5]

[1]*Department of Neurology, Philipps-University Marburg, Germany*

[2]*Department of Psychiatry and Psychotherapy, University Medical Center Goettingen, Germany*

[3]*Department of Pneumology, Werra-Meissner Clinic Eschwege, Germany*

[4]*Department of Medicine, Philipps-University Marburg, Germany*

[5]*Department of Neurology, Hephata Clinic Schwalmstadt-Treysa, Germany*

[*]**Corresponding Author:** Philipp Hessmann, Department of Psychiatry and Psychotherapy, University Medical Center Goettingen, Von-Siebold-Strasse 5, 37075 Goettingen, Germany, E-mail: p.hessmann@gmx.net

Abstract

Background: The aim of this study was to evaluate health-related quality of life (HrQoL) in patients with obstructive sleep apnea (OSA) and to investigate the impact of socio demographic and clinical parameters on HrQoL.

Methods: A total of 627 patients were consecutively recruited in 18 sleep laboratories in the state of Hessen, Germany. Standardized questionnaires were used to assess co-morbid disorders, depressive symptoms (Beck Depression Inventory) and daytime sleepiness (Epworth Sleepiness Scale). HrQoL was evaluated with the generic EuroQol-Instrument (EQ-5D-3L index and EQ VAS). Influencing factors were analyzed using bivariate and multiple linear regression analyses.

Results: The mean EQ-5D-3L index was 0.86 ± 0.19, and the mean EQ VAS score was 66.8 ± 19.3. Patients primarily reported problems in the domains of pain/discomfort (55.5%), anxiety/depression (33.5%), and usual activities (29.5%). Multivariate analyses explained 34.9% and 35.9% of the variance in the EQ VAS and the EQ-5D-3L index, respectively. Relevant predictors of HrQoL were patient age, daytime sleepiness, the presence of medical comorbidities and depression.

Conclusions: The results of our study suggest that depressive disorders and excessive daytime sleepiness have considerable effects on patient HrQoL and should be considered in the treatment of OSA patients to improve HrQoL.

Keywords: Obstructive sleep apnea; Quality of life; Excessive daytime sleepiness; Depression

Introduction

Obstructive sleep apnea (OSA) is a common sleep-related breathing disorder characterized by intermittent apneas and hypopneas, leading to nocturnal hypoxemia, hypercapnia, arous-als, and sleep fragmentation [1]. These nocturnal events negatively affect patients' daytime performance, resulting in fatigue and excessive daytime sleepiness, altered mood, diminished neurocognitive abilities, reduced work productivity as well as cardiovascular diseases [2-4]. These impairments often result in reduced functional and social capability and poor quality of life [5,6]. Due to the increasing prevalence of OSA worldwide (approximately 3-9% in women and 3-17% in men), the diagnosis and treatment of patients suffering from OSA result in high health care costs [1,7]. Therefore, OSA has a major impact on national healthcare systems. Patient-centered outcome variables, such as health-related quality of life (HrQoL), have be-come increasingly important in clinical and health service research. HrQoL can be defined as a multidimensional and subjective construct describing the physical, mental, and social dimensions of quality of life that immediately influence a person's health status [8].

Numerous earlier studies have explored HrQoL in patients with OSA showing poorer HrQoL compared with the general population. The associations between depression/daytime sleepi-ness and HrQoL have frequently been assessed using generic or disease-specific question-naires [9,10]. Several studies found daytime sleepiness, depressive disorders and reduced sleep quality to significantly diminish HrQoL [11]. However, it remains unclear whether dis-ease severity is significantly associated with patient HrQoL [12-14]. A longitudinal study over five years by Silva et al. did not demonstrate a relevant worsening of HrQoL according to an increase in the severity of sleep disorders [6]. Despite the importance of evaluating predictive variables of HrQoL to improve health care for patients with OSA, there is a lack of evidence for the German population. Therefore, the aim of the study was to evaluate the association between health-related quality of life (HrQoL) in OSA and sociodemographic and clinical parameters.

Methods

Study design

The study was performed in 18 (of 24) sleep laboratories accredited by the German sleep society (Deutsche Gesellschaft für Schlafmedizin, DGSM) in the state of Hessen during the 2nd quarter of 2009. Patients with a recently diagnosed OSA and persons scheduled for the sleep laboratory for evaluation of a possible OSA were included. Enrollment in the study required an age ≥ 18 years and written informed consent. Persons suffering from dementia were excluded. In total, 627 patients were consecutively enrolled [15].

Patients and the physician of the respective sleep laboratory had to fill in questionnaires concerning sociodemographic parameters, medical comorbidities, medication, previous medical appointments, and medical costs. Additionally, questionnaires concerning patients' HrQoL (EuroQol-Instrument) [8], daytime sleepiness (Epworth Sleepiness Scale) [16], and depression (Beck's Depression Inventory) [17] were used.

Clinical measurements and patient-reported outcomes

EuroQol-Instrument (EQ-5D-3L index and EQ VAS): The generic EuroQol-instrument is widely used for the assessment of HrQoL [18]. The EQ-5D-3L index comprises five domains: mobility, self-care, usual activities, pain/discomfort, and anxiety/depression. Each domain can be rated at three levels: no problems, some/moderate problems, and severe problems. As a result, 3^5 (=243) different conditions of HrQoL are computable. The single values are converted into preference-based indices with a range from -0.205 to 0.999 (indicating worst and best HrQoL, respectively) using German tariffs [8]. For an evaluation of patients' current health status, the EQ VAS was used with a minimum score of 0 points (lowest HrQoL) and a maximum score of 100 points (highest HrQoL).

Epworth Sleepiness Scale (ESS): The Epworth Sleepiness Scale (ESS) is a widely used, self-administered instrument for the assessment of daytime sleepiness, including in patients with sleep-related breathing disorders [16]. The ESS comprises eight questions that are answered on a four-point Likert scale (0-3), with a maximum score of 24 points and higher scores indicating a greater chance for daytime sleepiness. Patients are asked to estimate the probability to doze off or to fall asleep during eight different usual daily activities.

Beck Depression Inventory (BDI-II): The presence of depressive symptoms was evaluated using the second edition of the Beck Depression Inventory (BDI-II) [17], assessing depression in its cognitive, behavioral, emotional, and physical dimensions. The BDI-II consists of 21 items, which were self-rated by the patient on a scale from 0 to 3 points, with a maximum score of 63. In accordance with previous studies, patients were divided into five severity groups by means of the BDI-II sum score: no depression (0-8 pts.), minimal depression (9-13 pts.), mild depression (14-19 pts.), moderate depression (20-28 pts.), or severe depression (>28 pts.) [19].

Data entry and statistical analysis: Statistical analyses were performed using Microsoft Office Excel 2003 (Microsoft Corporation, Redmond, USA) and SPSS Version 22.0 (IBM SPSS Statistics, Armonk, USA). All data are presented as means with standard deviation (SD) or number of cases (percentages) as appropriate. Differences between indicated groups were investigated using parametric and non-parametric tests. A significance level of $\alpha=0.05$ was defined to determine associations between HrQoL and different parameters such as socio-demographic and clinical data. For the comparison between two groups, t-tests and Mann-Whitney U-tests were used. Comparisons of more than two groups were performed using the Kruskal-Wallis test and an analysis of variance (F-test). To control for confounding effects, independent predictors of HrQoL were assessed using multivariate linear regression analyses with the EQ-5D-3L index and the EQ VAS score as dependent variables. Therefore, we selected variables using Spearman's rank correlation or Pearson's test with regard to their possible impact on patients' HrQoL. Afterwards, multivariate linear regression analyses were performed to detect unique contributions to the explanation of the criterion variables.

Ethical approval: The study was approved by the local ethics committee of the Philipps-University of Marburg (Approval-No. 195/07). After screening for inclusion, potential participants were informed of the aims, the content, and the protocol of the study. Informed consent was obtained from all individual participants included in the study.

Results

Socio-demographic and clinical characteristics of the sample

The clinical and socio-demographic characteristics of the study sample are provided in Table 1. Among the 627 study completers, the majority (80.2%) was male; the mean age was 56.1 ± 11.8 years (range 20-89 years). Female participants were significantly older than male patients ($p<0.001$). Half of the patients worked as employee full-time or part-time. Additionally, 5.7% of the participants were unable to work, and 8.5% of the participants were prematurely retired.

	Total	Female	Male
	mean ± SD	mean ± SD	mean ± SD
Age (years)	56.1 ± 11.8	60.1 ± 12.1	55.2 ± 11.5
	n (%)	n (%)	n (%)
	627 (100.0)	124 (19.8)	503 (80.2)
Family status			
Living in a relationship	502 (80.1)	85 (68.5)	417 (82.9)
Not living in a relationship	123 (19.6)	38 (30.6)	85 (16.9)
Employment situation			
Employee	312 (49.8)	43 (36.7)	269 (53.5)

Self-employed	61 (9.7)	7 (5.6)	54 (10.7)
Old-age pension	146 (23.3)	45 (36.3)	101 (20.1)
Gross Income (per month)			
less than 1700 Euros	57 (9.1)	21 (16.9)	36 (7.2)
more than 1700 Euros	286 (45.6)	28 (22.6)	285 (56.7)
Health Insurance			
Statutory	541 (86.3)	115 (92.7)	426 (84.7)
Private	80 (12.8)	8 (6.5)	72 (14.3)
Comorbidities			
Hypertension	357 (56.9)	81 (65.3)	276 (54.9)
Diabetes mellitus type II	75 (12.0)	16 (12.9)	59 (11.7)
Thyroidal diseases	66 (10.5)	28 (22.6)	38 (7.6)
Cardiac arrhythmia	62 (9.9)	16 (12.9)	46 (9.1)
Pulmonary diseases	59 (9.4)	10 (8.1)	49 (9.7)
Musculoskeletal diseases	53 (8.5)	19 (15.3)	34 (6.8)
COPD	52 (8.3)	15 (12.1)	37 (7.4)
Stroke	38 (6.1)	9 (7.3)	29 (5.8)
Restless legs syndrome	32 (5.1)	8 (6.5)	24 (4.8)
Chronic heart failure	29 (4.6)	7 (5.6)	22 (4.4)
Gastro-oesophageal reflux	22 (3.5)	5 (4.0)	17 (3.4)
Depression (BDI-II)			
No depression	252 (40.2)	38 (30.6)	214 (42.5)
Minimal depression	97 (15.5)	18 (14.5)	79 (15.7)
Mild depression	77 (12.3)	19 (15.3)	58 (11.5)
Moderate depression	73 (11.6)	18 (14.5)	55 (10.9)
Severe depression	27 (4.3)	7 (5.6)	20 (4.0)
Daytime sleepiness (ESS Score)			
0 to 10	358 (57.1)	60 (48.4)	298 (59.2)
11 to 15	163 (26.0)	33 (26.6)	130 (25.8)
16 to 20	59 (9.4)	15 (12.1)	44 (8.7)
21 to 24	5 (0.8)	1 (0.8)	4 (0.8)
SD: Standard Deviation; COPD: Chronic Obstructive Pulmonary Disease; BDI-II: Beck Depression Inventory; ESS: Epworth Sleepiness Scale.			

Table 1: Socio-demographic and clinical characteristics of the study population (n=627).

The three most common medical comorbidities were hypertension (56.9%), diabetes mellitus type 2 (12.0%), and thyroidal diseases (10.5%). The results of the Beck Depression Inventory (BDI-II) indicated that 43.7% of the patients suffered from depressive symptoms. More female patients were affected by depressive symptoms than male participants.

Daytime sleepiness was evaluated with the Epworth Sleepiness Scale (ESS). A total of 10.2% of the patients were moderately to severely impaired by daytime sleepiness (ESS score 16 to 24 points).

Health-related quality of life

As shown in Figure 1, the majority of the patients were not affected in the domains of self-care and mobility. In contrast, 55.5% and 33.5% of the patients reported moderate or severe problems in the domains of pain/discomfort and anxiety/depression. Usual activities were affected moderately to severely in 29.5% of the sample. Compared with the general population in Germany, patients suffering from OSA were considerably more impaired in all domains of the EQ-5D-3L.

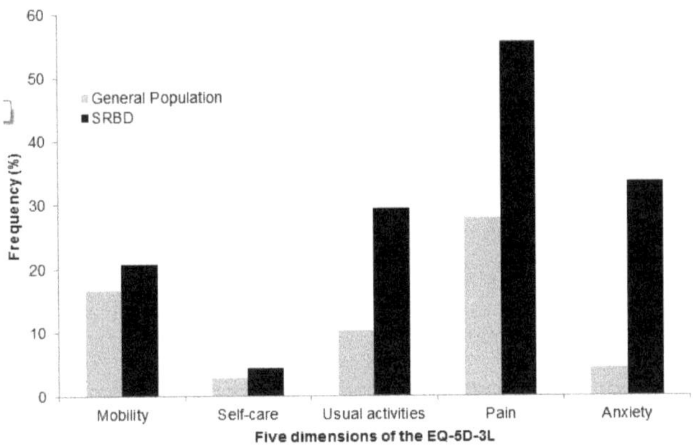

Figure 1: Frequency of moderate or severe problems in the five dimensions of the EQ-5D-3L in the study sample compared with the general population in Germany [20]. SRBD: Sleep-Related Breathing Disorder.

The mean EQ-5D-3L index was 0.86 ± 0.19 and the mean EQ VAS score was 66.8 ± 19.3. There was a decline in the EQ-5D-3L index and the EQ VAS score with increased patient age (p=0.016 and p=0.028). As shown in Table 2, male patients reported considerably higher HrQoL than female participants, as well as patients living in a relationship compared with those who were single, divorced or widowed. The EQ VAS score was reduced in patients with no or a lower/intermediate school degree compared with the EQ VAS score of those with better school education (p=0.013). The EQ VAS was also reduced in participants without a professional education or with non-academic degrees (p=0.007). Limitations in the professional career due to the disease substantially affected patient HrQoL (EQ-5D-3L index: p=0.007, EQ VAS: p=0.002). Additionally, the EQ-5D-3L index and the EQ VAS score were reduced in patients suffering from medical comorbidities such as hypertension, diabetes mellitus type 2, cardiac arrhythmias, pulmonary and musculoskeletal diseases or chronic obstructive pulmonary diseases. A diminished HrQoL was shown for patients with depressive symptoms (p<0.001 for both scores). The EQ-5D-3L index was 0.95 ± 0.10 in patients without depression and was 0.50 ± 0.32 in patients with severe depression. The EQ VAS score was 76.4 ± 15.4 for patients without depressive symptoms and was 45.5 ± 20.6 for severely depressed persons. Furthermore, a considerable association between diminished HrQoL and daytime sleepiness (evaluated with the Epworth Sleepiness Scale) was shown (EQ-5D-3L index and EQ VAS, p<0.001): the EQ VAS score was substantially decreased from 70.2 ± 18.0 (ESS score 0 to 10 points) to 48.0 ± 23.6 (ESS score 21 to 24 points) (Table 2).

	EQ-5D-3L index		EQ VAS	
	mean ± SD	p	mean ± SD	P
Overall Score	0.86 ± 0.19		66.8 ± 19.3	
Gender		p=0.001		p<0.001
Female	0.83 ± 0.20		61.4 ± 19.4	
Male	0.87 ± 0.19		68.1 ± 19.1	
Family status		p=0.025		p=0.018
Living in a relationship	0.87 ± 0.18		67.8 ± 18.7	
Not living in a relationship	0.69 ± 0.34		53.4 ± 27.6	
School Education		p=0.131		p=0.013
No degree	0.96 ± 0.08		58.3 ± 23.2	
Lower/intermediate degree	0.82 ± 0.24		62.9 ± 21.1	
Higher degree	0.89 ± 0.14		70.9 ± 17.6	
Professional education		p=0.063		p=0.007
None	0.74 ± 0.30		58.5 ± 24.2	
Academic degree	0.88 ± 0.18		69.6 ± 18.0	
Non-academic degree	0.86 ± 0.19		65.7 ± 19.0	

Professional Career		p=0.007		p=0.002
Limitations due to the disease	0.78 ± 0.25		50.0 ± 24.0	
No limitations	0.88 ± 0.18		68.4 ± 18.8	
Gross income (per month)		p=0.042		p=0.108
Less than 1700 Euros	0.84 ± 0.23		66.1 ± 18.2	
More than 1700 Euros	0.90 ± 0.16		69.8 ± 17.2	
Health insurance		p<0.001		p=0.001
Statutory	0.86 ± 0.20		65.8 ± 19.6	
Private	0.91 ± 0.16		73.6 ± 15.7	
Comorbidities				
Hypertension	0.85 ± 0.21	p=0.001	64.6 ± 19.7	p=0.001
No	0.89 ± 0.18		70.1 ± 19.0	
Diabetes mellitus type 2	0.81 ± 0.25	p=0.018	59.5 ± 21.9	p=0.001
No	0.87 ± 0.18		68.1 ± 18.8	
Cardiac arrhythmia	0.84 ± 0.18	p=0.029	60.8 ± 18.8	p=0.005
No	0.87 ± 0.19		68.1 ± 19.1	
Pulmonary diseases	0.82 ± 0.23	p=0.056	62.8 ± 18.6	p=0.045
No	0.87 ± 0.19		67.9 ± 19.5	
Musculoskeletal diseases	0.77 ± 0.25	p=0.002	57.1 ± 21.5	p<0.001
No	0.88 ± 0.18		68.0 ± 19.0	
COPD	0.77 ± 0.27	p=0.005	53.4 ± 20.2	p<0.001
No	0.87 ± 0.19		68.8 ± 18.8	
Depression (BDI-II)		p<0.001		p<0.001
No depression	0.95 ± 0.10		76.4 ± 15.4	
Minimal depression	0.90 ± 0.13		66.2 ± 16.5	
Mild depression	0.79 ± 0.19		57.1 ± 18.0	
Moderate depression	0.72 ± 0.24		54.0 ± 15.8	
Severe depression	0.50 ± 0.32		45.5 ± 20.6	
Daytime sleepiness (ESS Score)		p<0.001		p<0.001
0 to 10	0.89 ± 0.17		70.2 ± 18.0	
11 to 15	0.83 ± 0.22		62.0 ± 19.7	
16 to 20	0.82 ± 0.22		59.3 ± 18.3	
21 to 24	0.89 ± 0.04		48.0 ± 23.6	
SD: Standard Deviation; COPD: Chronic Obstructive Pulmonary Disease; BDI-II: Beck Depression Inventory; ESS: Epworth Sleepiness Scale				

Table 2: Bivariate associations between the EQ-5D-3L index and the EQ VAS score and socio-demographic data and clinical subscales.

Finally, patient age, gender, family status, school education, the presence of medical comorbidities, daytime sleepiness and the occurrence of depressive symptoms were included in the multivariate regression models. As shown in Table 3, the presence of depression as well as further medical comorbidities was considerably associated with lower EQ-5D-3L and EQ VAS values. Additionally, the results of the EQ VAS were significantly correlated with increasing age and daytime sleepiness. Multivariate regression analyses were able to explain approximately 35.9% (dependent variable: EQ-5D-3L index, model 1) and 34.9% (dependent variable: EQ VAS, model 2) of the variance.

	Model 1				Model 2			
	EQ-5D-3L index				EQ VAS			
	B	Bootstrap Std. Error	Lower bound	Upper bound	B	Bootstrap Std. Error	Lower bound	Upper bound
Age (years)	-0.001	0.001	-0.002	0.001	-0.144*	0.066	-0.273	-0.014
Gender	-0.001	0.021	-0.039	0.035	2.364	2.131	-2.027	6.518
Family Status	-0.022	0.013	-0.048	0.005	-1.517	1.262	-4.058	1.035
School Education	-0.004	0.01	-0.024	0.016	-0.306	1.006	-2.219	1.589
Presence of Comorbidities	-0.041*	0.019	-0.08	0	-6.726*	1.618	-9.869	-3.491
Daytime Sleepiness (ESS Score)	0.001	0.002	-0.003	0.005	-0.607*	0.212	-1.019	-0.197
Depression (BDI-II Score)	-0.013*	0.002	-0.016	-0.01	-1.013*	0.095	-1.198	-0.824
Constant	1.089	0.069	0.948	1.229	95.291	5.848	83.911	106.283
ESS: Epworth Sleepiness Scale; BDI-II: Beck Depression Inventory; B: Regression Coefficient; *Significant at $p<0.05$								

Table 3: Multivariate linear regression analyses to evaluate the association between selected socio-demographic and clinical factors with patients' HrQoL.

Discussion

The male/female ratio in this cohort showed a male preponderance as expected and as shown in large international studies [21]. Women are known to develop sleep apnea substantially later than men. Moreover, OSA is likely underdiagnosed in women. Only 36% of the patients reported daytime sleepiness as measured by the ESS. In the majority of patients, the ESS was between 0-10 points. This finding is typical for OSA patients. Many patients are not aware of their sleepiness despite falling asleep or dozing off in public. A large prospective review found that 21.8% of patients with OSA had a higher prevalence of depression than patients without OSA (9.4%) [22]. A longitudinal study in Taiwanese OSA patients by Chen et al. showed a 2.18-fold higher risk to develop depression within one year after the diagnosis for patients with OSA compared with that of the controls [23]. Further clinical investigations found a prevalence of depression in approximately 5%-63% of patients with OSA [24]. This wide range may be the result of confounders due to co-morbid disorders and the insufficient separation of the sequelae of depression and OSA.

The mean EQ VAS of patients in this study was 66.8 ± 19.3 and was similar to that of patients with narcolepsy as measured in a cohort of 75 patients with narcolepsy by Dodel et al. (mean EQ VAS: 60.7) [25]. This result is surprising because OSA is a disorder that has an excellent treatment outcome. Several previous studies evaluated the association between HrQoL in OSA patients and depression, as well as excessive daytime sleepiness (EDS). In general, an increase in depressive symptoms and excessive daytime sleepiness was associated with poorer HrQoL [10]. Thus, our results are in line with the majority of international evaluations. A cross-sectional study by Lee et al. evaluated the contributions of depression (Beck Depression Inventory), daytime sleepiness (Epworth Sleepiness Scale), apnea severity, and sleep quality to HrQoL in 793 incident and untreated OSA patients, as measured using the SF-36. It was found that 46.2% of the study sample suffered from depression [26]. The extent of depressive symptoms was the strongest variable influencing the physical and mental domains of HrQoL. However, excessive daytime sleepiness affected only the physical aspects of HrQoL. Silva et al. also used the SF-36 to prospectively assess HrQoL among 3,708 patients with sleep-related breathing disorders over five years. The authors reported a significant association between excessive daytime sleepiness and poorer HrQoL [6]. Akashiba et al. included 60 patients with severe OSA to evaluate the influence of depressive mood, excessive daytime sleepiness and polysomnographic parameters on HrQoL (SF-36) compared with healthy controls, resulting in lower HrQoL in OSA patients [10]. Furthermore, depression and excessive daytime sleepiness were the most important predictors of HrQoL in multivariate regression analysis.

The results of our study should be interpreted in the context of several limitations. Our study included 627 patients, which is a relatively small sample size compared with earlier evaluations [6,26]. Additionally, the study was conducted in a regional design, and the patients were consecutively recruited. Therefore, the study sample may not be representative of all German patients suffering from OSA or patients outside of Germany. To our knowledge, this is the first study evaluating HrQoL in patients with OSA in Germany that uses patients from specialized health care settings (sleep laboratories) in a regional study design. In conclusion, depressive disorders, excessive daytime sleepiness and the presence of medical comorbidities had a significant effect on patient HrQoL and should be considered in the treatment of OSA patients to improve the HrQoL of those patients.

Acknowledgements

We would like to thank the patients and colleagues who participated in the study from the following centers:

Schlafmedizinisches Zentrum Universitätsklinikum Marburg; Abteilung Innere Medizin/Schlafmedizin Ketteler Krankenhaus Offenbach; Abteilung Schlafmedizin St. Elisabethen Krankenhaus Frankfurt am Main; Neurologische Praxis Rabenau; Klinik für Neurologie Klinikum Weilmünster; Schlafzentrum Hephata Klinik Schwalmstadt-Treysa; Schlaflabor des Maingau-Krankenhaus Frankfurt am Main; Schlaflabor des Krankenhaus Sachsenhausen Frankfurt am Main; Fachbereich Pneumologie, Allergologie, Somnologie Deutsche Klinik für Diagnostik Wiesbaden; Schlaflabor Evangelisches Krankenhaus Elisabethenstift GmbH Darmstadt; Medizinische Klinik II Universitätsklinikum Gießen; Schlafmedizinisches Zentrum Kliniken des Main-Taunus-Kreises GmbH Hofheim; Abteilung Innere Medizin Krankenhaus Bad Arolsen GmbH; Innere Medizin Marien-Krankenhaus Kassel, Pneumologie Lungenfachklinik Immenhausen; Schlaf- und Atemzentrum Asklepioskliniken Bad Wildungen; Pneumologie Kreiskrankenhaus Eschwege, Pneumologische Gemeinschaftspraxis Fulda.

Funding

No funding was received for this research.

Conflicts of interest

All authors certify that they have no affiliations with or involvement in any organization or entity with any financial interest (such as honoraria; educational grants; participation in speakers' bureaus; membership, employment, consultancies, stock ownership, or other equity interest; and expert testimony or patent-licensing arrangements), or non-financial interest (such as personal or professional relationships, affiliations, knowledge or beliefs) in the subject matter or materials discussed in this manuscript.

Informed consent

Informed consent was obtained from all individual patients included in the study.

References

1. Punjabi NM (2008) The epidemiology of adult obstructive sleep apnea. Proc Am Thorac Soc 5: 136-143.
2. Ahn SH, Kim JH, Kim DU, Choo IS, Lee HJ, et al. (2013) Interaction between sleep-disordered breathing and acute ischemic stroke. J Clin Neurol 9: 9-13.
3. Chervin RD (2000) Sleepiness, fatigue, tiredness, and lack of energy in obstructive sleep apnea. Chest 118: 372-379.
4. Terán-Santos J, Jiménez-Gómez A, Cordero-Guevara J (1999) The association between sleep apnea and the risk of traffic accidents. Cooperative Group Burgos-Santander. N Engl J Med 340: 847-851.
5. Yang EH, Hla KM, McHorney CA, Havighurst T, Badr MS, et al. (2000) Sleep apnea and quality of life. Sleep 23: 535-541.
6. Silva GE, An MW, Goodwin JL, Shahar E, Redline S, et al. (2009) Longitudinal evaluation of sleep-disordered breathing and sleep symptoms with change in quality of life: the Sleep Heart Health Study (SHHS). Sleep 32: 1049-1057.
7. Pietzsch JB, Garner A, Cipriano LE, Linehan JH (2011) An integrated health-economic analysis of diagnostic and therapeutic strategies in the treatment of moderate-to-severe obstructive sleep apnea. Sleep 34: 695-709.
8. Greiner W, Claes C, Busschbach JJ, von der Schulenburg JM (2005) Validating the EQ-5D with time trade off for the German population. Eur J Health Econ 6: 124-130.
9. Stucki A, Cieza A, Schuurmans MM, Ustun B, Stucki G, et al. (2008) Content comparison of health-related quality of life instruments for obstructive sleep apnea. Sleep Med 9: 199-206.
10. Akashiba T, Kawahara S, Akahoshi T, Omori C, Saito O, et al. (2002) Relationship between quality of life and mood or depression in patients with severe obstructive sleep apnea syndrome. Chest 122: 861-865.
11. Baldwin CM, Griffith KA, Nieto FJ, O'Connor GT, Walsleben JA, et al. (2001) The association of sleep-disordered breathing and sleep symptoms with quality of life in the sleep heart health study. Sleep 24: 96-105.
12. Lacasse Y, Godbout C, Sériès F (2002) Health-related quality of life in obstructive sleep apnoea. Eur Respir J 19: 499-503.
13. Weaver EM, Woodson BT, Steward DL (2005) Polysomnography indexes are discordant with quality of life, symptoms, and reaction times in sleep apnea patients. Otolaryngol Head Neck Surg 132: 255-62.
14. Lopes C, Esteves AM, Bittencourt LR, Tufik S, Mello MT (2008) Relationship between the quality of life and the severity of obstructive sleep apnea syndrome. Braz J Med Biol Res 41: 908-913.
15. Mayer G, Apelt S, Hessmann P, Reese JP, Dodel R, et al. (2015) Versorgung von schlafapnoe-patienten in hessen. Somnologie 19: 145-153.
16. Johns MW (1991) A new method for measuring daytime sleepiness: the Epworth sleepiness scale. Sleep 14: 540-545.
17. Beck AT, Ward CH, Mendelson M, Mock J, Erbaugh J, et al. (1961) An inventory for measuring depression. Arch Gen Psychiatry 4: 561-571.
18. EuroQol Group (1990) EuroQol-a new facility for the measurement of health-related quality of life. Health Policy 16: 199-208.
19. Hautzinger M (1991) The Beck Depression Inventory in clinical practice. Nervenarzt 62: 689-696.
20. König HH, Bernert S, Angermeyer MC (2005) Health Status of the German population: results of a representative survey using the EuroQol questionnaire. Gesundheitswesen 67: 173-182.
21. Young T, Hutton R, Finn L, Badr S, Palta M, et al. (1996) The gender bias in sleep apnea diagnosis. Are women missed because they have different symptoms? Arch Intern Med 156: 2445-2451.
22. Sharafkhaneh A, Giray N, Richardson P, Young T, Hirshkowitz M, et al. (2005) Association of psychiatric disorders and sleep apnea in a large cohort. Sleep 28: 1405-1411.
23. Chen YH, Keller JK, Kang JH, Hsieh HJ, Lin HC, et al. (2013) Obstructive sleep apnea and the subsequent risk of depressive disorder: A population-based follow-up study. J Clin Sleep Med 9: 417-423.
24. Haynes P (2013) The link between OSA and depression: another reason for integrative sleep medicine teams. J Clin Sleep Med 9: 425-426.
25. Dodel R, Peter H, Spottke A, Noelker C, Althaus A, et al. (2007) Health-related quality of life in patients with narcolepsy. Sleep Med 8: 733-741.
26. Lee W, Lee SA, Ryu HU, Chung YS, Kim WS, et al. (2016) Quality of life in patients with obstructive sleep apnea: Relationship with daytime sleepiness, sleep quality, depression, and apnea severity. Chron Respir Dis 13: 33-39.

19

Herbal Drugs and Sleep: What can we Expect?

Antonio Joaquín Gomis Devesa*, Alfonso Martínez Martínez and Juan José Ortega-Albás

Clinical Neurophysiology, Sleep Disorders Unit, Hospital Universitario General de Castelló, Spain

***Corresponding author:** Antonio Joaquín Gomis Devesa, Antonio Joaquín Gomis Devesa Avda. Benicàssim, s/n, 12001, Castellón, Spain

Abstract

Herbal drugs are increasingly being used in our setting as an alternative to, or to supplement, the conventional medication used in sleep disorders. By reviewing different herbal drugs, a description of their therapeutic and adverse effects is established in order to recognise them in a sleep unit and thus be able to establish a more effective approach to them.

Keywords: Herbal drugs; Insomnia; Sleep disorders

Introduction

Phytotherapy is the use of natural plants or vegetable substances for the treatment of a wide range of symptoms and diseases, in order to improve organ and body system function. It is a widely used modality worldwide that forms part of other complete healthcare systems such as naturopathy, traditional Chinese medicine and homeopathy. Most of its widespread use is in the form of self-consumption. In many western countries like Spain, the production, authorisation, registration, distribution and dispensation of products of vegetable origin is regulated, either through food legislation or legislation applicable to plant-based traditional medicines. It is a natural therapy, in the subgroup called "biological practices", defined as those that use substances that are found in nature and used for their flavour, aroma or possible therapeutic properties, such as herbs, flowers, leaves, tree bark, fruit, seeds, stalks and roots, foodstuffs and vitamins. Some examples include the use of dietary supplements, some of them part of conventional medicine, herbal products and others known as "natural" [1].

The fourth section of Royal Decree 1345/2007 is related to traditional plant-based medicines, and establishes the requirement to register traditional plant-based medicines, the criteria to be met for the simplified procedure, the "per se" simplified registration procedure for traditional plant-based medicines, the causes for denial of registration and market recall when a substance or vegetable product, or a combination of the two, ceases to be included in the list edited by the European Medicines Agency Herbal Medicinal Products Committee.

According to the World Health Organisation, a medicinal plant is one which, in one or more of its organs, contains substances that can be used for preventive and/or therapeutic purposes, or are precursors for chemical-pharmaceutical synthesis. The Royal Spanish Pharmacopoeia establishes that "plants, parts of plants, fungi or lichens, whole, fragmented or cut, unprocessed, generally dried, although occasionally also fresh, are considered to be vegetable drugs. Some exudates that have not undergone specific treatment are also considered to be vegetable drugs". Medicinal or herbal products solely of vegetable origin are thus obtained from these plants and their active substances (drugs, understood as the part of a medicinal plant used for therapeutic purposes).

The growing use of phytotherapy in Spain, together with greater monitoring by pharmacies, has enabled us to detect, analyse and interpret the possible side effects and interactions of these products, especially in polymedicated patients. The saying "not all green is healthy" is pertinent to this context. Although the therapeutic margin of this type of product is very broad, they are not free from undesired reactions, whether cross-reactions or otherwise, and this could in some cases lead to life-threatening patient intoxication. As a general rule, these medicinal products should be taken with plenty of water, and those that affect the CNS should not be mixed with alcohol.

Background and Knowledge

In addition, in 2004, the Spanish Ministry of Health and Consumer Affairs published a Ministerial Order containing a list of plants for which sale to the public was restricted or forbidden because of their toxicity [2], which is part of Law 25/1990, of 20 December, on Medicinal Products, specifically section 2. The Spanish Society of Phytotherapy was consulted for the compilation of the list. However, in one of its journals, the society expressed its "surprise to find that our suggestions and proposals were not taken into consideration, and we would like to insist that the list should be reviewed by a committee of experts and updated at least once a year, based on scientific criteria" [3].

Medicinal plants, then, after the starting material has been collected in order to formulate and manufacture phytotherapy products, must be prescribed by a doctor, dispensed by a pharmacy and be subject to pharmacotherapeutic monitoring, to optimise the therapeutic results for a given condition in a target patient, thus preventing the side effects associated with their incorrect consumption.

In 1990, 2.5% of the population of the United States used one or more herbal drugs. In 1997, 42% of the American population was using some sort of medicine other than conventional medicine, and 12% were using herbal medicine concomitantly with other prescribed drugs or in monotherapy [4]. Despite the high documented prevalence of the use of herbal products by patients, less than half of them tell their doctors that they are taking them. It is therefore important for healthcare professionals to discuss herbal drugs with their patients [5].

But just as or even more important than discussing the use of herbal drugs in a GP practice, and in a sleep unit in particular, is the fact that pharmacists know enough to discern whether taking these drugs could be having an impact on the onset and/or perpetuation of the nosological conditions that caused the patient to seek medical care. So it is essential not to take a trivial or frivolous approach due to ignorance or limited knowledge of a socially accepted and increasingly widespread therapy.

As with any drug or chemically active ingredient, the toxicity of a herbal drug depends on dose, form, what it is taken with and the underlying condition being treated. In general, most commonly-used herbal drugs have a relatively good safety profile and a low incidence of adverse events. The U.K. Medicines Control Agency published a report establishing that, "in general, it is unlikely that a herbal drug will represent an important threat to human health" [6]. A 5-year study, conducted from 1991 to 1995, by the U.K. National Poisons Unit, on the side effects that could arise from the use of complementary medicines and food supplements, received 1,297 reports, but directly related adverse effects were only found on 38 occasions [7]. In addition, according to the World Health Organisation, there were approximately 8,000 reports of adverse events of herbal drugs from 1968 to 1997, although most of the signs were anecdotal and usually not due to the supplement itself, but to its contaminants [8].

The "modern" use of a herbal remedy may not reflect its use in "ancient" medicine. For example, an excellent safety record for an "ancient" oral product may have no relevance for the same product's use in a "modern" concentrated product at a high dose. On the other hand, herbal drugs that are apparently safe in healthy conditions, can be more dangerous in specific conditions (pregnancy, renal or hepatic function disorders, etc.), in special circumstances (during perioperative periods, etc.) or when combined with some conventional medicines [9].

Herbal Drugs and Sleep

There are numerous herbal drugs that affect the nervous system. Note that in most cases, the active substances in herbal drugs that affect the nervous system are very active even at very low doses, especially alkaloids. In general, they are potentially very toxic substances with numerous collateral effects, and dosage must be closely monitored in all cases [10].

Central stimulants

Central nervous system stimulants increase the activity of different nerve centres. From the perspective of their therapeutic application, and with the exception of antidepressants, they are not very widely used as they involve two important disadvantages: firstly, the central nervous system cannot effectively be stimulated for a long time, as temporary stimulation is followed by depression (except with some antidepressants) that can be even more intense than before the stimulant is administered; and secondly, stimulants usually present numerous side effects that limit their use. Pharmacologically, central stimulants can be divided into three groups:

predominantly cerebral stimulants.

predominantly bulbar stimulants.

predominantly medullary stimulants.

Stimulants that are predominantly cerebral or neocortical are also known as psychotropic drugs. They can be considered to have a tranquilliser antagonistic effect. They can cause seizures at high doses.

All psychic or psychomotor stimulant herbal drugs contain xanthic bases (caffeine, theophylline and theobromine) that act as stimulants of the cerebral cortex, and they can stimulate the spinal cord at high (toxic) doses [11]. At therapeutic doses, they stimulate mental function, increasing the ability to concentrate and pay attention, while at high doses they cause restlessness and insomnia, and can stimulate the respiratory, vasomotor and vagal bulbar centres, especially when they are depressed [12]. They also act as diuretics, as they increase glomerular filtration and reduce tubular resorption, thereby increasing the excretion of water and ions such as sodium, chlorine and, to a lesser extent, potassium.

Drugs rich in xanthic bases are:

Coffee (*Coffea arabica*)**:** It is also choleretic. Tree originating in Ethiopia. The seeds of the fruit constitute the drug. It contains up to 3% of xanthic bases, especially caffeine.

Tea (*Thea sinensis*)**:** Tree growing in tropical African and American countries. Its young leaves are used, which contain up to 4% caffeine bound to polyphenols (giving its characteristic delayed release in the body), tannins and flavonoids [13].

Mate (*Ilex paraguensis*)**:** Tree originating in Brazil and Paraguay. Its leaves contain up to 2.3% caffeine.

Cola (*Cola nitida*)**:** Tree originating in equatorial Africa. It contains up to 2.5% caffeine and also has a delayed effect [14].

Guarana (*Paullinia cupana*)**:** Native to the Amazon rain forest and grown in Brazil. Its seeds, which contain up to 5% caffeine, tannins and flavonoids, are chewed and used to make a social beverage; where they are consumed they represent a public health problem, as their high tannin content makes them highly carcinogenic [15].

Caffeine in particular, the most consumed in our setting, is used as a stimulating social beverage. In case of drunkenness due to excessive alcohol intake, they partially neutralise the effects of ethyl alcohol. Depending on the doses consumed, they can cause insomnia, anxiety, restlessness and vagal symptoms that should be considered in our medical history [16]. It causes addiction, and at low doses stimulates the CNS, reducing the sensation of fatigue and tiredness.

Predominantly bulbar stimulants are known as analeptic, and can also cause seizures at high doses. They act primarily on the bulbar respiratory centre and to a lesser extent on the vasomotor centre.

The following are analeptic drugs:

Camphor (*Cinnamomum camphora*)**:** Tree from the wood of which camphor is obtained.

Rosemary (*Rosmarinus officinalis*)**:** Mediterranean bush, the essential oil of which is also rich in camphor.

Lobelia (*Lobelia Inflata*)**:** North American herbaceous herb, the stalks and leaves of which contain lobeline as the most abundant alkaloid; a piperidine derivative that is used as a respiratory stimulant in bulbar syncope derived from epidural anaesthesia, and in barbiturate, morphine and carbon monoxide intoxication. The mechanism of action is caused by reflex bulbar excitation by stimulation of the cardio-aortic and carotid sinus nerve endings. Indeed, its overdose can cause respiratory centre paralysis [17].

The main predominantly medullary stimulant is strychnine (*Strychnos nux-vomica*).

Strychnine (*Strychnos nux-vomica*)**:** Asian tree, the seeds of which contain strychnine as the most abundant alkaloid, which causes hyperexcitability followed by reflex seizures in response to all kinds of external stimuli. Strychnine does not limit its effect to the spinal cord and at high doses it acts on the bulb, causing increased respiratory rate, vasoconstriction and bradycardia [18].

Central depressants

They are a heterogeneous group of drugs that are capable of reducing the activity of different nerve centres.

According to their effect, they are classified as:

1) Hypnotic agents.

2) Sedatives.

3) Tranquillisers (neuroleptic agents, minor tranquillisers and anxiolytic agents)

4) Antineuralgic agents.

5) Centrally-acting muscle relaxants.

6) Analgesics.

Hypnotic agents

These drugs induce sleep, and occasionally act synergically as sedatives, depending on the doses used. They are used in the treatment of psychophysiological or simple insomnia of undetermined cause, of which three modalities can be described: sleep onset insomnia or with elongated sleep onset latency, most common in middle-aged or young people with nervous hyperexcitability and an anxious component, and early-morning awakening insomnia and sleep-maintenance insomnia, related to a greater anxious-emotional burden and more common in older people.

A hypnotic agent is a drug capable of causing physiological-like sleep; that is, a state of unconsciousness that can be reversed by sensitive or sensory stimuli. In this respect, an ideal hypnotic agent must meet the following conditions:

1) Act rapidly, reducing sleep latency time.

2) Not qualitatively and quantitatively alter sleep macrostructure.

3) Not cause side effects that have an impact on the patient's health.

4) Provide a broad therapeutic safety margin.

5) Not cause drug addiction.

6) The most used hypnotic drugs are benzodiazepines, Z-drugs and chloral hydrate; according to the premises described above, they are far from ideal agents [19].

In phytotherapy, two drugs are basically used as hypnotic agents:

Kava-kava (*Piper methysticum*)**:** Bush originating in the Pacific Islands (Micronesia), the roots of which contain kavalactones that have a neurosedative and hypnotic effect, which appears to be due to their effect on the limbic structures, particularly the amygdala complex. At low doses it has an anxiolytic effect that, in double-blind trials, has been shown to be similar to that of oxazepam with no adverse reactions [20]; it is often used to treat benzodiazepine dependency. As a hypnotic agent, it is usually combined with magnesium orotate in order to enhance its effect. It also has a myorelaxant effect.

California poppy (*Eschscholzia californica*)**:** Herbaceous plant native to California. The whole of the plant is used as it contains a complex of different isoquinoline alkaloids belonging to 5 different series: protopine, pavine, aporphine, protoberberine and 5-benzyl tetrahydroisoquinoline. It has a hypnotic (100 mg/kg), sedative or anxiolytic (25 mg/kg) effect, depending on the administered dose [21]. It is also used in the treatment of benzodiazepine dependency.

Sedatives

These drugs are used in states of anxiety and nervous tension, as they cause sedation, and even occasionally a degree of analgesia, by mitigating nervous hyperexcitability. Sedation is usually accompanied by intellectual depression and "numbed" consciousness, with a tendency to sleep even with regular therapeutic doses. This characteristic differentiates sedatives from tranquillisers, as the latter calm nervous excitability with no tendency to sleep or mental numbness. There are numerous herbal sedatives, and they can be classified according to the chemical structure of the substance responsible for the sedative effect

Essential oil or oleoresins: hop, lavender, valeriana.

Alkaloids: passiflora

Glucosides, bitter substances or resins: motherwort.

Hop (*Humulus lupulus*)**:** Eurosiberian climbing herbaceous plant of which the female seed cones are used with an oleoresin in which the resinous fraction contains bitter substances (humulone and lupulone); its volatile or oily fraction is rich in methylbutenol, which experimentally has sedative effects [22] It is currently used in phytotherapy in the treatment of insomnia [23].

Lavender (*Lavandula angustifolia*)**:** Mediterranean bush, the flowers of which contain an essential oil rich in linalyl acetate and linalool. These products have been experimentally shown to inhibit caffeine stimulation by up to 50%, largely through olfactory receptors [24]. It is used in phytotherapy to treat neuroleptic and benzodiazepine dependency, especially in geriatric patients [25].

Valerian (*Valeriana officinalis*): Eurosiberian herbaceous plant, the roots of which contain 0.3-0.8% essential oil. The plant's characteristic "sweaty feet" smell is due to its high content of isovalerianic and acetoxy valerenic acids of essential oil. It also contains 1% valepotriates. It has a sedative and anti-seizure effect [26]. ***In vitro***, valerenic acid inhibits 3H-GABA uptake and stimulates its release in the synaptosomes, independently of Na-KATIasa activity and membrane potential [27]. GABA is considered to be an important neurotransmission inhibitor involved in processes that coincide with stress and anxiety. This causes the chloride channels to open, so its conductivity increases through the cell membranes, reducing the reaction to depolarising stimuli. Isovalerianic acid increases the affinity of GABA for their receptors, thus resulting in greater bonding with the receptor and a more intense effect. All this leads to a reduction in nerve cell excitability. Pharmacodynamic studies have shown that liquid valerian extract (1200 mg) has a sedative effect comparable to that of diazepam (10 mg) [28]. Valerian is currently basically used in the treatment of insomnia and as an alternative to hypnotic-sedative agents such as benzodiazepines and/or Z-drugs in patients with nervous disorders (anxiety, palpitations, tension migraines, etc.). It is important when guiding patients who are taking valerian to warn them that its continued use leads to dependency, so it should be prescribed discontinuously [29]. When administered immediately before going to bed to induce sleep, it creates some initial anxiety or restless sleep. To avoid these unpleasant effects, it is advisable to take the valerian-based product at least one hour before dinner.

Passiflora (*Passiflora incarnata*): North American creeper, the aerial part of which contains flavonoids, notably vitexin, orientin, lucenin, coumarin and umbelliferone. It also contains maltol, responsible for its myorelaxant effect [30]. In humans, both the oral and peritoneal administration of passiflora extracts causes a sedative or hypnotic effect, depending on the administered dose [31]. Its long-term use is not free from hepatotoxic and pancreotoxic effects, and the drug or its pharmaceutical derivatives can cause vomiting because of its strong bitter flavour. In a related plant, Passiflora coerulea, used ethnopharmacologically as a sedative, it has been shown that its anxiolytic and myorelaxant effect is due to its flavonoid content, especially chrysin (5- and 7-hydroxyflavone), which acts as a partial agonist of the central receptors for benzodiazepines [32]. It appears that the resulting sedative effect is due to the pharmacological interaction and synergy between flavonoids, maltol and indole alkaloids. Cardiac arrhythmias, long QTc, vomiting and hypersomnia have been described as side effects of this drug [33], hence the importance of learning whether our patients are self-medicating with the plant. It is currently used in phytotherapy in sedative, hypnotic, myorelaxant and anxiolytic products.

Motherwort (*Leonurus cardiaca*): Herbaceous plant native to Asia, the aerial part of which contains bitter glucosides with a structure similar to that of bufadienolides, alkaloids (leonurine) and essential oil. It is used as a sedative in the treatment of nervous disorders. It is contraindicated in patients treated with cardiotonic agents as it could enhance their effect, and the dose should be carefully calculated in all cases, due to these bufadienolides' high affinity for and effect on the myocardium.

Tranquillisers

Tranquillisers or ataraxic drugs are those that have a calming effect on nervous hyperexcitability, without "numbing" consciousness and without inducing sleep tendency at the usual doses. They are selective central nervous system depressants that primarily act on a subcortical level, particularly the hypothalamus, the mesodiencephalic activating system and the limbic system, with no predominant effect on the cerebral cortex. The patient can thus reorganise his or her superior neurological functions. In phytotherapy, this group of drugs is divided into:

1) Neuroleptic agents or major tranquillisers.

2) Minor tranquillisers.

3) Anxiolytic agents.

Neuroleptic agents (Rauwolfia alkaloids (*Rauwolfia serpentina*)): Bush native to Africa, the roots of which contain different alkaloids, primarily reserpine, which reduces irritability and anxiety without inducing sleep or "mental numbness". One side effect is clear extrapyramidal symptoms, even at therapeutic doses in long-term therapy. It is almost exclusively used on highly-agitated psychiatric patients in order to facilitate their cooperation and social reintegration.

Minor tranquillisers: They have a gentle calming effect. In phytotherapy, a series of drugs are used as minor tranquillisers, including: small-leaved lime (Tilia cordata and Tilia platyphyllos), sweet camomile (Matricaria chamomilla), Roman camomile (Chamaemelum nobile), lemon balm (Melissa officinalis), bitter orange (Citrus aurantium), boldo (Boldea fragrans) and bogbean (Menyanthes trifoliata).

Anxiolytic agents: In phytotherapy, both vegetable hypnotic agents and sedatives are used, occasionally in combination with antidepressants (St John's Wort, Hypericum perforatum). Examples are common hawthorn (Crataegus monogyna) and black horehound (Ballota nigra)

References

1. (June 2011) Ministry Of Health, Social Policy and Equality, Spain. Análisis de situación de las terapias naturales.
2. (2004) Ministry of Health and Consumer Affairs, Spain. 2225 Order SCO/190/2004, of 28 January, establishing the list of plants, the public sale of which is forbidden or restricted by reason of their toxicity. BOE, 32: 5051-5055.
3. (2004) Revista de Fitoterapia. 4: 69-76.
4. Eisenberg DM, Davis RB, Ettner SL, Appel S, Wilkey S, et al. (1998) Trends in alternative medicine use in the United States, 1990-1997: results of a follow-up national survey. JAMA 280: 1569-1575.
5. Leung JM, Dzankic S, Manku K, Yuan S (2001) The prevalence and predictors of the use of alternative medicine in presurgical patients in five California hospitals. Anesth Analg 93: 1062-1068.
6. U.K. Medicine & Healthcare Products Regulatory Agency, Medicines Control Agency: Safety of Herbal Medicinal Products.
7. Shaw D, Leon C, Kolev S, Murray V (1997) Traditional remedies and food supplements. A 5-year toxicological study (1991-1995). Drug Saf 17: 342-356.
8. Ernst E (2003) Serious adverse effects of unconventional therapies for children and adolescents: a systematic review of recent evidence. Eur J Pediatr 162: 72-80.
9. Kaufman DW, Kelly JP, Rosenberg L, Anderson TE, Mitchell AA (2002) Recent patterns of medication use in the ambulatory adult population of the United States: the Slone survey. JAMA 287: 337-344.
10. (1980) QUER, FONT. Plantas Medicinales.
11. Oei A, Hartley LR (2005) The effects of caffeine and expectancy on attention and memory. Hum Psychopharmacol 20: 193-202.
12. Drake C, Roehrs T, Shambroom J, Roth T (2013) Caffeine effects on sleep taken 0, 3, or 6 hours before going to bed. J Clin Sleep Med 9: 1195-1200.
13. Bhatti SK, O'Keefe JH, Lavie CJ (2013) Coffee and tea: perks for health and longevity? Curr Opin Clin Nutr Metab Care 16: 688-697.
14. Atawodi SE, Mende P, Pfundstein B, Preussmann R, Spiegelhalder B (1995) Nitrosatable amines and nitrosamide formation in natural stimulants: Cola acuminata, C. nitida and Garcinia cola. Food Chem Toxicol 33: 625-630.
15. Morton JF (1992) Widespread tannin intake via stimulants and masticatories, especially guarana, kola nut, betel vine, and accessories. Basic Life Sci 59: 739-765.
16. O'Keefe JH, Bhatti SK, Patil HR, DiNicolantonio JJ, Lucan SC, et al. (2013) Effects of habitual coffee consumption on cardiometabolic disease, cardiovascular health, and all-cause mortality. J Am Coll Cardiol 62: 1043-1051.
17. Crooks PA, Zheng G, Vartak AP, Culver JP, Zheng F, et al. (2011) Design, synthesis and interaction at the vesicular monoamine transporter-2 of lobeline analogs: potential pharmacotherapies for the treatment of psychostimulant abuse. Curr Top Med Chem 11: 1103-1127.

18. Katiyar C, Kumar A, Bhattacharya SK, Singh RS (2010) Ayurvedic processed seeds of nux-vomica: neuropharmacological and chemical evaluation. Fitoterapia 81: 190-195.
19. Ortega-Albás JJ, Gomis Devesa AJ (2014) Hypnotic-Sedating Drugs in the Treatment of Insomnia: Objective or Subjective Improvement? J Sleep Disorders Ther 3: 158.
20. Sarris J, Laporte E, Scholey A, King R, Pipingas A, et al. (2013) Does a medicinal dose of kava impair driving? A randomized, placebo-controlled, double-blind study. Traffic Inj Prev 14: 13-17.
21. Hanus M, Lafon J, Mathieu M (2004) Double-blind, randomised, placebo-controlled study to evaluate the efficacy and safety of a fixed combination containing two plant extracts (Crataegus oxyacantha and Eschscholtzia californica) and magnesium in mild-to-moderate anxiety disorders. Curr Med Res Opin 20: 63-71.
22. Schiller H, Forster A, Vonhoff C, Hegger M, Biller A, et al. (2006) Sedating effects of Humulus lupulus L. extracts. Phytomedicine 13: 535-541.
23. Maroo N, Hazra A, Das T (2013) Efficacy and safety of a polyherbal sedative-hypnotic formulation NSF-3 in primary insomnia in comparison to zolpidem: a randomized controlled trial. Indian J Pharmacol 45: 34-39.
24. Buchbauer G, Jirovetz L, Jäger W, Dietrich H, Plank C (1991) Aromatherapy: evidence for sedative effects of the essential oil of lavender after inhalation. Z Naturforsch C 46: 1067-1072.
25. Chioca LR, Ferro MM, Baretta IP, Oliveira SM, Silva CR, et al. (2013) Anxiolytic-like effect of lavender essential oil inhalation in mice: participation of serotonergic but not GABAA/benzodiazepine neurotransmission. J Ethnopharmacol 147: 412-418.
26. Schulz H, Jobert M, Hübner WD (1998) The quantitative EEG as a screening instrument to identify sedative effects of single doses of plant extracts in comparison with diazepam. Phytomedicine 5: 449-458.
27. Trauner G, Khom S, Baburin I, Benedek B, Hering S, et al. (2008) Modulation of GABAA receptors by valerian extracts is related to the content of valerenic acid. Planta Med 74: 19-24.
28. Felgentreff F, Becker A, Meier B, Brattström A (2012) Valerian extract characterized by high valerenic acid and low acetoxy valerenic acid contents demonstrates anxiolytic activity. Phytomedicine 19: 1216-1222.
29. Kirkwood CK (1999) Management of insomnia. J Am Pharm Assoc (Wash) 39: 688-696.
30. Bizet D, Et Roubaudi F, (1998) La Passiflore Passiflora incarnata L Passifloracées. Phytotherapy 26: 22-24.
31. Deng J, Zhou Y, Bai M, Li H, Li L (2010) Anxiolytic and sedative activities of Passiflora edulis f. flavicarpa. J Ethnopharmacol 128: 148-153.
32. Brown E, Hurd NS, McCall S, Ceremuga TE (2007) Evaluation of the anxiolytic effects of chrysin, a Passiflora incarnata extract, in the laboratory rat. AANA J 75: 333-337.
33. Fisher AA, Purcell P, Le Couteur DG (2000) Toxicity of Passiflora incarnata L. J Toxicol Clin Toxicol 38: 63-66.

20

Influence of Ramadan Observance on Sleep Pattern and Wakefulness at Work among Medical Trainer in Tunisia

Sameh Msaad*, **Nada Kotti, Sourour Abid, Mounira Hajjaji, Samia Sellami, Samy Kammoun, Ilhem Yangui and Arbi Masmoudi**

Department of Pulmonology, Hedi Chaker Hospital, University of Sfax, Sfax, Tunisia

***Corresponding author:** Msaad S, Department of Pulmonology, Hedi Chaker Hospital, University of Sfax, Sfax, Tunisia, E-mail: msaadsameh@yahoo.fr

Abstract

Introduction: Muslims practice intermittent Islamic fasting all over the globe each year during Ramadan. This practice induces several changes that may affect work performance. The aim of this study is to evaluate the impact of fast during Ramadan on eating behaviors, sleep habits, daytime sleepiness, and professional life.

Methods: Target population was medical trainees who were working since at least 4 months at the beginning of the study. They were invited to complete an anonymous self-administered questionnaire during and apart from Ramadan.

Results: Two hundred forty-three subjects (243) had correctly completed the questionnaire (mean age = 26.81 ± 2.17 years and sex-ratio = 0.69). During Ramadan, all Alcohol drinkers had stopped drinking (p<0.001), and daily tobacco consumption had significantly dropped from 14.82 ± 8.26 to 11.67 ± 8.64 cigarettes during Ramadan (0.002). Consumption of both coffee and tea was significantly reduced from 2.44 ± 1.3 to 1.03 ± 0.71 and from 1.06 ± 0.59 to 0.77 ± 0.66 cups a day, respectively (p<0.0001). The average number of meals per day dropped from 2.92 ± 0.49 before Ramadan to 1.79 ± 0.58 during Ramadan (p = 0.032). The average bedtime was significantly delayed until to 3.80 ± 5.37 am, while it was at 9.7 ± 10.93 pm during the previous month (p<0.0001).

The percentage of subjects who went to bed after midnight also had significantly increased from 57.1% to 93.1% (p<0.001). The degree of dissatisfaction about sleep quality had substantially increased from 18.9% at baseline to 54.7% during Ramadan (p<0.0001). Fasted Trainees found more difficult getting up in the mornings (74.1% versus 79% respectively, p<0.0001). The percentage of trainees who often arrived late for work or missed it increased significantly, from 3.7% at baseline to 11.9% during Ramadan (p<0.0001). The majority (81.1%) reported feeling extra sleepy during the daytime of Ramadan month as compared to 60.1% during the previous month (p<0.0001). It was also noted a higher frequency of digestive disorders (46.9% versus 29.6%, <0.001), morning headaches (15.2% versus 6.6%), excessive nervousness (65% versus 57.6%, p<0.001) and concentration and memory disturbances (88.9% versus 77%, p<0.001). Both daily and weekly working hours had significantly decreased during the month of Ramadan (p<0.001). Trainees started their daily work 15 minutes later and left 20 minutes earlier, which results in 35 less minutes worked per day, and around 3 and half hours less per week. Most of participants (88.1%) thought that Ramadan had a negative effect on their sleeping pattern and affected their daytime functioning. Although, the percentage of those who took sedative-hypnotics for sleep disorders had significantly dropped from 7% at baseline to 3.3% during this month (p = 0.0001).

Conclusion: The present study showed that Ramadan is associated with several changes in eating behaviors and sleep habits. These changes resulted in sleep pattern impairment, increased daytime sleepiness and reduced work performance. Healthy sleep and eating habits with a suitable work rhythm should be recommended to Fasted medical trainees to minimize the impact of Ramadan on their wellbeing and professional life.

Keywords: Sleep; Ramadan; Medical trainee; Wakefulness behavior; Eating

Introduction

Ramadan is the ninth lunar month of the Islamic calendar. Fasting during this month is obligatory on every adult, sane, and able Muslim and concerns around one and a half billion of people around the world. It involves abstinence from three primal physical needs of human beings- food, drink, and sexual intercourse from dawn to sunset during the entire month of Ramadan (for a period of 29 or 30 days) [1].

Eating is only allowed during the night. The pattern of meals changes as well. Usually two to three main meals are taken: the first called "Iftar", which means breakfast, is served right after sunset, the second one is served after night prayer, while the third one called "Suhur" is taken right before dawn. Besides, Muslims engage themselves in many religious activities such as offering voluntary prayers, and reciting the Quran particularly in the final third part of the night.

They also have larger and more frequent nocturnal collective gatherings and others ceremonies. As a result, most of people stay awake until the early hours of the morning, which can lead to diurnal sleepiness and affects alertness at work as was suggested by several previous studies [2].

Like in others Muslims countries [1], sleep and eating behavior changes during Ramadan in fasting individuals have been noticed increasingly in Tunisia but have not been well documented.

Medical trainees are particularly concerned by these problems. Actually, they represent the largest and the most active population in Tunisian university hospitals and they have to work nocturnal shifts. They need to maintain optimal alertness and function at peak levels during work to ensure that patients receive safe and effective care.

The present study aimed to investigate the effects of Ramadan fasting on sleep habits, daytime sleepiness and wakefulness among a group of Tunisian medical trainees.

Methods

Type of study

This was a prospective monocentric and cross-sectional study performed one week before Ramadan and during the last week of Ramadan, June-July 2014.

During the study period, fasting day was about 15 hours, dawn (beginning of fasting) was between 03:00 and 03:15 am, and sunset (end of fasting) was between 06:30 and 06:45 am. The weather was hot with an average ambient temperature around 38°C and a relative humidity of 70% at the city of Sfax.

The study was approved by the university ethics committee, and informed consent was obtained from each participant.

Participants

The study was carried out in the two University Hospitals of Sfax (Hedi CHAKER and Habib BOURGUIBA university hospitals) and included medical trainees who were working since at least 4 months at the beginning of the study.

Trainees who took leave from work during Ramadan and those who didn't fast were excluded as well as pregnant or nursing women. The average working hours for Tunisian medical trainees is 6 hours a day, 6 days a week.

They also work night shifts usually more than one time a week. Of 570 subjects approached at the beginning, 60 had immediately refused to participate because of lack of time or lack of interest in the studied subject. As a result, a total of 510 subjects had agreed to participate in this study.

Data collection

The participants were requested to complete an anonymous self-administered questionnaire with honesty, and were assured of absolute confidentiality of all of their responses. The questionnaire was adapted from a French sleep disorders network "reseau moprhée" and modified according to the specificities of our population.

It contained 51 questions concerning the following aspects: demographic parameters, socio-economic conditions, habits and pathological antecedents, working conditions, eating behaviors, sleep-wake schedule, quality of sleep, wakefulness at work and daytime performance.

Statistical analysis

The data were analyzed (SPPS 20.0 for windows, United States) using descriptive statistics and expressed in the text and tables as means ± standard deviation or as percentages, when appropriate. For continuous variables, comparisons were performed using one-way repeated measures ANOVA.

When the difference was significant, post hoc testing was performed using Dunn's multiple comparison tests. Chi-square test was used for discrete variables. The statistical significant level was set at $p<0.05$.

Results

Demographic characteristics

Of the 510 trainees who participated in the study, only 243 subjects had correctly completed the questionnaire, for a response rate of 47.64%. The mean age of these participants was 26.81 ± 2.17 years with a slight female predominance (sex-ratio = 0.69).

About two third of them were single (62.6%), and most of them lived in families (85.2%). Among married participants, 14.8% had one or more children. The average body mass index (BMI) was 23.18 ± 3.34 Kg/m2. Nearly the fifth of participants (21.3%) were overweight, while obesity was noted in 4.6% of cases.

A weight gain of 5.68 ± 3.9 kg during the last six months was reported by 71 participants (29.2% of cases). The most common medical conditions reported by participants were, by descending order, psychiatric disorders (n = 19, 7.8%), and cardio-respiratory diseases (n = 8 3.3%).

Table 1 summarizes the principal characteristics of our population.

Habits and eating behaviors

Ten point seven pour cent of participants (n = 26) were drinkers, with an average of 2.23 ± 2.8 drinks per days. During Ramadan, all of them had stopped drinking ($p<0.001$).

Likewise among the 39 smokers (16%), daily tobacco consumption had significantly dropped from 14.82 ± 8.26 to 11.67 ± 8.64 cigarettes during Ramadan ($p = 0.002$). However, no one had stopped smoking during this month. Eighty three point one per cent of participants (n = 202) were coffee drinkers consuming an average of 2.44 ± 1.3 per day, while 56% of them were tea drinkers with an average consumption of 1.06 ± 0.59 cups a day.

During Ramadan, consumption of both coffee and tea was significantly reduced at 1.03 ± 0.71 and 0.77 ± 0.66 cups a day, respectively ($p<0.0001$).

The average number of meals per day dropped from 2.92 ± 0.49 before Ramadan to 1.79 ± 0.58 during Ramadan ($p = 0.032$).

The time of the first meal changed as well, and it was between 07:00 pm and 08:00 pm in the majority of cases (95%). Nearly two third of participants (61.3%) used to take a second meal during Ramadan, and it was commonly between 12:00 am and 01:00 am.

The Suhur, the third meal, was taken by only one third of the participants (37.4%), and it was between 01:00 am and 03:00 pm (Table 2).

Age (years)	**Characteristics**	26.81 ± 2.17
Sex-ratio (Females/Males)		0.69
BMI	Mean (kg/m^2)	23.18 ± 3.34
	≤18.5 (%)	3.3
	18.5-25 (%)	70.7
	25-30 (%)	21.3
	≥30 (%)	4.6
Martial statue (%)	Single	62.6
	Married	33.7
	Free Relationship	3 .7
Number of children (%)	0 Child	85.2
	1 Child	11.5
	2 children	2.9
	3 children	0.4
Habitation (%)	Single	7.4
	In family	85.2
	In group of friends	7.4
Medical conditions (%)	Respiratory	4.1
	Arterial hypertension	2.5
	Cardio-vascular diseases	3.3
	Thyroid diseases	2.5
	Neurologic diseases	0.8
	Psychiatric diseases	7.8
	Others	5.8

Table 1: Characteristics of the 243 participants.

		Before Ramadan	**During Ramadan**	**p**
Smoking	16%	14.82 ± 0.42 (cigarettes /day)	11.67 ± 8.64	0.002
hookah	7%	0.94 ± 0.36 hookah /day	0.94 ± 0.65 hookah /day	0.705
Coffee	83.1%	2.44 ± 1.3 cups/day	1.03 ± 0.71 cups/day	<0.0001
Tea	56%	1.06 ± 0.59 cups/day	0.77 ± 0.66 cups/day	<0.0001
Alcohol	10.7%	2.23 ± 2.8cups/day	0 cups/day	<0.001
Number of meal per day		2.92 ± 0.49	1.79 ± 0.58	0.032
First meal		From 06 am to 07 am:13.2%	From 07 pm to 08 pm:95.5%	
		From 07 am to 08 am:61.7%	Beyond 08 pm:4.5%	
		From 08 am to 09 am:21.8%		

	Post prandial:3.3%		
Second meal	From 12 am to 01 pm:11.5%	From 09 pm to 10 pm:3.7%	
	From 01 pm to 02 pm:45.3%	From 10 pm to 11 pm:7%	
	Beyond 02 pm:41.2%	From 11 pm to 12 pm:10.7%	
		From 12:00 am to 01:00 am:39.5%	
	No second meal:2.1%	No second meal:	
Third meal	From 06 pm to 07 pm:1.6%	From 01 am to 02 am:4.1%	
	From 07 pm to 08 pm:26.7%	From 02 am to 03 am:33.3%	
	From 08 pm to 09 pm:39.1%	No third meal:62.6%	
	From 09 pm to 10 pm:19.8%		
	Beyond 10 pm:10.7%		
	No third meal:2.1%		

Table 2: Habits and eating behaviours in our population before and during Ramadan.

Sleep pattern

During Ramadan, the average bedtime was significantly delayed until to 3.80 ± 5.37 am, while it was at 9.7 ± 10.93 pm during the previous month (p<0.0001). The percentage of subjects who went to bed after midnight also had significantly increased from 57.1% to 93.1% (p<0.001). On the other hand, the sleep latency had slightly decreased during Ramadan, but this decrease did not reach statistical significance (from 18.98 minutes to 18.29 minutes, p = 0.508).

It had also noted that 48.1% of participants complained of insomnia at baseline versus 57.6% during Ramadan (p<0.0001). In response to the question "do you feel that you don't sleep enough at night", the percentage of participants who replied "yes" had significantly increased from 18.9% at baseline to reach 54.7% during Ramadan (p<0.0001). Most of participants (88.1%) thought that Ramadan had a negative effect on their sleeping pattern and affected their daytime functioning.

Although, the percentage of those who took a sedative-hypnotics for sleep disorders had significantly dropped from 7% at baseline to 3.3% during this month (p = 0.0001) (Table 3).

Daytime wakefulness

During Ramadan, participants found more difficult getting up in the mornings (74.1% versus 79% respectively, p<0.0001) (Table 4). The percentage of trainees who often arrived late for work or missed it increased significantly, from 3.7% at baseline to 11.9% during Ramadan (p<0.0001).

The majority (81.1%) reported feeling extra sleepy during the daytime of Ramadan month as compared to 60.1% during the previous month (p<0.0001). The time period of the day when trainees felt the sleepiest was the same for the two study periods. It was the end of the day, than in the morning (Figure 1).

With regard sleepiness at the wheel, the percentage was 4.5% at baseline, and has more than tripled over Ramadan to reach 13.6% (p<0.0001). Similar trends had been observed for concentration and memory disturbances which significantly increased to 88.9% during Ramadan as compared to 77% at baseline (p<0.0001).

		Before Ramadan	During Ramadan	P
Bedtime		9.7 ± 10.93 pm	3.80 ± 5.37 am	<0.0001
Bedtime after midnight (%)		57.1	93.1	0.001
Sleep latency (min)		18.98 ± 14.78	18.29 ± 16.61	0.508
Do you think you have insomnia (%)?	No	51.9	42.4	0.0001
	Small	33.3	28.4	0.0001
	Medium	10.7	16	0.0001
	Very	2.9	9.9	0.003
	Extremely	1.2	3.3	0.0001

Do you feel that you don't sleep enough at night (%)	Yes	18.9	54.7	0.0001
	Moderately satisfied	63.4	38.3	0.0001
	Highly satisfied	17.7	7	0.0001
Do you take sedative-hypnotics for sleep disorders (%)?	Yes	7	3,3	0.0001
	No	93	96.7	
Do you think Ramadan had a negative impact on your sleep pattern and daytime functioning (%)?	Yes	88.1		
	No	11.9		

Table 3: Pattern sleep before and during Ramadan.

		Before Ramadan (%)	**During Ramadan (%)**	**p**
Do you find more difficult getting up in the mornings?	Yes	74.1	79	0.0001
	No	25.9	21	
Do you arrive late for work or miss it?	Never	53.9	41.2	
	Hardly	42.4	46.9	
	Often	3.7	11.9	
Do you feel extra sleepy during the daytime?	Yes	60.1	81.1	
	No	39.9	18.9	
Do you feel sleepy sleepiness at the wheel?	Yes	4.5	13.6	
	No	95.5	86.4	
Do you have concentration and memory disturbances?	Yes	77	88.9	
	No	23	11.1	

Table 4: Daytime wakefulness before and during Ramadan.

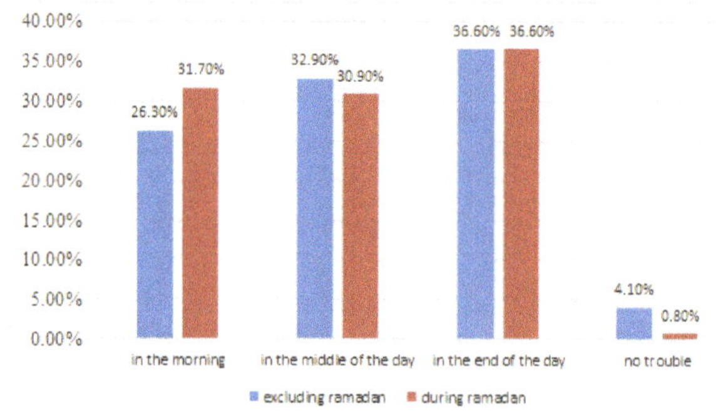

Figure 1: Time period of the day when trainees felt the sleepiest.

Somatic and psychiatric symptoms

Over Ramadan, the percentage of trainees who complained of excessive nervousness significantly increased to 65% as compared to 57.6% at baseline (p<0.001). Similarly, morning headaches were more than tripled during this month, as it were reported by 15.2% of trainees versus 6.6% before Ramadan (p<0.001). It was also noted a higher frequency of digestive disorders which concerned about the half of participants (46.9%) during Ramadan, while in the previous month, it was reported by only one third of them (29.6%) (p<0.009). Epigastralgia was the most common digestive complaint during the two study periods.

Working rhythm

Both daily and weekly working hours had significantly decreased during the month of Ramadan compared to the month prior (p<0.001). The number of night shifts per week had also decreased (p<0.001). Moreover, it was noted that trainees started their daily work 15 minutes later and left 20 minutes earlier, which results in 35 less minutes worked per day, and around 3 and half hours less per week.

Discussion

The present study explored the perception of young medical trainees in two Tunisian university hospitals regarding the impact of Ramadan fasting in their sleeping patterns, wakefulness and daytime functioning. A better understanding of this specific situation shall be helpful to propose suitable recommendations regarding working conditions, dietary habits and lifestyle behaviors adopted during Ramadan [3].

At baseline, smoking and alcohol consumption were notably less common than what was reported in general Tunisian population. In fact, smoking prevalence among Tunisian adults was estimated at 30.4% in 1996 as compared to 16% in our population [4]. Tunisians are also the heaviest drinkers in the Maghreb region, according to the World Health Organization. In contrast, only Ten point seven pour cent of our participants were drinkers, and most of them had low to moderate level drinking (average of 2.23 ± 2.8 cups per day). Coffee and tea were the preferred average by most of participants (respectively 83.1% and 56%) as they could potentially lead to an energetic impact, and improve wakefulness as well as mental performance.

During Ramadan, all these addictives behaviors were significantly reduced, which can be explained by a long fasting time, about 15 hours a day, while eating and drinking was allowed for only 9 hours a day [3]. Religious prohibition of alcohol was rigorously respected, and all drinkers had stopped drinking during the whole period of Ramadan. Similar result was reported in 2012 by Laraqui [5] in a cross-sectional study that concerned 2171 health care workers in a Moroccan hospital. However, no significant difference was found regarding coffee and tea consumption during Ramadan in comparison with the previous month. Likewise, in a Saudi study published in 2003 and including 56 Muslims healthy medical students, Bahammam [1] noted that there was no significant difference before and during Ramadan in the number of cups of tea, coffee, and chocolate or the number of cans of soda that subjects drank. In contrast with these findings, Laraqui [6], by asking 150 workers in a factory, reported a remarkable increasing consumption of energy drinks (coffee and tea) which was multiplied by four during Ramadan (from 12% to 50%).

Fasting during daytime leads to a sudden change in the circadian pattern of eating which concerns particularly meal schedule and frequency. As has been reported in previous study, the frequency of meals dropped significantly during Ramadan in our study [1,6]. Total food intake generally decreased [7] but a slight increase was reported in Moroccan and Saudi populations [8,9]. Similarly, in a study involving 147 Tunisian students from high health schools, Masmoudi [10] noted that Ramadan was notably associated with over-night eating and increasing consumption of sweet and anarchic food stuff. Eating such particular types of food at inappropriate times may be a factor in gastro-intestinal complaints and predisposes individuals to becoming overweight [11]. A significant correlation between the number of calories ingested during a meal and the duration of subsequent sleep has been reported in rats [12] but the relationship is less clear in humans. Similarly, eating at night after a day-time fast can disrupt sleep due to intestinal discomfort from eating too much or as sequel to hunger from having eaten too little earlier on [11].

Nearly two third of participants (61.3%) in our study used to take a second meal during Ramadan, and it was commonly late at night, before going to bed (commonly between 00:00 and 01:00 am). It has also been suggested that late occurrence of meals may be responsible for circadian rhythm changes in body temperature, and sleep onset latency, as a result. Actually, body temperature falls during sleep and rises at wake time [1]. In general, a falling body temperature induces sleep, whereas a rising temperature provokes wakefulness. During Ramadan, spicy nocturnal meals, the favorite food at Tunisian Ramadan table, can result in an increase in nocturnal body temperature which leads into delay in sleep onset [1,13-15]. Alternatively, the increased sleep latency could be explained by more specifically sleep-related mechanisms. Feedings has shown to induce an increase in the extracellular concentration of histamine in the hypothalamus. In turn, the hypothalamic administration of histamine is able to increase wakefulness [16]. The effect of Ramadan on sleep onset was also examined using the polysomnographic recordings before, at the beginning, at the end and after Ramadan. Sleep latency increased in the 10th and the 24th days of Ramadan. In our study, we didn't find any significant variation in the sleep latency.

The current study demonstrated a sudden and significant delay in bedtime and wake up during Ramadan, as compared to the month before, in agreement with previous works [1,5,10,14]. This delay occurred despite work commencement time did not change in Tunisian Hospitals during Ramadan, in contrast with others Muslims countries [15]. We hypothesize that, quite apart the changes in the circadian pattern of eating, several others factors may encourage participants to delay bedtimes, such as watching popular programs TV, gathering with families and friends, rising for the predawn meal and prayer, and many social activities that occur until late at night during Ramadan [14]. More than 60% of fasting individuals who stayed awake after 11:00 pm attributed their wakefulness to socializing with families and friends and watching TV [1,12].

As consequence of these nocturnal alterations, most of our study participants (88.1) thought that Ramadan had a negative effect on their sleeping pattern, and the frequency of dissatisfaction with sleep quality increased to 54.7% during Ramadan, as compared to 18.9% at baseline. In a sample of 734 Malaysian junior-level Muslim athletes, there was an equivocal opinion on whether Ramadan fast had any effect on their sleeping pattern. Of those who claimed that their sleep patterns were altered, about 45.9% complained of a reduction in sleeping duration and 45.4% reported that the quality and duration of their sleep were affected [17]. The same finding was reported by Bahammam [1], although, in this study, the total sleep time did not change before and during Ramadan. Rocky et al. [13] have demonstrated that the proportion of non-rapid eye movement sleep increased during Ramadan, particularly stage 2 which represents the light sleep; In contrast, Slow-wave sleep (deep sleep) duration and rapid eye movement sleep duration decreased. These disturbances of sleep structure may explain the subjective feeling of poor sleep quality during Ramadan even when getting the same amount of sleep as the previous month [1].

It appears that Ramadan has detrimental effects on daytime function and sleepiness. In support, it was observed that the majority (81.1%) of our study participants suffered from extra-daytime sleepiness during of Ramadan month as compared to 60.1% during the previous month. Several studies have assessed daytime sleepiness during Ramadan, subjectively, and objectively using the multiple sleep latency test (MSLTS) [15]. Among 734 Malaysian Muslim athletes, Singh et al. [17] noted that the majority of athletes (66.6%) reported feeling extra-sleepy during the daytime of the Ramadan month and 61.2% of these athletes took extra naps between 1-2 hours in the daytime during the fasting month. Likewise, in a sample including 2171 health care workers in Moroccan hospitals [5], sleepiness at work increased to 49.8% as compared to 9.8% at baseline, and the frequency of Epworth greater to 10 increased from 19.4% to 46%. Bahammam noted that the percentage of medical students who reported falling asleep in class increased from 15% at baseline to 36% during the first week of Ramadan [1]. The study of Roky [18] including 8 young Muslims showed an increase in daytime sleepiness, especially at 10:00

and 12:00 am at the end of Ramadan, and a decrease in daytime body temperature during Ramadan. Objective measure of alertness by the MSLT confirmed these results. Sleep latency, which is inversely proportional to sleepiness, increased during the daytime, particularly at 10:00 am, 12:00 am and 04:00 pm [19].

Conflicting results have been reported with regard to the effect of Ramadan fasting on daytime function. Several studies including university students [19-21] reported that fasting may cause mood swings, morning headaches, lethargic feelings, high overall fatigue-levels, decreased memory which in turn can lead to loosing of hours work and decreased work performance as was observed in our study [17]. Similarly, Bahammam noted that the percentage of subjects who exercise regularly dropped from 24% before Ramadan to 5% at the end of Ramadan without any clear reason of this decline [1]. During the first week of Ramadan, psychomotor performance indicators such as critical flicker fusion [21] and choice reaction time [22] have been reported to be impaired. These changes were more important in regular smokers and coffee consumers [7]. In contrast of these findings, Lotfi S reported that physical performance was not dramatically impairment during Ramadan in 9 male resistance athletes. A study in a Jordan population has reported that suicidal behavior decreased during Ramadan [23].

There are different hypothesis to explain sleepiness and daytime dysfunction during Ramadan. Some studies suggested that sleep deprivation or disruption, even modest may be responsible, as was the case in our study [24-28]. Based on this hypothesis, Bahammam demonstrated that if a regimen of a fixed sleep-wake schedule and a fixed caloric intake is followed during intermittent fasting, the effect of fasting on sleep architecture and daytime sleepiness will be minimal. Metabolic changes during the intermittent fasting have been also ruled out as possible factor for increase in subjective and objective sleepiness. Actually Ramadan diurnal fasting lead to decrease in the resting rate and energy expenditure, which in return bring about diurnal rectal temperature decrease as was observed by Roky [18]. It also induces increased cerebral theta activity [22].

Several strategies may be helpful to circumvent or reduce the adverse perturbations of Ramadan fasting. Trainees must realize the importance of sleep as part of their overall rest and recovery strategies, and prioritize sleep time over their evening social activities to increase sleep time. Taking a short afternoon nap is also recommended. Otherwise, fasted trainees can sleep ~1 hour earlier in the evening instead of taking naps during the day. In addition, taking three main meals especially the meal right before dawn is very important to have sufficient amount of calories over the 24 hours period during Ramadan. However, excessive eating at night, particularly prior to sleep should be ovoid. It also reasonable to improve training conditions as working in a hot and humid environment will result in a greater thermoregulatory challenge to the fasted trainees.

Our study has a few limitations that need to be addressed. First, the sample size of subjects recruited was small. The survey could only determine the subjective perception of participants, as no objective assessment methods was used. It was also difficult to distinguish the specific role of Ramadan in daytime sleepiness and functioning from others possible confounder factors such as sleep deprivation or disruption. Moreover, it must be noted that the findings of this study are specific to Tunisian Muslim medical trainees, and they are not necessarily valid as regards other countries observing Ramadan fasting. Further researches in Tunisia and adjacent Maghreb countries with polysomnographic recording is needed to objectively assess the effects of Islamic intermittent fasting on sleep architecture and daytime sleepiness.

Conclusion

Our study suggests that changes in lifestyle and eating behaviors during Ramadan may impact daytime sleepiness and functioning, which in return impair work performance. In contrast, the specific role of intermittent Islamic fasting is not supported by the available data. An approach to develop a tailored sleep health education and suitable nutritional behavior could be helpful to minimize adverse side effects on daytime function during fasting in medical trainees. Similarly, work rhythm should be adapted to specificities of this month.

References

1. BaHammam A (2003) Sleep pattern, daytime sleepiness, and eating habits during the month of Ramadan. Sleep Hypn 5: 165-174.
2. Laraqui CH, Tripodi D, Laraqui O, Rahhali A, Caubet A, et al. (2001) The effects of fasting and of the quality of sleep on work during the month of Ramadan. Arch Mal Prof 62: 115-120
3. Khalfallah T, Chaari N, Henchi MA, AbdallahB, Chikh RB, et al. (2004) Evaluation of the impact of Ramadan fasting on the physical workload. Archives des Arch Mal Prof 65: 564-570.
4. Fakhfakh R, Hsairi M, Maalej M, Achour N, Nacef T (2002) Tobacco use in Tunisia: behaviour and awareness. Bull World Health Organ 80: 350-356.
5. Laraqui S, Manar N, Laraqui O, Caubet A, Verger C, et al. (2012) Influence of Ramadan observance on wakefulness at work among health care workers in Morocco. Arch Mal Prof Env 73: 743-749.
6. Roky R, Houti I, Moussamih S, Qotbi S, Aadil N (2004) Physiological and chronobiological changes during Ramadan intermittent fasting. Ann Nutr Metab 48: 296-303.
7. Frost G, Pirani S (1987) Meal frequency and nutritional intake during Ramadan: a pilot study. Hum Nutr Appl Nutr 41: 47-50.
8. Adlouni A, Ghalim N, Benslimane A, Lecerf JM, Saile R (1997) Fasting during Ramadan induces a marked increase in high-density lipoprotein cholesterol and decrease in low-density lipoprotein cholesterol. Ann Nutr Metab 41: 242-249.
9. Reilly T, Waterhouse J (2007) Altered sleep-wake cycles and food intake: the Ramadan model. Physiol Behav 90: 219-28.
10. Masmoudi J, Trabelsi S, Elleuch A, Jaoua A (2008) Eating disorders during and outside ramadan. JTCC 18: 26-31.
11. Danguir J, Nicolaidis (1979) Dependence of sleep on nutrients' availability. Physiol Behav 22: 735-740.
12. BaHammam A, Alrajeh M, Albabtain M, Bahammam S, Sharif M (2010) Circadian pattern of sleep, energy expenditure, and body temperature of young healthy men during the intermittent fasting of Ramadan. Appetite 54: 426-429.
13. Roky R, Chapotot F, Hakkou F, Benchekroun MT, Buguet A (2001) Sleep during Ramadan intermittent fasting. J Sleep Res 10: 319-327.
14. Bahammam A (2006) Does Ramadan fasting affect sleep? Int J Clin Pract 60: 1631-1637.
15. BaHammam A (2006) Assessment of sleep patterns, daytime sleepiness, and chronotype during Ramadan in fasting and nonfasting individuals. Saudi Med J 26: 616-22.
16. Kadri N, Tilane A, El Batal M, Taltit Y, Tahiri SM, et al. (2000) Irritability during the month of Ramadan. Psychosom Med 62: 280-285.
17. Singh R, Hwa OC, Roy J, Jin CW, Ismail SM, et al. (2011) Subjective Perception of Sports Performance, Training, Sleep and Dietary Patterns of Malaysian Junior Muslim Athletes during Ramadan Intermittent Fasting. Asian J Sports Med 2: 167-176.

18. Roky RJ, Chapotot F, Benchekroun MT, Benaji B, Hakkou F, et al. (2003) Daytime sleepiness during Ramadan intermittent fasting: polysomnographic and quantitative waking EEG study. Sleep 12: 95-101.
19. Ennigrou S, Zenaidi M, Ben Slama F, Zouari B, Nacef T (2001) Ramadan and customs of life: investigation with 84 adult residents in the district of Tunis. Tunis Med 79: 508-514.
20. Ali MR, Amir T (1989) Effects of fasting on visual flicker fusion. Percept Mot Skills 69: 627-631.
21. Daradkeh TK (1992) Parasuicide during Ramadan in Jordan. Acta Psychiatr Scand 86: 253-254.
22. Devoto A, Lucidi F, Violani C, Bertini M (1999) Effects of different sleep reductions on daytime sleepiness. Sleep 22: 336-343.
23. Aziz AR, Png W (2008) Practical tips to exercise training during the Ramadan fasting month. ISN Bulletin 1: 13-19.
24. Paus T, Zatorre RJ, Hofle N, Caramanos Z, Gotman J, et al. (1997) Time-related changes in neural systems underlying attention and arousal during the performance of an auditory vigilance task. J Cogn Neurosci 9: 392-408.
25. Roky R, Iraki L, HajKhlifa R, Lakhdar Ghazal N, Hakkou F (2000) Daytime alertness, mood, psychomotor performances, and oral temperature during Ramadan intermittent fasting. Ann Nutr Metab 44: 101-107.
26. Lotfi S, Madani M, Abassi A, Tazi A, Boumahmaza M, et al. (2010) CNS Activation, reaction time, blood pressure and heart rate variation during Ramadan intermittent fasting and exercise. WJSS 3: 37-43.
27. Bahammam AS, Almushailhi K, Pandi-Perumal SR, Sharif MM (2014) Intermittent fasting during Ramadan: does it affect sleep? J Sleep Res 23: 35-43.
28. Aziz AR, Wahid MF, Png W, Jesuvadian CV (2010) Effects of Ramadan fasting on 60 min of endurance running performance in moderately trained men. Br J Sports Med 44: 516-521.

Mandibular Advancement Device Therapy in Obstructive Sleep Apnea and Snoring in Community Dental Care: Two-year Follow-up Study on Self-reported Sleep Quality, Side Effects, and Compliance

Tiina-Riitta Vuorjoki-Ranta[1*], Frank Lobbezoo[2], Henri Tuomilehto[3,4], Mauno Könönen[5], Antti Pihakari[1] and Jari Ahlberg[1,5]

[1]*Helsinki Health Centre, Unit for Specialized Oral Care in the Metropolitan Area and Kirkkonummi, Helsinki, Finland*

[2]*Department of Oral Kinesiology, Academic Centre for Dentistry Amsterdam (ACTA), University of Amsterdam and VU University Amsterdam, MOVE Research Institute Amsterdam, Amsterdam, The Netherlands*

[3]*Oivauni Sleep Clinic, Kuopio, Finland*

[4]*Institute of Public Health and Clinical Nutrition, Department of Clinical Nutrition, University of Eastern Finland*

[5]*Department of Stomatognathic Physiology and Prosthetic Dentistry, Institute of Dentistry, University of Helsinki, Finland*

[*]**Corresponding author:** Tiina-Riitta Vuorjoki-Ranta, Doctor of Dental Surgery, Helsinki Health Center, Toinen linja 4 C, 00530, Finland, E-mail: t.vuorjoki@kolumbus.fi

Abstract

Study background: Obesity is constantly increasing health problem worldwide and so are its detrimental consequences, including obstructive sleep apnea (OSA). Mandibular advancement devices (MADs) are proven to be efficient in treating mild to moderate OSA and snoring. We followed for two years 103 patients treated with a titrable MAD in a Community Dental Care setting.

Methods: A follow-up questionnaire was mailed in 2012 to 124 patients who had participated in a survey 2010 and given their consent for further study.

Results: Of all the 103 respondents 85% (n=88) still used MAD. Subjective tiredness ($p<0.05$) and the presence of any snoring ($p<0.01$) were reported more often in the long-term study than in the short-term study. In contrast, difficulty in initiating sleep with the device in situ was seen less often ($p<0.05$). According to the logistic regression, reduced loud snoring was significantly associated with the compliance of frequent wear of MAD ($p<0.05$). The majority (82%) of the patients also reported a positive impact of MAD in social (family) life due to reduced loud snoring.

Conclusion: Titrable MAD is a noteworthy treatment modality for mild to moderate OSA and especially snoring. Compliance in using MADs and reported subjective health seem to remain at good level. General dentists could probably perform a great part of the care. However, possible worsening of OSA and side effects of MADs should be borne in mind.

Keywords: Obstructive sleep apnea; Snoring; Oral appliance; Compliance; Community dental care; Long-term study

Introduction

The use of mandible advancement devices (MAD) in the treatment of obstructive sleep apnea (OSA) and snoring has increasingly become an alternative treatment modality for continuous positive airway pressure (CPAP) in patients with mild to moderate OSA. In these patients, clinical studies have shown equal efficacy between both modalities on ambulatory blood pressure, daytime sleepiness, and quality of life, among other things [1]. These results may also be explained by good clinical use of MAD, since particularly in mild OSA, the compliance with CPAP is frequently far from optimal [2-5].

Bearing in mind the increasing incidence of OSA worldwide [6,7] there is a need to improve clinical guidelines to be able to provide the best possible treatment option for each patient. In addition, the treatment modalities need to manage this condition cost-effectively. OSA is a chronic, progressive disease and particularly, the more severe stages of OSA have been linked to an increased risk of cardiovascular morbidity and mortality [8,9].

Obesity is the most important risk factor for OSA and based on current knowledge about the evolution of OSA, it is particularly the weight gain that represents a high risk for further progression towards more severe disease [10]. Recent studies have well-demonstrated that lifestyle intervention, including an early weight reduction program, represents a feasible and effective treatment for OSA and the achieved beneficial changes are sustained even four years after the active intervention, thus preventing the progression of the disease or even curing it in obese patients with OSA [11,12].

On the other hand, it has been shown that deviations in craniofacial morphology are much more common in normal weight than in overweight adult patients with OSA [13]. Together, these findings imply that there may be three different phenotypes of sleep-disordered breathing; one related to excess fat tissue, the other to craniofacial abnormalities and the third a combination of these two phenotypes.

Hence, especially in normal-weight patients with mild or moderate OSA and in the case of disturbing snoring, MAD could represent a first-line treatment strategy.

Not only the efficacy but also the possible side effects of a treatment play important roles when choosing one treatment over the other. MAD reportedly causes symptoms of temporomandibular disorders (TMD), tooth pain, and development of posterior open bite [14-16]. This may seriously affect the compliance, thus resulting in discontinuing of treatment. However, the adverse symptoms are often transient. Also, loss or frequent breakage of the device, along with the cost of repairing or replacing it, may lead to cessation of treatment [17].

Our recent pilot study, based on self-report on short-term MAD treatment among patients in Community Dental Care, showed good compliance and a fair treatment effect on sleep quality [18]. As many as four out of every five patients had worn their device at least three nights per week, while sleep was reported being significantly less disrupted and more restorative, leading to markedly less frequent daytime sleepiness.

To our knowledge, thus far no other study exists on the effects of MAD on OSA and snoring that has been performed among patients treated in Community Dental Care. The aim of this study was to evaluate self-reported longer-term effects and compliance of MAD treatment in this specific setting, perhaps presenting better the real-life setting of the treatment.

Materials and Methods

A pilot questionnaire study was performed in 2010 [18], comprising 142 patients who had received MAD treatment for OSA or snoring in the Unit for Specialized Oral Care in the Metropolitan Area in Finland. The unit is a part of the public dental care system with subsidy. All patients had been treated with a titrable Herbst-type MAD. To the participants of that study, a follow-up questionnaire was mailed in 2012. Altogether, 124 respondents who had completed the pilot questionnaire and gave written consent to the additional study were mailed the follow-up questionnaire.

From the questionnaire, data were categorized for the present study as follows:

Descriptive data: gender, age, weight, length, tobacco use, alcohol consumption (equivalent doses of beer, wine, or spirits), aspects of general health, and orofacial pain experience during the past month [18-20]. The body mass index (BMI) was calculated from the weight and length data. Data on treatment decision-making, prior dental treatment, adaptation to the treatment, device maintenance need, and various subjective side effects were also included.

Compliance in using the oral appliance: self-assessed frequency of wearing the MAD (never or less than once a month, less than weekly, 1-2 nights per week, 3-5 nights per week, every night or almost every night).

Insomnia symptoms [7,21]: difficulties initiating sleep (DIS), disrupted sleep (DS), and early morning awakenings (EMA) (symptoms present at least 3 nights per week).

Perceived consequences of sleep: non-restorative sleep (NRS) (sustained>1 month), and tiredness (at least 3 days per week).

Snoring: as perceived or reported by a bed partner (every night or almost every night).

Type of snoring: as reported and confirmed by bed partner (smooth and quiet, smooth and rather loud, smooth and loud, intermittent and very loud)

Statistical analysis

For the demographic data, the Chi square test was used to study the associations between the categorical variables. Student's t-test was used to compare the group means when the data were normally distributed, and when not, the Mann-Whitney U-test was applied. McNemar change test was used to compare the insomnia symptoms and perceived consequences of sleep between short-term and long-term studies. Logistic regression was used to study the probability of the compliance of frequent wearing of the MAD ('every night' or 'almost every night'=1, else=0). Independent variables entered into the model, adjusted by BMI, age, and gender, were; NRS (yes=1, no=0), DS (yes=1, no=0), intermittent very loud snoring (yes=1, no=0). The method enter was used, i.e., all independent variables were entered in the model as a single step.

Results

The response rate of eligible subjects of the second questionnaire was 83% (n=103). The flow chart of the study is shown in Figure 1. Of all the respondents, 85% still used the MAD (n=88), 67% of them were male (n=59). Mean lifetime of devices i.e. the mean time period between oral appliance put to use and the return date of long-term survey was 35 months (2.9 years) (SD=11.0), the longest period being 67 months (5.6 years) and the shortest 23 months (1.9 years). As compared with the short-term study [18], there were no significant differences in the demographic data, viz., age, gender, BMI, alcohol consumption, and smoking status.

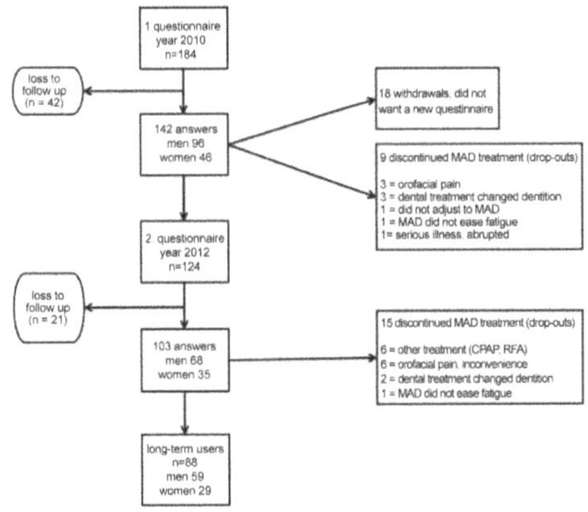

Figure 1: Flow chart of the study

OSA was diagnosed in 77.3%, the rest 22.7% was diagnosed as snorers. In both genders, health was more often reported as 'very good' or 'good' than in the pilot study ($p<0.05$) (45% of women and 54% of men). None of the respondents in the present study reported their health as 'very poor'. Compared to the pilot study (figures in parentheses), diagnosed illnesses were: hypertension blood pressure 36 % (35%), allergic rhinitis 28% (25%) and cardiac arrhythmia 17%

(18%) (NS). Cardiac arrhythmia was more common in women, viz. 28%, than in men (12%.) Other diagnosed illnesses were not related to gender.

The subjects had significantly less difficulty in initiating sleep with MAD in situ than what they reported earlier ($p<0.05$). Altogether 82% of patients claimed that MAD has a positive impact on personal life due to reduced loud snoring. Whereas subjective tiredness ($p<0.05$) and snoring ($p<0.01$) were reported more often than in the short-term study. Table 1 shows perceived insomnia symptoms and snoring and related daytime consequences between baseline and the present study.

n=88	%	Baseline	Long-term	p value
DIS		10.2	2.3	0.039
DS		39.8	52.3	0.072
EMA		11.4	13.6	0.774
NRS		4.5	6.8	0.727
Tiredness		15.9	27.3	0.021
Snoring		14.8	36.4	0.002

Table 1: Overall occurrence of perceived insomnia symptoms and their awake consequences at baseline and two-year long-term. McNemar change test (DIS: difficulties initiating sleep, DS: disrupted sleep, EMA: early morning awakening, NRS: non-restorative sleep).

The treatment of OSA was initiated by a physician for the majority (81%) and the rest by a dentist. None of the subjects had received treatment by their own request. Prior dental check-up to the treatment was performed in 36%. Most often reported problems with wearing the MAD were sore teeth (39%), soreness in masticatory muscles (37%), and experience that the teeth do not fit (27%) upon awakening. Orofacial pain experience within the past month was reported more often (31% vs. 22%, $p<0.01$) in the present study than in the short-term study.

Within a short period after initiating the treatment altogether 75% of patients had well adapted to the MAD. Logistic regression, adjusted by BMI, age and gender, revealed a significant association between good compliance (frequent use of MAD) and less loud snoring ($p<0.05$) (Table 2).

n=88	Odds Ratio	91% confidence interval	p-value
NRS	0.5	0.1-5.1	0.51
DS	0.9	0.2-4.0	0.26
Loud snoring	0.6	0.3-0.9	0.04

Table 2: The compliance of frequent wear of the MAD Logistic regression (NRS: non-restorative sleep, DS: disrupted sleep Model adjusted by BMI, age, and gender).

Discussion

The present study is the first long-term study on the treatment of OSA with MADs in Community Dental Care. Main reason for carrying out this study was to clarify possibilities in treating the increasing amount of patients with sleep-disordered breathing [22] in common dental practice. Long-term studies in such real-life setting are lacking according to our knowledge.

The main finding of the present study was that treatment of OSA with MAD is well tolerated and its compliance remains good. This is also supported in studies carried out in specialist settings [16,17,23-25]. MAD was found to reduce loud snoring. Also, the occurrence of early morning awakenings (EMA) and non-restorative sleep (NRS) remained at low level among respondents in the follow-up period. In addition, morning sleepiness remained minor in follow-up.

Some of the subjective benefits that emerged initially in our short-term study were less prevalent. Daytime tiredness was more often reported. Similarly, disrupted sleep (DS) and the frequency of snoring were reportedly increased. This set back of longer-term subjective benefits has also been shown in a study by Ghazal et al. [26]. Although half of the respondents stated their health as 'good' or 'very good' (in our short-term study 41%), and none continuously as 'poor' or 'very poor', our results indicate that long-term follow-up and, when needed, adjustment of the device may be necessary to obtain the best possible result.

In the present study orofacial pain was reported more frequently than in our short-term study. This is contradictory to what has been reported earlier regarding TMD, i.e., TMD having a transient nature in association with MAD [14,16]. However, we only used a single question to evaluate this (derived from the Finnish translation of the RDC/TMD): "Have you had pain in the face, jaw, temple, in front ear or in the ear in the past month?") [19,20]. Bearing in mind the quasi-static nature of TMD, our findings have to be interpreted cautiously. Also, posterior open bite (POB) as a complication has been reported in clinical studies earlier [15,16], which due to the study design cannot be evaluated here.

Limitation of the present study is that it is based on a questionnaire without objective evidence. Yet, only few longer-term studies exist in this field [27,28]. Also, the sample size (n=103) in our study may be considered fair [23]. Nevertheless, larger-scale studies that include clinical evidence are certainly needed. However, few follow-up studies have concentrated on subjective results of sleep quality. In fact, most existing studies have focused on the influence of MAD on aspects of the masticatory system, namely, TMD-problems [14-16].

When evaluating an impact of treatment long-term evidence is essential. Unfortunately, most published studies have been concentrating only on short-time use of MADs. As seen in the present study, the long-term effects of MAD on sleep quality weakened to some extent, which was a disappointment, as the results in our previous study [18] as well as in other short-term studies [29,30] have been promising. On the other hand, Jauhar et al. reported only modest improvement in sleep quality in their ten-year follow-up study [25]. Nevertheless, McGown et al. and Wiman Eriksson et al. found improved daytime tiredness compared to baseline in a long-term design [27,28]. This all may be summoned that more intensive control of effect of the treatment, i.e. regular checkups of the symptoms and if needed, the devices, may be advisable for better results.

Since the treatment of OSA is demanding, there are no simple solutions and the treatment must always be planned individually. It is important to keep on improving the current treatment modalities and, in addition, trying to find new guidelines for better treatment of OSA patients. There seems to be several phenotypes of OSA patients i.e. related to obesity or cranio-facial anatomy. Furthermore, it may be a combination of different factors and treatment may modulate the underlying mechanisms. Tuomilehto et al showed that weight loss of obese OSA patients could reduce the amount of respiratory events in both supine and non-supine positions [11]. However, the reduction in the number of events was higher in the non-supine position. Especially for positional OSA, where most of the respiratory events occur in supine position, oral appliances are shown to be particularly effective and may offer an important alternative to CPAP [31,32]. However, it seems that regular follow-up and support for MAD users may be essential.

Acknowledgement

This study was supported by grants from the City of Helsinki Health Centre and the Finnish Association of Women Dentists.

References

1. Phillips CL, Grunstein RR, Darendeliler MA, Mihailidou AS, Srinivasan VK, et al. (2013) Health outcomes of continuous positive airway pressure versus oral appliance treatment for obstructive sleep apnea: a randomized controlled trial. Am J Respir Crit Care Med 187: 879-887.
2. Health Quality Ontario (2009) Oral appliances for obstructive sleep apnea: an evidence-based analysis. Ont Health Technol Assess Ser 9: 1-51.
3. White DP, Shafazand S (2013) Mandibular advancement device vs. CPAP in the treatment of obstructive sleep apnea: are they equally effective in Short term health outcomes? J Clin Sleep Med 9: 971-972.
4. Marklund M, Verbraecken J, Randerath W. (2012) Non-CPAP therapies in obstructive sleep apnoea: mandibular advancement device therapy. Eur Respir J 39: 1241-7.
5. Gagnadoux F, Fleury B, Vielle B, Pételle B, Meslier N, et al. (2009) Titrated mandibular advancement versus positive airway pressure for sleep apnoea. Eur Respir J 34: 914-920.
6. Lam JC, Sharma SK, Lam B (2010) Obstructive sleep apnoea: definitions, epidemiology & natural history. Indian J Med Res 131: 165-170.
7. Ohayon MM, Partinen M (2002) Insomnia and global sleep dissatisfaction in Finland. J Sleep Res 11: 339-346.
8. Punjabi NM, Caffo BS, Goodwin JL, Gottlieb DJ, Newman AB, et al. (2009) Sleep-disordered breathing and mortality: a prospective cohort study. PLoS Med 6: e1000132.
9. Marin JM, Carrizo SJ, Vicente E, Agusti AG (2005) Long-term cardiovascular outcomes in men with obstructive sleep apnoea-hypopnoea with or without treatment with continuous positive airway pressure: an observational study. Lancet 365: 1046-1053.
10. Berger G, Berger R, Oksenberg A (2009) Progression of snoring and obstructive sleep apnoea: the role of increasing weight and time. Eur Respir J 33: 338-345.
11. Tuomilehto HP, Seppä JM, Partinen MM, Peltonen M, Gylling H, et al. (2009) Lifestyle intervention with weight reduction: first-line treatment in mild obstructive sleep apnea. Am J Respir Crit Care Med 179: 320-327.
12. Tuomilehto H, Seppä J, Uusitupa M, Tuomilehto J, Gylling H on behalf of the Kuopio Sleep Apnea Group. (2013) Weight reduction and increased physical activity prevent the progression of obstructive sleep apnea: A 4-year observational postintervention follow-up of a randomized clinical trial. JAMA Intern Med 173: 930-2.
13. Pahkala R, Puustinen R, Tuomilehto H, Ahlberg J, Seppä J (2011) Risk factors for sleep-disordered breathing: the role of craniofacial structure. Acta Odontol Scand 69: 137-143.
14. Doff MH, Veldhuis SK, Hoekema A, Slater JJ, Wijkstra PJ, et al. (2012) Long-term oral appliance therapy in obstructive sleep apnea syndrome: a controlled study on temporomandibular side effects. Clin Oral Investig 16: 689-697.
15. Perez CV, de Leeuw R, Okeson JP, Carlson CR, Li HF, et al. (2013) The incidence and prevalence of temporomandibular disorders and posterior open bite in patients receiving mandibular advancement device therapy for obstructive sleep apnea. Sleep Breath 17: 323-32.
16. Fransson AM, Tegelberg A, Johansson A, Wenneberg B (2004) Influence on the masticatory system in treatment of obstructive sleep apnea and snoring with a mandibular protruding device: a 2-year follow-up. Am J Orthod Dentofacial Orthop 126: 687-693.
17. Brette C, Ramanantsoa H, Renouardiere J, Renouardiere R, Roisman G, et al. (2012) A mandibular advancement device for the treatment of obstructive sleep apnea: long-term use and tolerance. Int Orthod 10: 363-376.
18. Vuorjoki-Ranta TR, Lobbezoo F, Tuomilehto H, Könönen M, Pihakari A, et al. (2013) Mandibular advancement devices in the treatment of obstructive sleep apnea and snoring in community dental care: a pilot study on self-reported sleep quality. Health 5: 1-5.
19. Schiffman E, Ohrbach R, Truelove E, Look J, Anderson G, et al. (2014) Diagnostic Criteria for Temporomandibular Disorders (DC/TMD) for Clinical and Research Applications: Recommendations of the International RDC/TMD Consortium Network and Orofacial Pain Special Interest Group. J Oral Facial Pain Headache 28: 6-27.
20. Suvinen T, Rantala M, Könönen M, Ahlberg J, Bergen D. et al. (2010) Research Diagnostic Criteria for Temporomandibular Disorders (RDC/TMD. Finnish Translation 2010.
21. American Academy of Sleep Medicine (AASM). (2001) ICSD – International classification of sleep disorders, revised: Diagnostic and coding manual. American Academy of Sleep Medicine.
22. McClean KM, Kee F, Young IS, Elborn JS (2008) Obesity and the lung: 1. Epidemiology. Thorax 63: 649-654.
23. Marklund M, Sahlin C, Stenlund H, Persson M, Franklin KA (2001) Mandibular advancement device in patients with obstructive sleep apnea : long-term effects on apnea and sleep. Chest 120: 162-169.
24. Tison C, Sébille-Elhage S, Ferri J (2011) [Mandibular advancement device: a 5-year long experience in obstructive sleep apnea/hypopnea syndrome]. Rev Stomatol Chir Maxillofac 112: 80-86.
25. Jauhar S, Lyons MF, Banham SW, Cameron DA, Orchardson R (2008) Ten-year follow-up of mandibular advancement devices for the management of snoring and sleep apnea. J Prosthet Dent 99: 314-321.
26. Ghazal A, Sorichter S, Jonas I, Rose EC (2009) A randomized prospective long-term study of two oral appliances for sleep apnoea treatment. J Sleep Res 18: 321-328.
27. McGown AD, Makker HK, Battagel JM, L'Estrange PR, Grant HR, et al. (2001) Long-term use of mandibular advancement splints for snoring and obstructive sleep apnoea: a questionnaire survey. Eur Respir J 17: 462-466.
28. Wiman Eriksson E, Leissner L, Isacsson G, Fransson A (2014) A prospective 10-year follow-up polygraphic study of patients treated with a mandibular protruding device. Sleep Breath .
29. Aarab G, Lobbezoo F, Hamburger HL, Naeije M. (2011) Oral appliance therapy versus nasal continuous positive airway pressure in obstructive sleep apnea: a randomized, placebo-controlled trial. Respiration 81: 411-19.
30. Petri N, Svanholt P, Solow B, Wildschiødtz G, Winkel P (2008) Mandibular advancement appliance for obstructive sleep apnoea: results of a randomised placebo controlled trial using parallel group design. J Sleep Res 17: 221-229.
31. Yoshida K (2001) Influence of sleep posture on response to oral appliance therapy for sleep apnea syndrome. Sleep 24: 538-544.
32. Marklund M, Persson M, Franklin KA (1998) Treatment success with a mandibular advancement device is related to supine-dependent sleep apnea. Chest 114: 1630-1635.

Obstructive Sleep Apnea as a Risk Factor for Atrial Fibrillation

Irini Youssef[1], Haroon Kamran[1], Mena Yacoub[2], Nirav Patel[3], Clive Goulbourne[1], Shweta Kumar[1], Jesse Kane[1], Haley Hoffner[1], Moro Salifu[1] and Samy I McFarlane[1*]

[1]Department of Medicine, Divisions of Endocrinology, Cardiology and Renal Medicine, State University of New York, Downstate Medical Center, Brooklyn, NY, USA

[2]Department of Cardiology, Northside Hospital, St. Petersburg FL, USA

[3]Department of Cardiology, Hartford Hospital, Hartford, CT

[*]**Corresponding author:** Samy I. McFarlane, Department of Medicine, Divisions of Endocrinology, Cardiology and Renal Medicine, State University of New York, Downstate Medical Center, Brooklyn, NY, USA, E-mail: smcfarlane@downstate.edu

Abstract

Objectives: To conducted a meta-analysis assessing the relationship between Obstructive Sleep Apnea (OSA) and the risk of Atrial Fibrillation (AF)

Methods: We searched PUBMED, Medline, and Cochrane Library using the keywords “atrial fibrillation”, “obstructive sleep apnea” and “sleep disordered breathing (SDB)”. All subjects included had established diagnosis of OSA/SDB. We then compared the occurrence of AF versus no AF. Analysis done with Comprehensive Meta-Analysis package V3 (Biostat, USA).

Results: A total of 579 results were generated. Duplicates were removed and 372 records were excluded based on irrelevant abstracts, titles, study design not consistent with the stated outcome, or full-text unavailable. Twelve studies meeting the inclusion criteria were reviewed in full-text; 2 of these articles were eventually removed due to unconfirmed OSA diagnostic modality, and one was also removed based on a control group inconsistent with the other studies. Therefore, a total of 9 studies were included (n=19,837). Sample sizes ranged from n=160 patients to n=6841 patients. The risk of AF was found to be higher among OSA/SDB versus control group (OR; 2.120, C.I: 1.845- 2.436, Z; 10.598 p: <0.001). The heterogeneity observed for the pooled analysis was Q-value; 22.487 df (Q); 8 P-value; 0.004, I-squared; 64.424 Tau2; 0.098, suggesting appropriate study selection and moderate heterogeneity.

Conclusion: OSA/SDB is strongly associated with AFib confirming the notion that OSA/SDB populations are high risk for development of AF. Prospective studies are needed to ascertain the effect of the treatment of OSA/SDB for the prevention of AF, a growing health burden with serious consequences.

Keywords: Sleep Apnea; Atrial Fibrillation; Meta-analysis; Health; Cardiac arrhythmias

Introduction

AF is a growing health problem worldwide, estimated to affect 5.6 million to 15.9 million people in the United States by 2050 [1]. It is associated with an increased risk for morbidity and mortality [2], Modifiable risk factors for AF have been delineated, and include hypertension, obesity and alcohol consumption [3]. As the incidence of AF continues to rise, it is imperative to identify and treat potentially modifiable risk factors for the disease. OSA/SDB has been identified as potentially modifiable risk factors for AF. OSA is generally under-diagnosed medical problem, estimated to affect as many as 1 in 5 adults with the incidence on the rise as the obesity epidemic continues to grow [4]. OSA is associated with a myriad of negative health consequences including hypertension, heart disease, depression, and premature mortality [5]. Growing evidence suggests that OSA may be implicated in providing both a substrate and maintenance factor for AF [6]. There have been several proposed hypothesis as well as animal models attempting to clarify the role of the underlying pathophysiological mechanisms of OSA on the genesis of AF; however, there are little or no controlled studies of all relevant available data, showing a direct impact of OSA on the incidence of AF.

We now aim to extend prior work explaining the relationship between OSA and AF by performing a comprehensive meta-analysis reporting the association between OSA and AF.

The objective of this meta-analysis is to integrate all available data in an effort to identify a role, if any, of OSA on the development or progression of AF.

Methods

We searched databases including PUBMED, Medline, and Cochrane Library for relevant studies using the keywords “atrial fibrillation” and “obstructive sleep apnea”. Relevant references cited in other studies were also scrutinized for the study objective. Studies included in our meta-analysis provided odds-ratio or relative-risk values with 95% confidence intervals (CIs).

The OSA group, included an apnea-hypopnea index of ≥ 5 as diagnostic of OSA or 3% oxygen desaturation index (ODI) of >15 events, or a respiratory disturbance index (RDI) of >30 events. The Control group for all studies was defined as no recent or prior diagnosis of OSA by history or diagnostic testing (all indices <5 events).

To qualify for inclusion, the study must have (1) designated OSA as the exposure; (2) have a proper control group (no OSA) as mentioned; (3) have atrial fibrillation as the primary outcome, or an outcome amongst other diagnosed arrhythmia; (4) must have mentioned its criteria for diagnosing OSA, and the method of diagnosis. Studies excluded were studies not answering the objective. Additional exclusion criteria included (1) studies identifying atrial fibrillation as the exposure; (2) studies failing to clarify their definition of obstructive sleep apnea; (3) studies that did not specify atrial fibrillation in their arrhythmias of interest; (4) studies including patients treated with CPAP; (5) absence of a "non-exposed" (control) group; and (6), data only reported in abstract form Figure 1.

The following data was collected from each study (1) OSA criteria; (2) total study population; (3) number of subjects in "exposed" and "non-exposed" group; (4) number of subjects who developed AF per group;(4) P values and CI's.

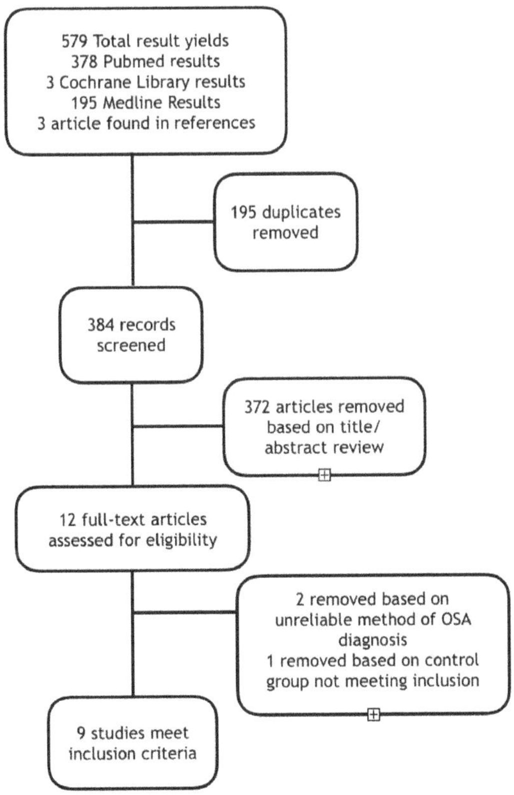

Figure 1: Flow diagram explaining the process of selections of the studies included in our meta-analysis.

Data analysis

The search of the databases and references yielded a total of 579 results. After removing duplicate studies, there were 384 studies left for screening and 372 of these records were excluded (Figure 1), based on not meeting the inclusion criteria. Twelve studies were read by full-text; 2 of these articles were removed due to unmentioned or unreliable OSA diagnostic modality, and 1 was removed based on a control group inconsistent with other studies (e.g. AHI >15 diagnostic for OSA). This left us with 9 studies of 19,837 patients that met all inclusion criteria, 12,255 exposed, and 7582 non-exposed. Sample sizes ranged from n=160 patients to n=6841 patients. Characteristics of these studies were as follows: 4 cross sectional studies, 3 prospective cohort studies, and 2 retrospective cohort studies.

For the purpose of this analysis the OSA group included any severity of OSA; namely mild, moderate or severe OSA. This was important to minimize the variability of data among individual studies, as some studies included mild *vs.* no OSA while others reported moderate to severe *vs.* no OSA.

We used Comprehensive Meta-Analysis package V3 (Biostat, USA). Mantel-Haenszel method (Mantel & Haenszel) for calculating the weighted pooled odds ratio under the fixed effects model. We incorporated heterogeneity statistics to calculate the summary odds ratio under the random effects model (Der Simonian & Laird). The data is reported as odds ratios with 95% Confidence intervals using the random effects model.

Results

There were a total of 9 studies included in this meta-analysis for the random pooled effects. In the main pooled analysis, the control group included 7582 subjects, of which 461 developed AF and the OSA group included 12255 subjects out of which 943 developed AF. The risk of AF was found to be higher among OSA versus control group (OR; 2.120, C.I: 1.845-2.436, Z; 10.598 p<0.001). These results suggest higher incidence of AF among patients with an established diagnosis of OSA *vs.* no OSA (Figure 2).

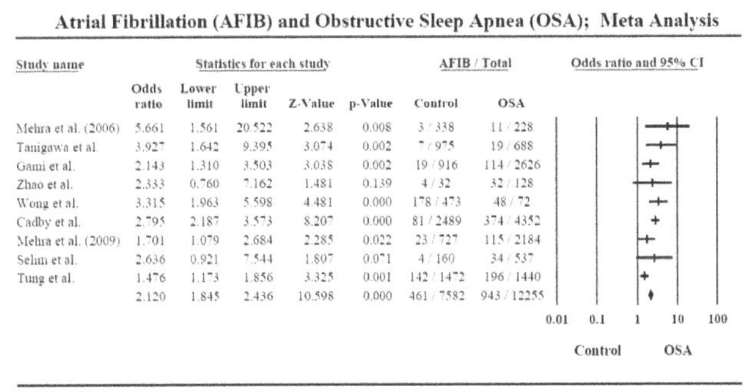

Figure 2: Forrest plot depicting the odds ratio of having AFIB associated with OSA.

2 out of the 9 studies showed no difference between OSA and no OSA and incidence of AF (Zhao et al. (OR: 2.333, C.I: 0.760- 7.162, Z: 1.481 p<0.139) and Selim et al. (OR; 2.636, C.I: 0.921-7.544, Z; 1.807 p<0.071).

The Heterogeneity observed for the pooled analysis was Q-value; 22.487 df (Q); 8 P-value; 0.004, I-squared; 64.424 Tau2; 0.098, suggesting appropriate study selection and moderate heterogeneity (Table 1).

Study	Type of Study	Number of patients	Number of exposed	Number of non-exposed	Total Afib	AF in non-exposed	AF in exposed	P value/CI
Mehra et al. [7]	Cross-sectional	566	228	338	14	3	11	1.03-15.74
Tanigawa et al. [8]	Prevalence	1663	688	975	26	7	19	P<0.001
Gami et al. [9]	Retrospective cohort	3542	2626	916	133	19	114	1.34 to 3.54
Zhao et al. [10]	prospective	160	128	32	36	4	32	p=0.07
Wong et al. [11]	Retrospective	545	72	473	226	178	48	1.3-2.58
Cadby et al. [12]	Prospective	6841	4352	2489	455	81	374	2.06-3.34
Mehra et al. [13]	cross-sectional	2911	2184	727	138	23	115	P<0.001
Selim et al. [14]	Cross-sectional	697	537	160	38	4	34	P>0.05
Tung et al. [15]	Prospective	2912	1440	1472	338	142	196	P>0.05

Table 1: Study characteristics.

Discussion

The results of our study demonstrate that OSA/SDB is strongly associated with atrial fibrillation. Our results are consistent with other large-scale studies that have found an independent and strong association between SDB and cardiac arrhythmias. Cadby et al. studied patients attending a sleep clinic referred for in-laboratory polysomnography for possible OSA between 1989 and 2001. After adjustment for multivariate predictors, the authors found that OSA diagnosis (AHI>5), OSA severity (using AHI clinical cut points), log (AHI+1), and log (SaO2t<90%+1) were all independently predictive of developing AF. Their adjusted HR for AHI>5 *vs.* AHI<5 was 1.55 (95% CI, 1.21-2.00).

Gami et al. is another large-scale retrospective cohort study, which determined the incidence of AF in patients referred for polysomnography. In their study of 3,542 patients, AF occurred in 114 of 2,626 patients (4.3%) with OSA and in 19 of 916 patients (2.1%) without OSA. Moreover, OSA (defined by an apnea-hypopnea index 5) was a strong predictor of incident AF (HR 2.18, 95% CI 1.34 to 3.54, p 0.002). Additionally, the authors also found that the severity of OSA was associated with higher incidence of incident AF.

Of the nine studies included in this analysis, two did not reach statistical significance. The Sleep apnea and Atrial fibrillation after Bypass OperaTion (SABOT) study was a prospective observational study conducted on 160 patients without AF who underwent elective CABG. The authors of the study measured the prevalence of OSA in patients prior to CABG then followed the patients post-operatively for the occurrence of incident AF.

There have been several postulated mechanisms for the role of obstructive sleep apnea as a promulgator of atrial fibrillation. Hypoxia induced chemo-reflexive tachycardia and hypertension may increase myocardial oxygen demand resulting in repeated atrial ischemia and subsequent AF [16]. Animal models have shown that hypoxia induces transient prolongation and an increase in heterogeneity of refractory periods, depressed conduction velocity, and increased heterogeneous conduction, causing expanded vulnerability to re-entrant arrhythmias [17]. Increased sympathetic tone and decreased parasympathetic tone have been found to precede generation of paroxysmal AF. These autonomic changes are secondary to recurrent nocturnal apneas and chemoreceptor induced decrease in parasympathetic tone, manifesting as impaired cardiac vagal input and parasympathetic components of heart rate variability [18].

Upper airway collapse during sleep also generates major drops in intrathoracic pressure that are transmitted to the thin-walled atria, contributing to atrial chamber enlargement secondary to increased transmural forces. These changes are associated with greater left atrial volumes and a greater degree of left ventricular diastolic dysfunction in controls without OSA, even after matching for BMI [19]. These same forces may be important in tissue stretching at the level of pulmonary vein ostia, foci commonly implicated in development of AF [20].

Repeated cycles of hypoxia and deoxygenation also lead to the formation of reactive oxygen species, and oxidative stress has been implicated as a substrate of AF initiation and maintenance [21]. Markers of inflammation, including CRP, IL-6 and IL-8, are also increased in chronic OSA, and have been associated with a greater risk of AF, post-CABG AF, and AF recurrence after cardio version and ablation [22].

Finally, elevated levels of Angiotensin II and Aldosterone, found in human and animal studies during increased sympathetic activation, and completely mitigated by renal sympathetic denervation, in combination with reactive oxygen species, potentially contribute to atrial tissue fibrosis and arrhythmogenesis [23].

Despite the rapidly growing epidemic of obesity and attendant risk of OSA, the US Preventive Services Task Force conclude that the current evidence is insufficient to assess the balance of benefits, and harms of screening for OSA in asymptomatic adults. Given the increasing prevalence of OSA risk factors including obesity, the current prevalence of OSA may be underestimated. Thus, further research on subclinical OSA and its risk factors (male sex, older age, postmenopausal status, higher BMI, cranio-facial and upper airway abnormalities) is required in order to select patients most likely to benefit from screening, and early treatment, to prevent or decrease likelihood of AF development or progression [24].

Limitations

There are some limitations to our meta-analysis. A few of our studies were cross-sectional data, limiting the ability to draw conclusions about temporality and incident risk. One of the studies in our meta-analysis determined exposure status based on review of subject medical records. The authors did not specifically mention the diagnostic test used to determine the presence of OSA in these patients. Nevertheless, removal of this study during data-analysis did not alter the results of our study, and so it was still included. Mehra et al. sampled the extremes of the SDB spectrum (SDB defined as RDI>30 events/h and non-SDB defined as RDI<5), which increased the efficiency of the study, but limited the ability to evaluate an intermediate threshold (between RDI of 5 and 30). Moreover, some studies consisted of samples of patients referred to sleep clinics because of suspected sleep disorders. This may lead to a potential ascertainment bias. Another limitation is that patients in prospective cohort studies have greater follow-up compared to patients with OSA in the general population, which could have led to increased diagnosis of AF in study patients compared to symptomatic AF patients. Finally, the Mehra et al. study included a population of purely males, precluding the opportunity of extending the results to female populations.

The utility of the apnea-hypopnea index as an accurate assessment of OSA has its inherent limitations; the mean time of each apneic and hypopneic episode is not included in the index. Moreover, due to the combination of both episodes into one index, the comparability of patients with more apneic versus hyopneic episodes may lead to an underestimation of OSA severity in those with more or longer apneic episodes due to longer and greater reductions in airflow and arterial oxygen saturation [15].

In all, this study brings to light an important risk factor for one of the most common and globally burdening cardiac arrhythmia. An increased awareness of this association is tantamount to identification and treatment of OSA to decrease its impact on the development of AF.

Funding

This work was sponsored, in part, by the Brooklyn Health Disparities Center NIH grant #P20 MD006875.

References

1. Miyasaka Y, Barnes ME, Gersh BJ, Cha SS, Bailey KR, et al. (2006) Secular trends in incidence of atrial fibrillation in Olmsted County, Minnesota, 1980 to 2000, and implications on the projections for future prevalence. Circulation 114: 119-125.
2. Benjamin EJ, Wolf PA, D'Agostino RB, Silbershatz H, Kannel WB, et al. (1998) Impact of atrial fibrillation on the risk of death: the Framingham Heart Study. Circulation 98: 946-952.
3. Du X, Dong J, Ma C (2017) Is Atrial Fibrillation a Preventable Disease? J Am Coll Cardiol. 69: 1968-1982.
4. Young T, Peppard PE, Gottlieb DJ (2002) Epidemiology of obstructive sleep apnea: A population health perspective. Am J Respir Crit Care Med 165: 1217-1239.
5. Motamedi KK, McClary AC, Amedee RG (2009) Obstructive sleep apnea: A growing problem. Ochsner J 9: 149-153.
6. Al-Falahi Z, Williamson J, Dimitri H (2017) Atrial fibrillation and sleep apnoea: Guilt by association? Heart Lung Circ 26: 902-910.
7. Mehra R, Benjamin EJ, Shahar E (2006) Association of nocturnal arrhythmias with sleep-disordered breathing: The Sleep Heart Health Study. Am J Respir Crit Care Med 173: 910-916.
8. Tanigawa T, Yamagishi K, Sakurai S (2006) Arterial oxygen desaturation during sleep and atrial fibrillation. Heart 92: 1854-1855.
9. Gami AS, Hodge DO, Herges RM, Olson EJ, Nykodym J, et al. (2007) Obstructive sleep apnea, obesity, and the risk of incident atrial fibrillation. J Am Coll Cardiol 49: 565-571.
10. Zhao LP, Kofidis T, Lim TW (2015) Sleep apnea is associated with new-onset atrial fibrillation after coronary artery bypass grafting. J Crit Care 30: 1418.e1-5.
11. Wong JK, Maxwell BG, Kushida CA (2015) Obstructive sleep apnea is an independent predictor of postoperative atrial fibrillation in cardiac surgery. J Cardiothorac Vasc Anesth 29: 1140-1147.
12. Cadby G, Mcardle N, Briffa T (2015) Severity of OSA is an independent predictor of incident atrial fibrillation hospitalization in a large sleep-clinic cohort. Chest 148: 945-952.
13. Mehra R, Stone KL, Varosy PD, Hoffman AR, Marcus GM, et al. (2009) Nocturnal Arrhythmias across a spectrum of obstructive and central sleep-disordered breathing in older men: outcomes of sleep disorders in older men (MrOS sleep) study. Arch Intern Med 169: 1147-1155.
14. Selim BJ, Koo BB, Qin L, Jeon S, Won C (2016) The association between nocturnal cardiac arrhythmias and sleep-disordered breathing: The dream study. J Clin Sleep Med 12: 829-837.
15. Tung P, Levitzky YS, Wang R, Weng J, Quan SF, et al. (2017) Obstructive and central sleep apnea and the risk of incident atrial fibrillation in a community cohort of men and women. J Am Heart Assoc 6: e004500.
16. Skalidis EI, Hamilos MI, Karalis IK, Chlouverakis G, Kochiadakis GE, et al. (2008) Isolated atrial microvascular dysfunction in patients with lone recurrent atrial fibrillation. J Am Coll Cardiol. 51: 2053-2057.
17. Lammers WJ, Kirchhof C, Bonke FI, Allessie MA (1992) Vulnerability of rabbit atrium to reentry by hypoxia. Role of inhomogeneity in conduction and wavelength. Am J Physiol 262: H47-55.
18. Baranchuk A, Simpson CS, Redfearn DP, Fitzpatrick M (2008) It's time to wake up! Sleep apnea and cardiac arrhythmias. Europace 10: 666-667.
19. Otto ME, Belohlavek M, Romero-Corral A, Gami AS, Gilman G, et al (2007) Comparison of cardiac structural and functional changes in obese otherwise healthy adults with versus without obstructive sleep apnea. Am J Cardiol 99: 1298-1302.
20. Caples SM, Somers VK (2009) Sleep-disordered breathing and atrial fibrillation. Prog Cardiovasc Dis 51: 411-415.
21. Korantzopoulos P, Kolettis TM, Galaris D, Goudevenos JA (2007) The role of oxidative stress in the pathogenesis and perpetuation of atrial fibrillation. Int J Cardiol 115: 135-143.
22. Wu N, Xu B, Xiang Y, Wu L, Zhang Y, et al (2013) Association of inflammatory factors with occurrence and recurrence of atrial fibrillation: A meta-analysis. Int J Cardiol 169: 62-72.
23. Goudis CA, Ketikoglou DG (2017) Obstructive sleep and atrial fibrillation: Pathophysiological mechanisms and therapeutic implications. Int J Cardiol 230:293-300.
24. Asghari A, Mohammadi F (2013) Is Apnea-Hypopnea Index a proper measure for Obstructive Sleep Apnea severity? Med J Islam Repub Iran 27: 161-162.

23

Parkinson's Disease

Vadivelan M*

Department of Medicine, Jawaharlal Institute of Postgraduate Medical Education and Research, Pondicherry, India

***Corresponding author:** Vadivelan M, No. E-2, Jawaharlal Institute of Postgraduate Medical Education and Research (JIPMER) Quarters, JIPMER Campus, Dhanvantari Nagar P.O., Pondicherry - 605 006, India, E-mail: vadivelan.m@jipmer.edu.in

Abstract

Parkinson's disease is a neurodegenerative condition that commonly afflicts the elderly population. It is responsible for high morbidity and disabilities in old age. Understanding the pathophysiology of the disease will help in better management of patients with Parkinsonism. Newer anti-parkinsonian drugs achieve better control of symptoms with fewer side effects. Complications of the disease include hypostatic pneumonia and head injuries due to frequent falls.

Keywords: Parkinsonism; Levodopa; Dopamine; Agonists

Introduction

Parkinson's disease is a neurodegenerative condition that presents clinically as rest tremor, rigidity and bradykinesia. Apart from these cardinal symptoms, a gamut of motor and non-motor features can be attributed to this condition. The motor features are mask like facies, reduced eye blinking and hypophonia. The non-motor features include mood changes, sleep disturbance, autonomic dysfunction and cognitive impairment.

The disease is commonly seen in individuals above the age of 60 years. There is no gender predilection in Parkinson's disease. Complications like immobility and tendency to fall are responsible for morbidity due to parkinsonism.

Pathophysiology

The basic pathologic change that occurs in Parkinson's disease is degeneration of dopaminergic neurons in the substantia nigra. This leads to a reduction in dopamine production from the nigral cells. Apart from this, there is deposition of Lewy bodies (intra-cytoplasmic hyaline inclusions) in the substantia nigra. Reduced dopamine synthesis is responsible for symptoms like bradykinesia in Parkinson's disease.

Nuclei in the basal ganglia are connected to neurons in the motor cortex and help in the regulation of motor function. Input to the basal ganglia occurs from the striatum. The output regions of the basal ganglia include the substantia nigra and globus pallidus. There is an inhibitory effect on neurons in the brainstem and thalamus due to output from the basal ganglia. The brainstem and thalamic neurons are also connected to the motor neurons of the spinal cord and the cerebral cortex. Thus, they also play a role in the regulation of motor function.

Due to dopamine depletion in the basal ganglia, there is an excitatory effect on the subthalamic nucleus and globus pallidus. This leads to thalamic and motor cortical inhibition which is responsible for the clinical features of Parkinson's disease.

Etiology and Pathogenesis

A majority of cases of Parkinson's disease are sporadic in nature and their cause is not known. A small number of cases are familial in nature. In familial cases, genetic mutations have been identified that can cause disease in association with exposure to an environmental factor.

There is currently no evidence to link any environmental factor in the pathogenesis of Parkinson's disease. However, studies have suggested that there is an increased risk of the disease in persons who have been exposed to pesticides, while there is a reduced risk in those consuming nicotine and caffeine.

A compound called methyl-phenyl-tetrahydropyridine (MPTP) was implicated in the causation of severe Parkinsonism in young drug addicts. MPTP is metabolized to a mitochondrial toxin in the central nervous system. This toxin causes damage to the dopaminergic neurons. However, there is no current evidence to demonstrate the role of MPTP in sporadic cases of Parkinson's disease.

The factors responsible for neuronal cell death in Parkinson's disease are oxidative stress, inflammation, protein aggregation, excitotoxicity and mitochondrial dysfunction. Cell death occurs due to signal-mediated apoptosis. A proper understanding of the mechanisms leading to neuronal cell death can help in the development of neuroprotective drugs in the future for better management of the disease.

Clinical Features

The symptoms of Parkinson's disease are unilateral in the early stages of the disease. Bilateral involvement is common in the advanced stages of the disease. Resting tremor is a common symptom and it is usually seen as flexion/extension of the fingers and abduction/adduction of thumb in the upper limb. Tremor can involve the lower limbs and tongue over a period of time. The tremor is usually present at rest and is decreased on movements.

Another common symptom is bradykinesia which is defined as slowness in the initiation of movements. There is difficulty in performing fine movements with fingers. Patients with Parkinson's disease have a typical gait. They find difficulty in initiation of walking, take short steps and have reduced arm swing while walking. They can lose balance while turning which may result in falls during walking.

The cardinal finding in patients with Parkinson's disease is cogwheel rigidity that is usually seen in the upper limbs. Patients also have a mask-like expressionless face and reduced blinking. Glabellar tap sign is positive in such patients. Speech becomes soft and difficult to understand, which becomes indistinct gradually. As the disease progresses, postural reflexes become impaired that can lead to inadvertent falls and subsequent injuries.

Investigations

The diagnosis of Parkinson's disease is based only on clinical findings. Investigations are indicated if patients have unusual features of the disease. In such cases, investigations are needed to rule out other causes of parkinsonism.

Wilson's disease needs to be ruled out if patients present with parkinsonian features before the age of 40 years. Neuro-imaging of the brain (MRI brain) may show degenerative changes in the basal ganglia in patients with Wilson's disease.

MRI of the brain is indicated in patients with primary parkinsonism if there are signs of pyramidal or cerebellar involvement.

Management

Management of Parkinson's disease can be broadly divided as follows-

Pharmacologic therapy

Surgical management

Physiotherapy and speech therapy

Management of non-motor and non-dopaminergic features

Pharmacologic therapy

Levodopa: Levodopa is a precursor of dopamine and is the drug of choice in the management of Parkinson's disease. Usually, it is combined with a peripherally acting dopa-decarboxylase inhibitor. On oral administration, levodopa undergoes peripheral decarboxylation to release dopamine. As a result, only a small amount of dopamine reaches the brain. Also, side effects like nausea and vomiting occur due to peripheral decarboxylation of the drug.

Hence, levodopa is combined with a peripheral decarboxylase inhibitor like carbidopa or benserazide to prevent the occurrence of side effects and to ensure that adequate amount of dopamine reaches the brain. Nausea and vomiting due to levodopa can be minimized with the help of domperidone.

Levodopa provides symptomatic improvement of the motor features of the disease. There is improvement of bradykinesia, rigidity and tremor in patients with levodopa. It helps in improving the quality of life in patients with Parkinson's disease. Carbidopa/levodopa combination is available as 10/100 and 25/100 mg. It can be given orally 3-4 times in a day. The maximum dose of levodopa that can be administered is 1000 mg/day.

Long-term treatment with levodopa leads to the development of motor complications and involuntary movements. These are termed as dyskinesias. Dyskinesias can occur as choreiform movements, dystonia or myoclonus. They are seen commonly when the drug reaches its peak plasma concentration (peak-dose phenomenon).

Diphasic dyskinesias occur when the action of levodopa begins and when it starts wearing off. They manifest as transient, stereotypic, rhythmic movements predominantly involving the lower limbs. Management is by increasing the dose of levodopa in such patients.

There can be sudden and unpredictable changes in response to levodopa therapy over a period of time due to progression of the disease. This is manifested as complex motor fluctuations. Here, there is an alternation of disabling dyskinesias and severe Parkinsonism (on-off phenomenon). The exact cause of levodopa-induced motor fluctuations is not known. They are more commonly seen in patients with severe disease and with higher doses of levodopa.

Levodopa induced dyskinesias can be due to non-physiologic levodopa replacement in the striatum. In the normal individual, dopamine in the striatum is maintained at a constant level. In patients with Parkinsonism, there is degeneration of dopamine producing neurons in the striatum. As a result, striatal dopamine level becomes dependent on the peripheral availability of levodopa. Oral levodopa does not lead to physiologic levels of dopamine in the striatum. This causes the dopamine receptors to be exposed to alternating high and low concentrations of dopamine. Ultimately, this leads to molecular changes in the striatal neurons that is responsible for levodopa induced motor complications. Management of levodopa induced dyskinesias is by administration of levodopa in smaller but more frequent doses.

Common side effects of levodopa are nausea and vomiting. Behavioural changes can be seen in patients taking levodopa. They can manifest as drug (levodopa) craving and hypersexuality.

Dopamine agonists: This group of drugs act on the dopamine receptors in the brain. They are less efficacious than levodopa. They can be used to improve motor function and decrease the 'off' period in patients with motor fluctuations. These drugs are less likely to induce dyskinesias or cause dose fluctuations as seen with levodopa.

Dopamine agonists can be ergot derivatives like bromocriptine, pergolide and cabergoline. These can be associated with fibrosis of the cardiac valves and hence are not preferred for the management of Parkinsonism.

Non-ergot dopamine agonists include pramipexole, ropinirole and rotigotine. Ropinirole and pramipexole can be given orally thrice daily or once daily as an extended-release preparation. Rotigotine is available as a trans-dermal patch and can be applied to the skin once daily. Apomorphine is a parenteral dopamine agonist and can be administered subcutaneously or as a continuous infusion. It has the advantage of reducing the 'off' period and dyskinesias in patients with advanced disease.

Pramipexole can be started as 0.25 mg tablets thrice daily and increased to a maximum dose of 1 mg thrice daily. Ropinirole is started at a dose of 6 mg/day and can be given till the maximum dose of 24 mg/day.

Side effects of dopamine agonists are nausea and vomiting that can be controlled with domperidone. Serious side effects include hallucinations, cognitive impairment, sleep attacks, pathologic gambling and hypersexuality.

COMT inhibitors: Catechol-O-methyltransferase (COMT) is an enzyme that is responsible for the metabolism of levodopa. Inhibition of COMT will increase the half-life of levodopa and its availability in the striatum. Hence, COMT inhibitors decrease the 'off' period and increase the 'on' period in patients with motor fluctuations.

Examples of COMT inhibitors are entacapone and tolcapone. Entacapone is given orally as 200 mg in combination with levodopa. Tolcapone is initiated as 100 mg thrice daily orally and can be increased to a maximum dose of 200 mg thrice daily.

Side effects due to COMT inhibitors are nausea, vomiting and an increase in dyskinesias. Serious side effects like hepatotoxicity and diarrhea are commonly seen with tolcapone, but not with entacapone.

MAO-B inhibitors: Monoamine oxidase type B (MAO-B) inhibitors block the metabolism of dopamine in the brain and lead to increased concentration of dopamine in the neuronal synapses. They can be used alone in patients with early disease or can be combined with levodopa in patients with motor fluctuations to decrease the 'off' period. This group of drugs has some neuro-protective effect. It prevents further oxidative stress to the surviving dopamine producing neurons in the substantia nigra.

Drugs that belong to this group are selegiline and rasagiline. Selegiline is given orally as 5 mg twice daily while rasagiline is administered orally as 1 mg/day.

Surgical management: The commonly employed surgical technique for management of patients with Parkinson's disease is deep brain stimulation (DBS). In this procedure, an electrode is placed in the sub-thalamic nucleus or the globus pallidus. This electrode is then connected to a stimulator that is inserted subcutaneously over the chest wall. The technique mimics the effects of a brain lesion without causing an actual lesion.

DBS is relatively safe and can be used for performing procedures bilaterally as it does not involve creation of any lesion in the brain. It helps in improving dyskinesias and 'off' period in patients with Parkinsonism. However, there is no improvement in clinical features that do not show any response to levodopa. Also, DBS does not prevent the development or progression of non-dopaminergic features of the disease like dementia and falls.

DBS is indicated in patients with levodopa-induced motor complications that cannot be controlled with modification of the drug. Complications of the procedure are hemorrhage and infection during surgical insertion of the electrode, lead displacement, speech abnormalities and paresthesias.

Physiotherapy and speech therapy

Active and passive physiotherapy leads to an improvement in the functional physical capacity of patients with Parkinson's disease. Physiotherapy helps in decreasing muscle rigidity while speech therapy is helpful for patients with dysarthria and dysphonia.

Management of non-motor and non-dopaminergic features

The common non-dopaminergic features of Parkinson's disease are depression, psychosis, dementia, autonomic dysfunction and sleep disturbances.

Depression is seen in approximately 50% of patients with Parkinson's disease. It can be treated with anti-depressants like selective serotonin reuptake inhibitors (SSRIs).

Psychosis in patients with Parkinson's disease commonly manifests as visual hallucinations. It can be managed with the help of atypical neuroleptics like clozapine or quetiapine.

Dementia is a common problem in a large majority of patients with Parkinson's disease. Such patients usually have impairment of cognitive function and attention. All drugs used in the management of Parkinson's disease can cause cognitive impairment. Levodopa in the lowest possible dose is recommended for patients with cognitive dysfunction. Anticholinesterase drugs like donepezil and rivastigmine can be useful for improving cognitive function in patients with dementia.

Autonomic disturbances seen in patients with Parkinson's disease are constipation, sexual dysfunction and orthostatic hypotension. Constipation can be managed with a high fibre diet and plenty of oral fluids. If the problem persists, then laxatives can be tried. Sexual dysfunction in males can be treated with 5-phosphodiesterase inhibitors like sildenafil. Management of orthostatic hypotension can be done by addition of extra salt in the diet or by administration of low doses of fludrocortisone.

Sleep disturbances like fragmentation of normal sleep, daytime somnolence and disturbances in rapid eye movement (REM) sleep are commonly encountered in patients with parkinsonism. Benzodiazepines like clonazepam can help in the management of sleep abnormalities in such cases.

Stem cell therapy in Parkinson's disease

Transplantation of new dopamine generating cells into the substantia nigra can be an important treatment option in Parkinson's disease. This concept has formed the basic premise for stem cell therapy in Parkinsonism [1,2].

Embryonic stem (ES) cells can undergo in vitro proliferation and differentiation into various cell lineages in various cell culture conditions [3,4]. In this regard, mouse ES cells have been used as a source of transplantable tissue in various studies [5].

Deacon et al showed that ES cells have a capacity to undergo differentiation into dopamine producing neurons when they are grafted to the brain [6]. However; it was not possible to study the functional effects of the engrafted cells. This was because a large number of cells were used in the study which proliferated into big teratomas. These teratomas outgrew the target areas.

Mc Kay et al described the in vitro generation of dopaminergic neurons from mouse ES cells [7]. In this study, 30% dopamine differentiation was achieved by subjecting the stem cells to treatment with fibroblast growth factor 2 (FGF2), sonic hedgehog (SHH), fibroblast growth factor 8 (FGF8) and ascorbic acid. These dopamine producing neurons have been shown to have functional effects in rodent models of Parkinson's disease [8,9].

Neural progenitor cells (NPCs) are multipotent cells which can give rise to neurons, astrocytes and oligodendrocytes. They are usually obtained from the fetal or adult brain [10,11]. Some NPCs can undergo differentiation into dopamine producing neurons, but they have shown no benefits in a rodent model of Parkinson's disease [12].

In a majority of studies conducted on stem cell therapy for Parkinson's disease, cells have been grafted in an ectopic target area instead of the substantia nigra. This type of engraftment was necessitated because the dopamine producing neurons did not show positive effects when they were placed in the substantia nigra. New investigational techniques that are being tried are grafting of stem cells to many target sites in the basal ganglia region [13].

Atypical and secondary Parkinsonism

Atypical Parkinsonism is a group of neurodegenerative disorders that are characterized by extensive neurodegeneration as compared to primary Parkinson's disease. Features of atypical parkinsonism include absence of rest tremor and early speech impairment. These clinical features show little or no improvement with levodopa.

Atypical parkinsonism includes the entities of multiple-system atrophy, progressive supranuclear palsy, corticobasal ganglionic degeneration and frontotemporal dementia.

Multiple-system atrophy (MSA) is an entity that presents as a combination of parkinsonian, cerebellar and autonomic features. It can be divided into a cerebellar type (MSA-c) or a parkinsonian type (MSA-p). Patients with MSA present with signs of cerebellar disease and early autonomic dysfunction.

Progressive supranuclear palsy (PSP) manifests as eyelid apraxia and restriction of eye movements. Gait disturbance, dysphagia, dysphonia and dementia are also commonly seen in patients with PSP.

Corticobasal ganglionic degeneration and frontotemporal dementia are less common forms of atypical parkinsonism.

Causes of secondary parkinsonism are head trauma, toxins, encephalitis and drugs. Toxins implicated in the development of secondary parkinsonism include manganese and carbon monoxide. Infections of the central nervous system (CNS) like viral encephalitis can be responsible for secondary parkinsonism. Drugs that are anti-dopaminergic or have dopamine-blocking action can lead to secondary parkinsonism. Examples of drugs which can cause secondary parkinsonism are neuroleptics, metoclopramide and chlorperazine.

Summary

Parkinson's disease is a common neurodegenerative disorder. It usually presents as tremor in patients above the age of 60 years. Rigidity and bradykinesia are common findings on neurologic examination. The basic pathology in Parkinson's disease is depletion of dopamine producing neurons in the substantia nigra due to a variety of reasons.

Levodopa is the drug of choice in the management of patients with Parkinsonism. Newer groups of drugs like COMT inhibitors and dopamine agonists are also helpful in relief of symptoms. Physiotherapy and speech therapy help can decrease the morbidity of patients suffering from Parkinson's disease.

References

1. Olanow WC, Schapira AHV (2012) Parkinson's disease and other movement disorders. In: Longo DL, Fauci AS, Kasper DL, Hauser SL, Jameson JL, et al. (eds) Harrison's Principles of Internal Medicine, Vol. 2, (18thedn) New York: The Mc-Graw Hill Companies 3317-3326.
2. Allen CMC, Lueck CJ, Dennis M (2010) Neurological disease-Neurodegenerative diseases. In: Colledge NR, Walker BR, Ralston SH, editors. Davidson's Principles & Practice of Medicine, 21st ed. China: Elsevier Limited 1199-1202.
3. Evans MJ, Kaufman MH (1981) Establishment in culture of pluripotential cells from mouse embryos. Nature 292: 154-156.
4. Martin GR (1981) Isolation of a pluripotent cell line from early mouse embryos cultured in medium conditioned by teratocarcinoma stem cells. Proc Natl Acad Sci U S A 78: 7634-7638.
5. Pedersen RA (1999) Embryonic stem cells for medicine. Sci Am 280: 68-73.
6. Deacon T, Dinsmore J, Costantini LC, Ratliff J, Isacson O (1998) Blastula-stage stem cells can differentiate into dopaminergic and serotonergic neurons after transplantation. Exp Neurol 149: 28-41.
7. Lee SH, Lumelsky N, Studer L, Auerbach JM, McKay RD (2000) Efficient generation of midbrain and hindbrain neurons from mouse embryonic stem cells. Nat Biotechnol 18: 675-679.
8. Bjorklund LM, Sánchez-Pernaute R, Chung S, Andersson T, Chen IY, et al. (2002) Embryonic stem cells develop into functional dopaminergic neurons after transplantation in a Parkinson rat model. Proc Natl Acad Sci U S A 99: 2344-2349.
9. Kim JH, Auerbach JM, Rodríguez-Gómez JA, Velasco I, Gavin D, et al. (2002) Dopamine neurons derived from embryonic stem cells function in an animal model of Parkinson's disease. Nature 418: 50-56.
10. Johe KK, Hazel TG, Muller T, Dugich-Djordjevic MM, McKay RD (1996) Single factors direct the differentiation of stem cells from the fetal and adult central nervous system. Genes Dev 10: 3129-3140.
11. Reynolds BA, Weiss S (1992) Generation of neurons and astrocytes from isolated cells of the adult mammalian central nervous system. Science 255: 1707-1710.
12. Svendsen CN, Caldwell MA, Shen J, ter Borg MG, Rosser AE, et al. (1997) Long-term survival of human central nervous system progenitor cells transplanted into a rat model of Parkinson's disease. Exp Neurol 148: 135-146.
13. Ramachandran AC, Bartlett LE, Mendez IM (2002) A multiple target neural transplantation strategy for Parkinson's disease. Rev Neurosci 13: 243-256.

Psychological and Emotional Stress among the Students Living in Dormitory: A Comparison between Normal and Depressive Students

Seoyoun Kim[1*], Hyojae Kim[1] and Jong-Chul Yang[2]

[1]*Korea International High School (KIS), Jeju, Korea*

[2]*Department of Psychiatry, Chonbuk National University Hospital, Jeonju, Korea*

***Corresponding author:** Seoyoun Kim, 8-Global edu-ro 260 beon-gil, Daejeong-eup, Seogwipo-si, Jeju-do-699-931, Korea

Abstract

Background: Students' mental stability can be restored by comfort from a familiar home environment and support from their parents. However, many boarding students face various psychological and physical problems by themselves and cannot benefit from home care. The goal of this study is to examine psychological and emotional stress among students living in a dormitory.

Methods: Between October and November 2014, 124 students (74 male, 50 female) were enrolled at Korea International School (KIS) in Jeju, South Korea. By the Zung Selfrating Depression Scale (ZSDS), they were divided into two groups: the normal group and the depression group. I evaluated each group under the following circumstances: (1) individual school life, (2) physical health, (3) factor analysis of ZSDS. The Statistical Package for Social Sciences Software (SPSS-version 21) was used to analyze the data.

Results: 45.9% of all enrolled students scored in the mild to moderated depression range. Female students had a more prevalent depression rate (female: 54%, male: 41%). There was nearly no statistical difference in physical symptoms, except for dyspepsia, arthralgia, and lower back pain in the normal and depression groups respectively ($P<0.05$). The normal range group students had more study and exercise time. In the factor analysis of ZSDS, the depressive group had a more manifest depressed mood and 50 percentage higher ZSDS items score than the normal group: core depressive factor, anxiety factor.

Conclusions: Our study showed there was nearly no difference in physical symptoms between both groups. However, it informed that the group having depression has more problems with motor symptoms because the group lacks an adequate amount of exercise due to psychological instability. In addition, this study also showed that mood disturbance was clearly more intense while the cognitive functions related to academic performance were proven not to be problematic in the depressive group.

Keywords: Stress; Zung self-rating depression scale; High school students; Dormitory

Introduction

Famous private boarding high schools are granted privileges to university entrance. However, since these boarding students are exposed to uncertainties in the future, they experience emotional instability and are more reserved and inward looking during the period of university entrance examinations, manifesting feelings of anxiety and distress. Furthermore, senior year of high school is a transition time from being an adolescent to being an adult, and they seek to fulfill individuality, as well as seek and build close and social relationships with other students [1].

Most students regain their psychological stability while living at home with their parents. However, boarding school students have to adjust to living away from the security of a family and away from parental guidance. Therefore, boarding students find psychological and physical problems because they do not receive care from home. For many boarding students, the separation from home for the first time may create feelings of doubt, confusion, and anxiety [2]. In the harassed mental symptom of boarding students, loneliness is the most terrible problem. They were overwhelmed by a longing for warm-hearted family loving. If they get over this process, loneliness leads an individual to achieve deeper self-awareness, a time to be creative, and an opportunity to attain self-fulfillment and to explore the meaning of life [3]. However, not every boarding student is psychologically mature enough to convert their loneliness to positive outcomes. Most outstanding students learn how to deal with the attachment and separation processes of interpersonal situations in normal psychological growth and to create a unique self-identity. However, those who fail to learn how to manage stressful situations suffer from unpleasant and distressing consequences due to their social and emotional loneliness [4].

In addition, unresolved loneliness can provide a source for depressive episodes. Depression can be manifested with a loss of interest, depressed mood, psychic anxiety, somatic anxiety, altered appetite and sleep, and painful physical symptoms [5]. Students with depressive symptoms can affect all areas of functioning including motivation, concentration, feelings of self-worth and mood [6].

During one's senior year, which is considered to be the most crucial period of one's life, various symptoms induced from depression may cause detrimental results. Thus, it is crucial to examine the psychological status of students who are in this important period of their lives. In this respect, the importance of this study lies in understanding differences between normal and depressive groups of students and intervening major issues for them.

The aim of this study was to investigate the prevalence of depressive students and the physical and mental symptoms difference among normal and depressive students within a dormitory.

Methods

A cross-sectional study design was applied. The research population consists of 9th, 10th and 11th grade residential students in Korea International High School (KIS) students in Korea. A total of 124 dormitory students were enrolled in this study between October and November 2014. During the first stage, we conducted the presentation of written informed consent. For the second stage, we received the Zung Self-rating Depression Scales (ZSDS). Students were then divided into the normal and depression groups. Individual groups answered a questionnaire comprised of questions covering individual school life style (breakfast, snack, daily sleep time, daily class study time, daily self-study time, daily exercise time), physical status (neurologic, ophthalmic, auditory, respiratory, cardiovascular, gastrointestinal, urologic, dermatologic), and mental status.

We developed individual school life style items [7] and a physical symptom checklist based on a previous research study [8]. The ZSDS is a self-reported 20-item measure of the symptoms of depression. Items are ranked from 1-4, with higher scores corresponding to more frequent symptoms. Depression items score were scored as follows; 1=a little of the time, 2=some of the time, 3=a good part of the time, 4=most of the time [9,10]. The worst psychological condition is defined to have the highest score of 80 and the best condition is interpreted as the lowest score of 20. Total scores on the ZSDS indicated the level of depressive symptoms that may be of clinical relevance. The ZSDS were interpreted as follows: normal range (20-44), mildly depressed (45-59), moderately depressed (60-69), severely depressed (70 and above). A ZSDS score of ≥50 was considered indicative of clinical depression.

Normal and depressive groups were analyzed by 4 subgroups of ZSDS. The subgroups were divided with factor 1 to factor 4 [11]. Factor 1 was composed of 8 questionnaire items of ZSDS: item 1 (depressed affect), item 3 (crying spells), item 6 (decreased libido), item 14 (hopelessness), item 17 (personal devaluation), item 18 (emptiness), item 19 (suicidal rumination), item 20 (dissatisfaction). Factor 2 was composed of 4 questionnaire items of ZSDS: item 11 (confusion), item 12 (psychomotor retardation), item 16 (indecisiveness), item 10 (fatigue). Factor 3 was composed of 3 questionnaire items of ZSDS: item 4 (sleep disturbances), item 13 (psychomotor agitation), item 15 (irritability). Factor 4 was composed of 3 items of ZSDS: item 5 (decreased appetite), item 7 (weight loss), item 9 (tachycardia).

The Statistical Package for Social Sciences Software (SPSS-version 21), chi-square test was used to analyze the data. Means and standard deviations were calculated for sub-scale scores of each group. The p-value of <0.05 were considered the level of statistical significance difference.

Results

A total of 124 KIS students answered the study survey. The study subjects' stratified characteristics are shown in Figures 1 and 2.

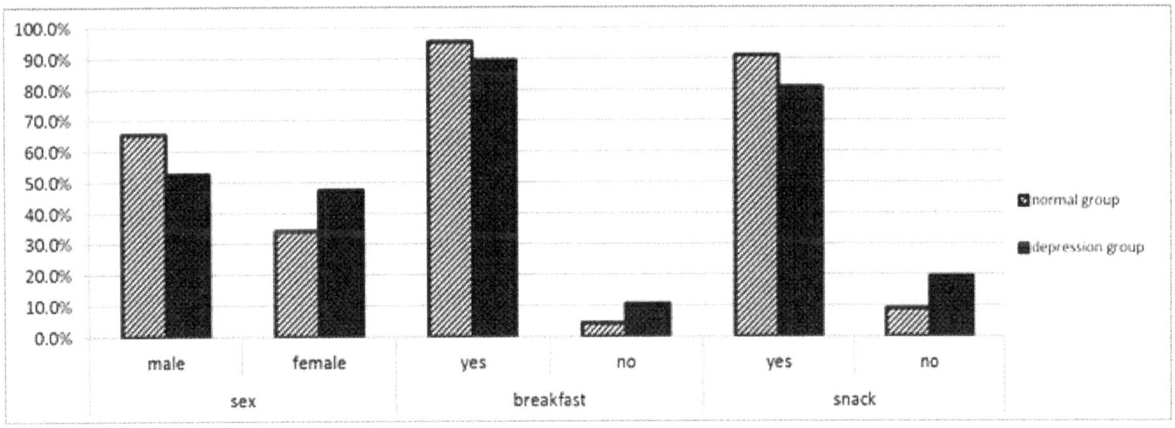

Figure 1: Characteristics of the normal and depressive group

50 students (40.3%) were females. Male to female student in normal ZSDS range were 44 (65.7%)/23 (34.3%) and male to female student in depressive ZSDS range were 30 (52.6%)/27 (47.4%).

These results showed that female students had a more depressive tendency than male students. There was no significant difference of school life characteristics in the groups. The only minimal differences in the normal range group rather than the depressive group were more breakfast eating habits (95.5%/89.5%) and more daily exercise time (77.24 ± 51.69/67.37 ± 49.37).

Other students' characteristics were similar with the normal to depressive group, respectively: daily sleep time (390.82 ± 63.06/389.65 ± 73.89 minute), daily class study time (7.08 ± 1.24/7.18 ± 1.02 hour) and daily self-study time (3.18 ± 1.53/2.98 ± 1.19 hour).

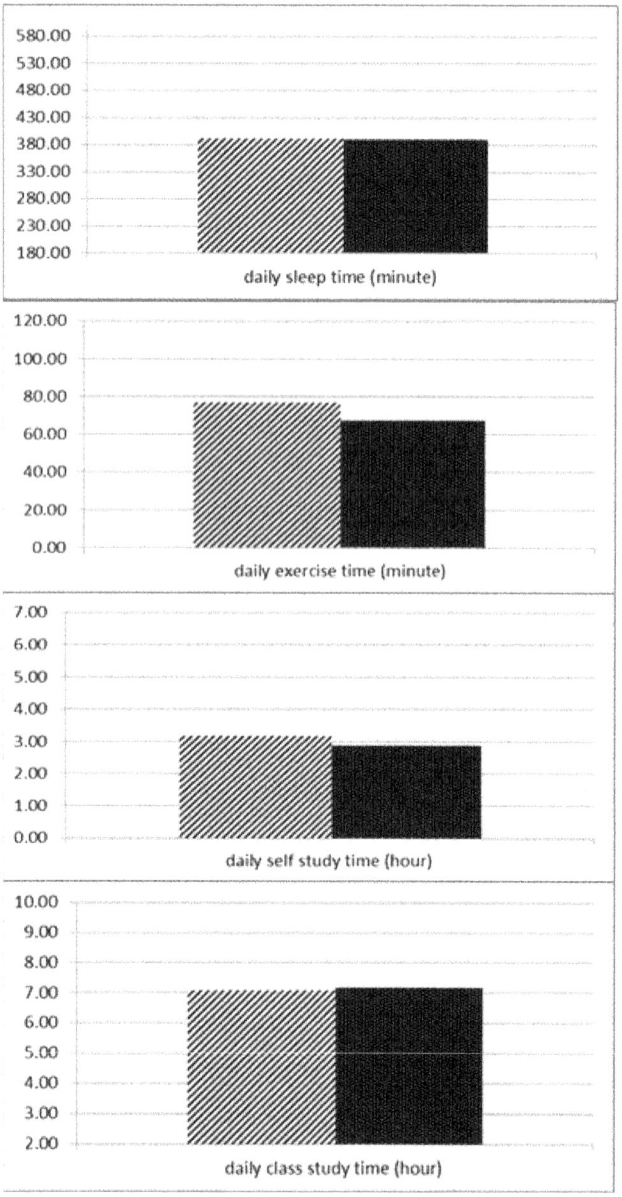

Figure 2: Individual school life characteristics of the normal and depressive group.

Tables 1 and 2 report the results for the prevalence of physical symptoms in both groups. There were no physical symptoms difference in the groups, except for more dyspepsia (47.4%), joint pain (36.8%), and back pain (59.6%) in the depressive group (p<0.05).

	Normal range; N (%)	**Depression range; N (%)**	**P value**
Neurologic symptoms			
Headache	22 (32.8%)	28 (49.1%)	>0.05
dizziness	16 (23.9%)	21 (36.8%)	>0.05
Tremor	10 (14.9%)	10 (17.5%)	>0.05
Abnormal body sensation	1 (1.5%)	4 (7.0%)	>0.05
Ophthalmic symptoms			
Blurred vision	15 (22.4%)	20 (35.1%)	>0.05
Eyeball pain	11 (16.4%)	16 (28.1%)	>0.05
Decreased visual acuity	22 (32.8%)	24 (42.1%)	>0.05
Eyeball strain	33 (49.3%)	36 (63.2%)	>0.05
Auditory symptoms			
Tinnitus	21 (31.3%)	25 (43.9%)	>0.05
Decreased auditory function	9 (13.4%)	9 (15.8%)	>0.05
Deafness	4 (6.0%)	9 (15.8%)	>0.05

Table 1: Prevalence of physical symptoms in head and neck.

	Normal range; N (%)	**Depression range; N (%)**	**P value**
Cardio-pulmonary symptoms			
Chest pain	14 (20.9%)	13 (22.8%)	>0.05
Palpitation	13 (19.4%)	19 (33.3%)	>0.05
Arrhythmia	3 (4.5%)	2 (3.5%)	>0.05
Tachycardia	3 (4.5%)	4 (7.0%)	>0.05
Edema	7 (10.4%)	3 (5.3%)	>0.05
Common cold	36 (53.7%)	32 (56.1%)	>0.05
Coughing	35 (52.2%)	33 (57.9%)	>0.05
Sputum	25 (37.3%)	31 (54.4%)	>0.05
Dyspnea	8 (11.9%)	3 (5.3%)	>0.05
Hoarseness	18 (26.9%)	13 (23.2%)	>0.05
Gastrointestinal symptoms			
Epigastric pain	13 (19.4%)	12 (21.1%)	>0.05
Dyspepsia	19 (28.4%)	27 (47.4%)	<0.05*
Difficulty swallowing	4 (6.0%)	4 (7.0%)	>0.05
Nausea, vomiting	12 (17.9%)	18 (31.6%)	>0.05
Diarrhea	16 (23.9%)	20 (35.1%)	>0.05
Abdominal pain	13 (19.4%)	19 (33.3%)	>0.05
Melena	6 (9.0%)	1 (1.8%)	>0.05

Constipation	12 (17.9%)	16 (28.1%)	>0.05
Frequent loose stool	7 (10.4%)	9 (15.8%)	>0.05
Voiding and skin symptoms			
Painful urination	3 (4.5%)	2 (3.5%)	>0.05
Tenesmus	5 (7.5%)	3 (5.3%)	>0.05
Frequent urination	5 (7.5%)	7 (12.3%)	>0.05
Diminished urine stream	3 (4.5%)	3 (5.3%)	>0.05
Itching sensation	17 (25.4%)	15 (26.3%)	>0.05
Skin eruption	7 (10.4%)	12 (21.1%)	>0.05
Skeletal symptoms			
Joint pain	12 (17.9%)	21 (36.8%)	<0.05*
Joint stiffness and motion limit	3 (4.5%)	8 (14.0%)	>0.05
Back pain	27 (40.3%)	34 (59.6%)	<0.05*

Table 2: Prevalence of physical symptoms in body and extremity.

Table 3 presented the ZSDS score in both groups. The mean ZSDS score in the normal and depressive groups were 38.16 ± 4.60 and 51.11 ± 4.27, respectively. Mild depressed range ZSDS students were 44.7% and moderately depressed range ZSDS students were 1.6%.

	Normal group	Depressive group
I feel down hearted and blue	1.49 ± 0.63	2.23 ± 1.01
Morning is when I feel the best	3.27 ± 0.86	3.60 ± 0.65
I have crying spells or feel like it	1.13 ± 0.34	1.74 ± 0.79
I have trouble sleeping at night	1.42 ± 0.76	2.12 ± 0.96
I eat as much as I used to	2.36 ± 1.04	2.67 ± 1.00
I still enjoy sex	2.94 ± 1.14	3.40 ± 0.99
I notice that I am losing weight	1.48 ± 0.68	1.81 ± 0.95
I have trouble with constipation	1.37 ± 0.62	1.65 ± 0.95
My heart beats faster than usual	1.28 ± 0.62	1.63 ± 0.87
I get tired for no reason	1.84 ± 0.86	2.70 ± 1.05
My mind is as clear as it used to be	2.46 ± 0.99	3.37 ± 0.67
I find it easy to do the things I used to	2.33 ± 0.89	2.98 ± 0.89
I am restless and can't keep still	1.67 ± 0.63	1.98 ± 0.91
I feel hopeful about the future	2.01 ± 0.84	3.44 ± 0.65
I am more irritable than usual	1.66 ± 0.75	2.07 ± 0.99
I find it easy to make decisions	2.55 ± 0.82	3.21 ± 0.84
I feel that I am useful and needed	2.03 ± 0.73	3.16 ± 0.81
My life is pretty full	1.93 ± 0.70	3.11 ± 0.88
I feel that others would be better off if I were dead	1.22 ± 0.51	1.54 ± 0.65
I still enjoy the things I used to do	1.72 ± 0.69	2.70 ± 0.94
Mean scale (sum)	38.16 ± 4.60	51.11 ± 4.27

Table 3: Comparison of the Zung self-rating depression sale score in both group.

Figure 3 provides a four factor of the Zung Self-rating Depression Scale; core depressive factor (factor 1), cognitive factor (factor 2), anxiety factor (factor 3) and somatic factor (factor 4). There are 7 items which demonstrated a gap exceeding 50 percent in item scores between two groups. Additionally, six items were from factor 1 (items 1: depressed affect, items 3: crying spells, items 14: hopelessness, items 17: personal devaluation, items 18: emptiness, items 20: dissatisfaction). These results indicate that the major problem in the depressive group is a depressive mood. The last one is item 4 (sleep disturbance) of factor 3. This result is identified with the result of daily sleep time, the only category which showed a difference among school life characteristics in the two groups.

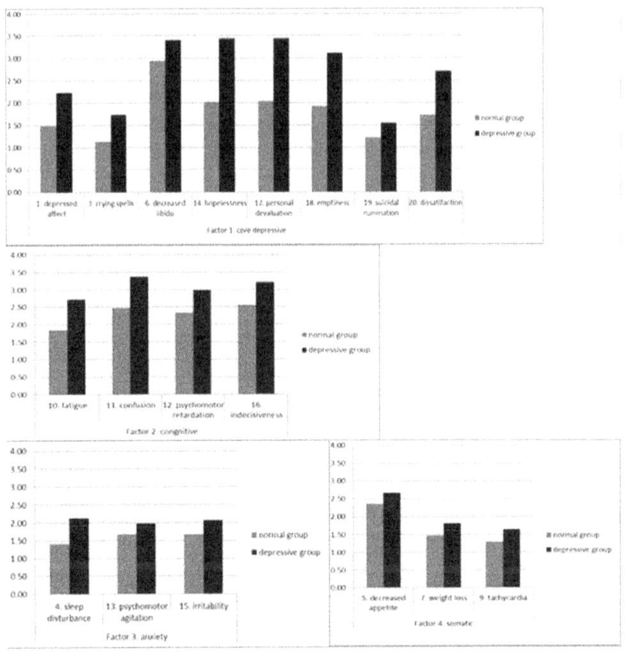

Figure 3: Relationships between factor analysis of the ZSDS in both groups.

Discussion

According to an investigation conducted by the Ministry of Health and Welfare in Korea in 2007, the depression rate (when is defined as depression influencing even daily life for more than two weeks in one year) of middle school students and high school students increased from 29.9% in 2005 to 41.3% in 2007 [12]. The studies about the increase in depression of Korean teenagers demonstrate that academic stress from studying, prospects, future, and school life based on an educational system that only focuses on college entrance exams is the main factor of depression besides developmental features during the adolescent period [13,14] According to a recent study, the academic stress level of Korean students was 50.5%, the highest among the 30 countries in the Organization for Economic Cooperation and Development (OECD). This is a rather high figure compared to the total average of 33.3% [15].

In Korea, in order to make a good college entrance result, high school students want to live in famous high school dormitories in order to study hard. However, because of the strict school life and the massive amounts of studying students do, they have huge physical and mental problems. Residency is a time when future work habits and self-care behaviorisms can be strongly influenced. However, most boarding schools are located far away from students' homes. There may be various problems because students' homes differ. These stressors can impact mental health, such as family disconnections, community dysfunctions, and social disadvantages [16]. Parents are usually the most meaningful source of social support in early life, and the perception of parental love and caring have important effects on biological and psychological health and illness throughout life [17]. In previous studies of psychological health of the resident and day students, full boarding students were more likely to experience obsessive-compulsive disorder, sensitivity in relationships, depression, anxiety, paranoia, and psychosis symptoms compared to day students [18]. Residency in dormitory school is a time when future work habits and self-care behaviors can be strongly influenced. If residents are provided opportunities to develop self-care practices to help cope with the stress of the future profession, it may mitigate more severe mental dysfunction and burnout later. Wellness health behaviors that buffer stress reactivity include physical activity, exercise, a nutritious diet, mind-body activities, prayer, seeking social support, getting restful sleep [19].

Depression is a seriously disabling health problem with a life time prevalence of 16% and with a female to male ratio of about 5:2 [20]. Studies suggest gender differences in residents' experience of distress; female residents have higher levels of anxiety and depression while males experience higher levels of depersonalization [21,22]. The tendency of females to report more depressive symptoms than males might be responsible for their greater likelihood of meeting criteria for a depressive disorder, even though males and females with depressed mood reports similar levels of subjective, social and occupational impairment. Several studies have shown that a female preponderance in rates of depression occurs at low symptom thresholds and becomes more pronounced as the number of symptoms increase [23]. According to the findings in our study, female students in the depression ZSDS range were a more prevalent ratio (47.4%) than the normal range (34.3%). Typical depressive symptoms include depressed mood, decreased interest, diminished pleasure, feeling of worthlessness, inappropriate guilt, decrease appetite and libido, and insomnia [24]. Moreover, clinical manifestations of depression differ by gender, with females more often reporting disturbances of appetite and sleep, fatigue, somatic anxiety and hypochondriasis [25]. Menstruation disorders are especially more prevalent in early puberty among girls. These severe menstruation disorder signs affect quality of life [26]. Throughout adolescence, these disorders increase with a steep slope and are more prevalent among girls who are more vulnerable to various psychosocial factors, so the ration of girls' involvement in these disorders compared to boys is 1.3:1 [27].

Depressive symptoms have been grouped into psychological and somatic or into affective, somatic and cognitive symptoms [5,28] In the primary care setting, approximately two thirds of patients with depression report somatic symptoms solely as the reason for consultation [5]. Depression is mostly difficult to recognize in such patients, being the major reason for under-diagnosis and under-treatment of depression [11]. Traditionally, the heterogenous symptoms of depression have been grouped into different symptomatic dimensions according to their clinical significance but there is no consensus on how this is best done. We decided to evaluate the status and degree of depression among boarding students by using a ZSDS questionnaire and factor analysis of the ZSDS. The ZSDS has been used as a prevalent method to evaluate depression disorders among different nationalities. Tens items are worded positively and the the other 10 are worded negatively. The four factors were divided into core depressive factor (factor 1), cognitive factor (factor 2), anxiety factor (factor 3) and somatic factor (factor 4), according to the nature of the symptoms [11]. Core depressive factor (factor 1) appears to primarily reflect emotional or affective symptoms of depression. Cognitive factor (factor 2) appears to reflect symptoms related to difficulty in concentration, decision making, confusion or loss of mental clarity, and psychomotor retardation. Anxiety factor (factor 3) appears to reflect symptoms related to irritability, psychomotor agitation, restlessness, and sleep disturbance. Somatic factor (factor 4) includes 3 ZSDS items: items 5 (decreased appetite), items 7 (weight loss), and items 9 (tachycardia). Remnant 2 ZSDS items were not classified: items 2 (diurnal variation), items 8 (constipation). In our study, there are 7 items which showed a gap exceeding 50 percent of item score between two groups. Since 6 items were from factor 1 representing depressed mood, it was indicated that emotional and affective disorder were the most evident issues in the depressive group.

Conclusion

The study was commenced to investigate the physical and mental status of senior high school students who are endeavoring to resolve the uncertainty of their future, and was designed to understand the changes of psychological status among boarding students who are facing university entrance and trying to achieve their dream but cannot gain support from their home environment. Unlike other general high schools in Korea, which only focus on students' academic performance, KIS emphasizes various extracurricular activities (sports, art, field trips, etc.), as well as academic achievement. This tendency would probably affect the students and in fact there was no significant difference between the normal and depressive groups in terms of physical symptoms. However, emotional stress can be a great burden for adolescents living in a dormitory who should manage their lives by themselves. This study also showed that mood disturbance was clearly more intense while the cognitive functions related to academic performance were proven not problematic in the depressive group. In the adolescent period, neglected depressive mood can be converted to major depressive disorder. Major depressive disorder not only produces decrement in health that are equivalent to those of other chronic disease, but also worsens mean health scores substantially more when comorbid with these diseases. To solve this problem, it seemed that difficulty in talking to parents, teachers and issues arising from peer relations should first be managed. For this, good social support from school administrative officers, teachers, parents, and classmates may help individuals and provide relief to distressed students, nourishing them to maintain sound mentality. To deal with specific issues among boarding students, a comparison study between boarding and day students would be helpful in the future.

References

1. Ozdemir U, Tuncay T (2008) Correlates of loneliness among university students. Child Adolesc Psychiatry Ment Health 2: 29.
2. Weiss RS Loneliness (1973) The experience of emotional and social isolation. London: MIT Press.
3. Borys S, Perlman D (1985) Gender differences in loneliness. Personality and Social Psychology Bulletin 11: 63-74.
4. Cutrona CE (1982) Transition to college: Loneliness and the process of social adjustment. In: Peplau LA, Perlman D (eds) Loneliness: A sourcebook of theory, research, and therapy. New York, Wiley: 291-309.
5. Tylee A, Gandhi P (2005) The importance of somatic symptoms in depression in primary care. Prim Care Companion J Clin Psychiatry 7: 167-176.
6. Andrews B, Wilding JM (2004) The relation of depression and anxiety to life-stress and achievement in students. Br J Psychol 95: 509-521.
7. Miller R (1933) Some medical aspects of boarding-school life. Br Med J 1: 863-866.
8. Sakurada I, Kido T, Suwazono Y, Kobayashi E, Kinouchi N, et al. (1999) Health status of male preparatory school students loding at a dormitory in Japan. Environmental Health and Preventive Medicine 4: 30-33.
9. Zung WW (1965) A self-rating depression scale. Arch Gen Psychiatry 12: 63-70.
10. Zung WW (1971) A rating instrument for anxiety disorders. Psychosomatics 12: 371-379.
11. Romera I, Delagado-Cohen H, Perez T, Caballero L, Gilaberte I (2008) Factor analysis of the Zung self-rating depression scale in a large sample of patients with major depressive disorder in primary care. BMC Psychiatry 8: 1-8.
12. Kandel DB, Jonhson JG, Bird HR, Canino G, Goodman SH, et al. (1997) Psychiatric disorders associated with substance use among children and adolescents: finding from the methods for the epidemiology of child and adolescent mental disorders study. J Abnorm Child Psychol 25: 121-132.
13. Hong YS (2004) The effects of life stress and self-esteem for adolescent suicidal behaviors. Studies on Korean Youth 15(2): 153-182.
14. Hong SO, Eum KS, Bae OH (2003) A study on social support and stress of adolescent. Korea Association of Family Relations 8(1): 139-155.
15. Kim M (2015) The subjective well-being of korean children and its policy implications. Health-welfare policy forum; Korea institute for health and social affairs 2: 16-28.
16. Ozdemir U, Tuncay T (2008) Correlates of loneliness among university students. Child Adolesc Psychiatry Ment Health 2: 29.
17. Russek LG, Schwartz GE (1997) Perceptions of parental caring predict health status in midlife: a 35-year follow-up of the Harvar Mastery of Stress Study. Psychosom Med 59: 144-149.
18. Nikanami S, Zamani-Alavijeh F, Shafiee A, Seifi M (2011) Comparison of psychological status of full boarding and dya students in boarding schools. Asian J Psychiatry S41-S90.
19. Lebensohn P, Dodds S, Benn R, Brooks AJ, Birch M, et al. (2013) Resident wellness behaviors: relationship to stress, depression, and burnout. Fam Med 45: 541-549.
20. Duval F, Lebowitz BD, Macher JP (2006) Treatments in depression. Dialogues Clin Neurosci 8: 191-206.
21. Peterlini M, Tibério IF, Saadeh A, Pereira JC, Martins MA (2002) Anxiety and depression in the first year of medical residency training. Med Educ 36: 66-72.
22. Michels PJ, Probst JC, Godenick MT, Palesch Y (2003) Anxiety and anger among family practice residents: a South Carolina family practice research consortium study. Acad Med 78: 69-79.
23. Piccinelli M, Wilkinson G (2000) Gender differences in depression. Critical review. Br J Psychiatry 177: 486-492.
24. Dannon PN, Lowengrub K, Gonopolski Y, Kotler M (2006) Current and emerging somatic treatment strategies in psychotic major depression. Expert Rev Neurother 6: 73-80.
25. Silverstein B (1999) Gender difference in the prevalence of clinical depression: the role played by depression associated with somatic symptoms. Am J Psychiatry 156: 480-482.
26. Houston AM, Abraham A, Huang Z, D'Angelo LJ (2006) Knowledge, attitudes, and consequences of menstrual health in urban adolescent females. J Pediatr Adolesc Gynecol 19: 271-275.
27. Jane Costello E, Erkanli A, Angold A (2006) Is there an epidemic of child or adolescent depression? J Child Psychol Psychiatry 47: 1263-1271.
28. Zacher A (2003) [3 basic symptoms: affective--somatic--cognitive. Recognizing the faces of depression]. MMW Fortschr Med 145: 44-45.

Relationships between Airway Morphology and Sleep Breathing Indices in Jaw Deformity Patients

Hiroyuki Nakano[1], Katsuaki Mishima[2*], Asuka Nakano[2], Hokuto Suga[3], Yuichiro Miyawaki[4], Takamitsu Mano[2], Shintaro Nakagawa[2], Mayumi Matsumura[2], Yoshihide Mori[1] and Yoshiya Ueyama[2,5]

[1]*Section of Oral and Maxillofacial Surgery, Division of Maxillofacial Diagnostic and Surgical Sciences, Faculty of Dental Science, Kyushu University, Japan*

[2]*Department of Oral and Maxillofacial Surgery, Graduate School of Medicine, Yamaguchi University, Japan*

[3]*Department of Pediatric Dentistry, Kagoshima University Graduate School of Medical and Dental Sciences, Japan*

[4]*Miyawaki Orthodontic Clinic, Japan*

[5]*Division of Oral and Maxillofacial Surgery, Graduate School of Dental Science, Kyushu University, Japan*

[*]**Corresponding author:** Katsuaki Mishima, Department of Oral and Maxillofacial Surgery, Graduate School of Medicine, Yamaguchi University, Minami-kogushi 1-1-1, Ube City, Yamaguchi-755-8505, Japan, E-mail: kmishima@yamaguchi-u.ac.jp

Abstract

Purpose: The purpose of this study was to clarify how sleep breathing indices and airway morphology vary according to skeletal classification and the relationships between airway morphology and sleep breathing indices.

Method: Forty-four non-syndromic female Japanese patients, who were diagnosed with jaw deformities and underwent surgical orthodontic treatment were enrolled in this study. Using the Alice 5 diagnostic sleep system (Philips Respironics; Murrysville, PA), the apnea hypopnea index (AHI), apnea index (AI), and 4% oxygen desaturation index (4%ODI) were evaluated in each patient before they underwent orthognathic surgery. The following dimensions were measured on 2D CT images: the cross-sectional area at the level of the hard palate (HP), the cross-sectional area at the top of the uvula (TU), the cross-sectional area at the base of the tongue (BE). The following volumes were measured on 3D CT images: the volume of the upper airway (total volume), the volume of the region between the level of the hard palate and the top of the uvula (HP- TU volume), the volume of the region between the top of the uvula and the base of the epiglottis (TP-BE volume).

Result: There were no significant differences in airway morphology or sleep breathing indices among the three groups. Negative correlations were detected between HP-TU volume and 4%ODI, and between the HP area and AHI ($p<0.05$).

Conclusion: Our results establish that upper airway morphology also has important effects on the nocturnal breathing of jaw deformity patients.

Keywords: Sleep breathing indices; Jaw deformities; Airway

Introduction

Orthognathic surgery is performed to correct congenital and acquired jaw deformities. Guilleminault et al. [1] reported that obstructive sleep apnea syndrome (OSAS) can occur after mandibular setback surgery. Subsequently, several researchers have described the airway changes that occur after orthognathic surgery [2-4]. For example, mandibular setback surgery can narrow the pharyngeal airway space (PAS). However, it is unclear how jaw deformities affect sleep breathing indices.

It is generally considered that patients with mandibular retrognathism (skeletal class 2) have smaller airways than patients with mandibular prognathism (skeletal class 3). However, no detailed consensus has been reached regarding how airway morphology differs among patients with skeletal class 1, 2, and 3 relationships [5,6].

Computed tomography (CT) enables us to evaluate airway morphology three-dimensionally. We have already reported the optimal threshold levels for evaluating airway morphology with CT [7]. The purpose of this study was to clarify how sleep breathing indices and airway morphology vary according to skeletal classification and the relationships between airway morphology and sleep breathing indices.

Materials and Methods

Forty-four non-syndromic female Japanese patients, who were diagnosed with jaw deformities and underwent surgical orthodontic treatment at Yamaguchi University Hospital from July 2008 to December 2011, were enrolled in this study.

Their mean age at the time of the CT acquisition was 23.7 ± 8.2 years (Table 1), and their mean body mass index (BMI) was 19.9 ± 2.0 kg/m^2. The patients were divided into three groups based on their ANB angles; i.e., 14 patients whose ANB angles ranged from 0° to 4° were placed in the skeletal class 1 group, 17 patients whose ANB angles were greater than 4° were categorized into the skeletal class 2 group, and 13 patients whose ANB angles were less than 0° were included in the skeletal class 3 group.

Patients with a history of breathing problems were excluded from the study. The study was approved by the Ethics Committee of Yamaguchi University Hospital, and all participants signed informed consent forms.

	Gender	Age(y)	BMI(kg/m^2)
Skeletal 1 (n=14)	female	25.5 ± 9.3	18.9 ± 1.9
Skeletal 2 (n=17)	Female	22.6 ± 6.1	19.6 ± 1.9
Skeletal 3 (n=13)	Female	23.1 ± 9.4	21.2 ± 1.8

Table 1: Distribution of subjects.

Examination of breathing during sleep

Using the Alice 5 diagnostic sleep system (Philips Respironics; Murrysville, PA), the apnea hypopnea index (AHI), apnea index (AI), and 4% oxygen desaturation index (4%ODI) were evaluated in each patient before they underwent orthognathic surgery. The indices were defined according to standard criteria.

The AI and HI measure the number of pre-defined events per hour of sleep. The pre-defined events were as follows: AI: a ≥90% drop in the air temperature detected by an oronasal thermal sensor compared with the baseline, lasting for ≥ 10 sec; HI: a ≥50% reduction in nasal pressure from the baseline and an associated ≥4% desaturation from the pre-event baseline. AHI was defined as the sum of the AI and HI [8]. The indices were measured in various body postures.

Measurements of airway morphology

A CT machine (SOMATOM Definition SIEMENS Co. Forchheim, Germany) and a multi-slice helical technique were employed in this study. All CT scans were acquired with the subjects in centric occlusion, and the slice plane was oriented parallel to the Frankfort horizontal (FH) plane.

The CT images were taken before the patients underwent orthognathic surgery. The slice thickness of the reconstructed images was 0.6 mm. The CT images were imported into a personal computer, and the airway was reconstructed using CT analysis software (Mimics version 14.12). The upper and lower thresholds used to produce 3D images from the CT data were -470 HU and -1024 HU, respectively [7].

The level of the hard palate and the base of the epiglottis were used as the upper and lower boundaries of the airway, respectively. The pharyngeal walls were used as the lateral and posterior boundaries of the model. The anterior boundary was defined by the soft palate, the base of the tongue, and the anterior wall of the pharynx.

The following dimensions were measured on 2D CT images: the cross-sectional area at the level of the hard palate (HP), the cross-sectional area at the top of the uvula (TU), the cross-sectional area at the base of the tongue (BE) (Figure 1).

The following volumes were measured on 3D CT images: the volume of the upper airway (total volume), the volume of the region between the level of the hard palate and the top of the uvula (HP-TU volume), the volume of the region between the top of the uvula and the base of the epiglottis (TP-BE volume) (Figure 2).

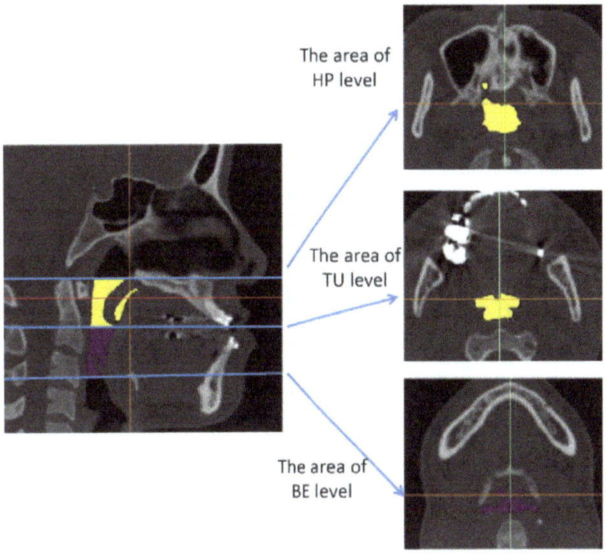

Figure 1: The method used to assess airway morphology (2D images) (The cross-sectional areas at the level of the hard palate, the top of the uvula, and the base of the tongue were measured).

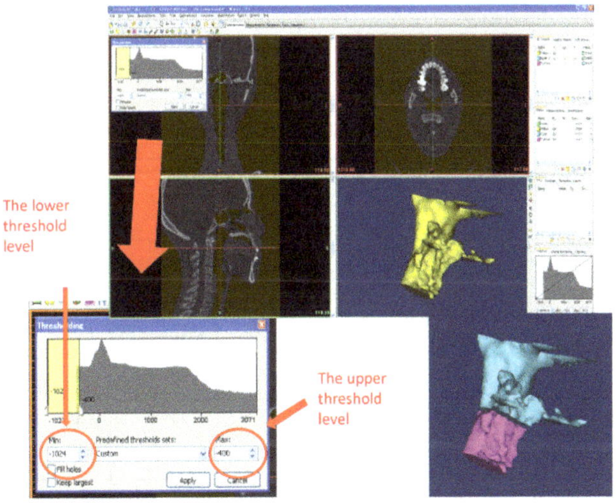

Figure 2: The method used to assess airway morphology (3D images) (The total volume, HP-TU volume, and TP-BE volume were measured).

Statistical analysis

SPSS software for Windows, version 11.0 (SPSS, Chicago, IL), was used for all statistical analyses. Descriptive statistics, including means and standard deviations for each group, were calculated. One-way analysis of variance was used to compare the airway morphologies and sleep breathing indices of the skeletal class 1, 2, and 3 groups. In addition, Spearman's rank correlation coefficients were used to evaluate the correlations between airway morphology and the sleep breathing indices. Values of $p<0.05$ were considered statistically significant.

Results

There were no significant differences in airway morphology or sleep breathing indices among the three groups (Tables 2 and 3). Negative correlations were detected between HP-TU volume and 4%ODI and between the HP area and AHI ($p<0.05$) (Table 4).

	skeletal 1	skeletal 2	skeletal 3	P value
The total volume (mm^3)	15669.9 ± 5248.2	13088.7 ± 6059.8	11970.5 ± 4892.4	0.2
The volume of HP-TU (mm^3)	8474.2 ± 3725.5	6143.5 ± 2811.6	5906.4 ± 3265.4	0.08
The volume of TP-BE (mm^3)	7083.6 ± 2237.2	6733.1 ± 3432.2	5970.6 ± 1970.4	0.55
The area of HP level (mm^2)	590.9 ± 172.5	511.9 ± 170.3	442 ± 238.2	0.14
The area of TU level (mm^2)	242.5 ± 115.6	180.1 ± 103.7	216.6 ± 112.6	0.29
The area of BE level (mm^2)	298.6 ± 77.3	273 ± 89.8	240.8 ± 97.6	0.24

Table 2: The relationship between airway morphology and skeletal morphology (one-way analysis of variance).

	skeletal 1	skeletal 2	skeletal 3	P value
AI (/hr)	0.8 ± 1	1.3 ± 1.6	0.8 ± 0.8	0.4
HI (/hr)	0.007 ± 0.03	0.006 ± 0.02	0.6 ± 1.2	0.05
AHI (/hr)	0.8 ± 1	1.3 ± 1.6	1.3 ± 1.4	0.55
4%ODI (/hr)	0.2 ± 0.2	0.5 ± 0.6	0.6 ± 0.9	0.16

Table 3: The relationship between skeletal morphology and SBI (one-way analysis of variance).

	AI	HI	AHI	4%ODI
The total volume	0.13 0.39	0.05 0.74	0.17 0.24	0.22 0.14
The volume of HP-TU	0.23 0.12	0.12 0.4	0.26 0.08	0.33 0.02*
The volume of TU-BE	0.05 0.71	0.03 0.82	0.08 0.58	0.16 0.28
The area of HP level	0.23 0.12	0.18 0.22	0.29 0.04*	0.19 0.2
The area of TU level	0.2 0.17	0 0.96	0.22 0.13	0.28 0.06
The area of BE level	0 0.98	0.09 0.55	0.06 0.67	0.15 0.3

Table 4: The correlation between airway morphology and SBI (Spearman's correlation coefficient by rank *$p<0.05$).

Discussion

A number of reports have described the airway morphology of Asian patients with jaw deformities [5,6]. Kikuchi [5] reported that the volume of the lower part of the pharyngeal space is increased in patients with mandibular prognathism (skeletal class 3). On the other hand, Hong et al. [6] reported that the volume of the upper part of the pharyngeal space is greater in patients with skeletal class 3 malocclusion than in those with other malocclusions and that the volume of the upper part of the pharyngeal airway is significantly correlated with the anterior position of the mandible. Hence, previous studies have reported different findings regarding the relationship between airway morphology and mandibular position. In our study, neither airway volume nor any of the sleep breathing indices displayed significant differences among the skeletal class groups. We think that this was because most patients with jaw deformities are young. However, mandibular retrognathism is a morphological feature of OSAS patients; therefore, we will continue to follow-up the airway morphology of the patients in this study.

Secondly, the relationships between airway morphology and sleep breathing indices were examined in the whole subject population because there were no significant differences in sleep breathing indices or airway volume among the skeletal class groups. Many studies have evaluated the airway morphology of OSAS patients [9-12]. There are two methods for assessing the airway morphology of OSAS patients using CT. The first method is to examine the distance from the level of the hard palate to the base of the epiglottis [9-11]. The second method is to evaluate the position of the cervical spine [4,12]. Muto et al. [13] reported that the degree of craniocervical inclination affected the dimensions of the PAS. Although it is important to understand this relationship, investigating it raises ethical problems because it requires the acquisition of several CT scans. In addition, we considered that craniocervical inclination would not vary much in our study because all of the CT scans were taken in the supine position; therefore, we evaluated airway morphology by measuring the distance from the level of the hard palate to the base of the epiglottis.

As a result, we found that the HP-TU volume displayed a negative relationship with 4%ODI, a sleep breathing index. Some other researchers have reported similar results [14,15]. Tsuiki et al. [14] reported that the success of oral appliance therapy for OSAS depended on anterior titration of the patient's mandibular position to enlarge the upper airway. Similarly, Gao et al. [15] reported that oral appliance therapy for OSAS works by enlarging the upper airway, mainly the region at the back of the soft palate, and keeping the airway open. Accordingly, many researchers have reported that upper airway morphology is closely related to OSAS. However, these studies only involved OSAS patients. Our results establish that upper airway morphology also has important effects on the nocturnal breathing of jaw deformity patients.

Acknowledgments

This work was supported by Grant-in-Aid for Scientific Research (C) (25293410) and Young Scientists (B) (25861954) from the Ministry of Education, Culture, Sports, Science and Technology (MEXT) and Japan Society for Promotion of Science (JSPS) KAKENHI Grant Number (25293410 and 25861954).

References

1. Kikuchi Y (2008) Three-dimensional relationship between pharyngeal airway and maxillo-facial morphology. Bull Tokyo Dent Coll 49: 65-75.
2. Hong JS, Oh KM, Kim BR, Kim YJ, Park YH (2011) Three-dimensional analysis of pharyngeal airway volume in adults with anterior position of the mandible. Am J Orthod Dentofacial Orthop 140: e161-169.
3. Guilleminault C, Riley R, Powell N (1985) Sleep apnea in normal subjects following mandibular osteotomy with retrusion. Chest 88: 776-778.
4. Kawamata A, Fujishita M, Ariji Y, Ariji E (2000) Three-dimensional computed tomographic evaluation of morphologic airway changes after mandibular setback osteotomy for prognathism. Oral Surg Oral Med Oral Pathol Oral Radiol Endod 89: 278-287.
5. Degerliyurt K, Ueki K, Hashiba Y, Marukawa K, Nakagawa K, et al. (2008) A comparative CT evaluation of pharyngeal airway changes in class III patients receiving bimaxillary surgery or mandibular setback surgery. Oral Surg Oral Med Oral Pathol Oral Radiol Endod 105: 495-502.
6. Park SB, Kim YI, Son WS, Hwang DS, Cho BH (2012) Cone-beam computed tomography evaluation of short- and long-term airway change and stability after orthognathic surgery in patients with Class III skeletal deformities: bimaxillary surgery and mandibular setback surgery. Int J Oral Maxillofac Surg 41: 87-93.
7. Nakano H, Mishima K, Ueda Y, Matsushita A, Suga H, et al. (2013) A new method for determining the optimal CT threshold for extracting the upper airway. Dentomaxillofac Radiol 42: 26397438.
8. [No authors listed] (1999) Sleep-related breathing disorders in adults: recommendations for syndrome definition and measurement techniques in clinical research. The Report of an American Academy of Sleep Medicine Task Force. Sleep 22: 667-689.
9. Caballero P, Alvarez-Sala R, García-Río F, Prados C, Hernán MA, et al. (1998) CT in the evaluation of the upper airway in healthy subjects and in patients with obstructive sleep apnea syndrome. Chest 113: 111-116.
10. Chen NH, Li KK, Li SY, Wong CR, Chuang ML, et al. (2002) Airway assessment by volumetric computed tomography in snorers and subjects with obstructive sleep apnea in a Far-East Asian population (Chinese). Laryngoscope 112: 721-726.
11. Abramson Z, Susarla S, August M, Troulis M, Kaban L (2010) Three-dimensional computed tomographic analysis of airway anatomy in patients with obstructive sleep apnea. J Oral Maxillofac Surg 68: 354-362.
12. Degerliyurt K, Ueki K, Hashiba Y, Marukawa K, Simsek B, et al. (2009) The effect of mandibular setback or two-jaws surgery on pharyngeal airway among different genders. Int J Oral Maxillofac Surg 38: 647-652.
13. Muto T, Takeda S, Kanazawa M, Yamazaki A, Fujiwara Y, et al. (2002) The effect of head posture on the pharyngeal airway space (PAS). Int J Oral Maxillofac Surg 31: 579-583.
14. Tsuiki S, Lowe AA, Almeida FR, Fleetham JA (2004) Effects of an anteriorly titrated mandibular position on awake airway and obstructive sleep apnea severity. Am J Orthod Dentofacial Orthop 125: 548-555.
15. Gao XM, Zeng XL, Fu MK, Huang XZ (1999) Magnetic resonance imaging of the upper airway in obstructive sleep apnea before and after oral appliance therapy. Chin J Dent Res 2: 27-35.

Reported Nightmares and Trait Anxiety Among Arab Children, Adolescents and Adults

Ahmed M Abdel-Khalek*

Department of Psychology, University of Alexandria, Egypt

***Corresponding author:** Ahmed M Abdel-Khalek, Department of Psychology, Faculty of Arts, University of Alexandria, Egypt, E-mail: aabdel-khalek@hotmail.com

Abstract

Background: Research on the association between nightmares and anxiety has reached conflicting results. Further, the Arabic studies in this domain are scarce.

Objective: This study sought to investigate the relation between reported nightmares and trait anxiety among a large sample of Arab students.

Methods: A convenience sample of non-clinical 8,218 school and university Arab students took part in this study. They were classified into 13 age groups (from 12 to 24). A self-rating scale was used to assess nightmares based on the participant's perceived frequency during the last month. A 5-point Likert type scale was used as follows: 0: No; 1: A little; 2: Moderate; 3: Much and 4: Very much. The Kuwait University Anxiety Scale was also used.

Results: All the Pearson correlation coefficients between reported nightmares and trait anxiety were statistically significant and positive in all of the 13 age groups, and ranged between 0.38 and 0.53, with a median of 0.44.

Conclusion: On the basis of a large sample of Arab students, and two scales with good psychometric properties, we can suggest that anxiety level should be considered in participants who experiencing nightmares.

Keywords: Nightmares; Anxiety; Children; Adolescents; Adults; Arabs

Introduction

We spend one third of our life asleep. Sleep is an active state critical for our physical, mental, and emotional well-being. In fact, sleep is a basic necessity of life, as fundamental for the maintenance of human health as air, food, and water. Sleep disorders represent pathophysiology, which causes an overriding the active processes that are probably homeostatic and circadian [1]. More than 90 sleep pathologies have been identified, one of them is nightmares. It is important to differentiate between nightmares in the non-institutionalized samples and nightmare disorder with specific diagnostic criteria. The present study was carried out with non-clinical participants.

The ICSD-R [2] defined the nightmare as a long, complicated dream that becomes increasingly frightening toward the end. Similarly, the first diagnostic criterion of the nightmare in the DSM5 [3] is as follows: "repeated occurrence of extended, extremely dysphoric, and well- remembered dream that usually involve efforts to avoid threats to survival, security, or physical integrity and generally occur during the second half of the major sleep episode". Zadra and Donderi [4] define a nightmare as "a very disturbing dream in which the unpleasant visual imagery and/or emotions wake the person up". They indicated that there is a continuum between bad dreams (without awakening) and nightmares (with awakening) with nightmares exhibiting the strongest correlations to psychopathology measures.

Prevalence of nightmares increases through childhood into adolescence from 1.3% to 3.9% among preschool children. Then, prevalence increases from ages 10 to 13 for both boys and girls but continues to increase to ages 20-29 for females, while decreasing for males. Prevalence decreases steadily with age for both sexes, but the gender difference remains. Among adults, prevalence for frequent nightmares is 1% to 2% [3].

Schredl and Reinhard [5] carried out a meta-analytic research based on 111 independent studies to estimate the gender differences in nightmare frequency. Overall, the effect sizes of these gender differences differed significantly from zero in three age groups of healthy persons (adolescents, young adults, and middle-aged adults), whereas for children and older persons no substantial gender difference in nightmare frequency could be demonstrated. They found that women tend to report nightmares more often than men but this gender difference was not found in children and older persons. Studies with binary coded items showed a markedly smaller effect size for the gender difference in nightmare frequency compared to the studies using multiple categories in a rating scale.

Using a large non-clinical probability Arab sample (N=11,334) aged 10 to 55, the prevalence rates (Much+Very much) according to perceived severity during the past month ranged from 4.5% (male adults) to 14.3% (female adolescents) [6]. With another sample of Arab children and adolescents (N=6,727), it was found that in the ages 15 to 18, females obtained a significantly higher mean scores on reported nightmares than did their male counterparts [7]. Generally speaking, the Arabic studies in this domain are scarce.

Considerable controversy has surrounded the association between nightmares and both psychopathology and lack of well-being. As early as 1980, Kales et al. [8] found that frequency of nightmares has been related to high scores on the neurotic and psychotic scales of the Minnesota Multiphasic Personality Inventory. With a sample of 148 Australian school students aged 12 and 18 years, Roberts and Lennings [9] found that all psychopathology scores were associated with the nightmare measures. Anxiety was the most commonly reported correlate of all three nightmare measures. Nightmare sleeping distress was more likely to be associated with high levels of neuroticism and with lower levels of psychoticism, but not with extraversion.

Several studies have demonstrated the association between nightmares and both neuroticism and anxiety [4,10-16]. Schredl et al. [15] concluded from the association between nightmares and neuroticism that this relationship fits in the general continuity hypothesis of dreaming, i.e., current waking - life experiences (stress) is incorporated into subsequent dreams. Picchioni et al. [17] demonstrated a positive association between nightmares and coping with stress. This association bolsters the supposition that nightmares may help to alleviate stress. Krakov et al. [18] noted that nightmares are secondary to another disorder, e.g., PTSD or anxiety disorder. In this psychiatric view, nightmares are a symptom of a larger syndrome: a nightly symptom of anxiety [16].

On the other hand, some studies failed to find an association between nightmares and both anxiety and neuroticism [19-22]. Beullens [23] stated that there is no indication of an elevated anxiety level in the daytime or of psychopathology in nightmares. On the other hand, Lancee et al. [24] concluded that nightmare frequency is associated with subjective sleep quality but not with psychopathology.

Given the conflict in the literature, the main objective of the present study was to investigate the association between reported nightmares and trait anxiety among non-clinical Arab samples: an under studied and underrepresented population in the literature of sleep disorders. It was hypothesized that participants who experience nightmares would be more anxious, i.e., a positive correlation between reported nightmares and trait anxiety. In addition to this main objective, the present study sought to explore the sex-related differences in nightmares and trait anxiety.

Materials and Methods

Participants

A convenience sample of 8,218 school and university Arab students took part in this study (49% males). They were classified into 13 subgroups according to their ages from 12 to 24 years. This sample was selected from the regular schools and university. It is important to note that the participants in this study were not diagnosed institutionalized patients. No exclusion criteria on psychiatric or neurological grounds were applied.

Assessment tools

Reported nightmares: A self-rating scale item was used to assess nightmares. The statement was as follows. "I have nightmares that wake me up scared". Participants were requested to respond to this item on a 5-point Likert-type scale as follows, 0: No; 1: A little; 2: Moderate; 3: Much and 4: Very much, so the possible range of scores is 0-4. Participants were instructed to answer this item, according to their subjective evaluation, on the basis of their perceived frequency during the past month, and not intensity.

It is important to note that the concept of nightmare is quite clear to, and assimilated by, Arab participants even young children in the present study (i.e., 12 years). The Arabic word to refer to this concept is well defined, i.e., "Kaboos". Unlike the "value neutral" English term, the "Kaboos" implies "pressure" or "stress" [6,7].

The Kuwait University Anxiety Scale (KUAS): It [25] consists of 20 brief statements, each answered on a four-point intensity scale, anchored by 1: Rarely, and 4: Always. The total score could range from 20 to 80, with a higher scores indicating higher anxiety. In previous studies on Arab samples, reliabilities of the scale ranged from 0.88 to 0.92 (Cronbach's alpha), and between 0.70 and 0.93 (test-retest), indicating good internal consistency and temporal stability. The criterion-related validity of the scale ranged between 0.70 and 0.88 (five criteria), while the loadings of the scale on a general factor of anxiety were 0.93 and 0.95 in two factor analyses, demonstrating the scale's criterion-related and construct validity. Discriminant validity of the scale has also been demonstrated. Factor analysis of the scale items yielded three factors labelled "cognitive/Affective", "Subjective", and "Somatic anxiety". The scale has displayed good psychometric properties in different Arabic and Western samples of college students [26]. The KUAS has four comparable Arabic, English, German, and Spanish versions.

Procedure

The Arabic versions of the nightmare item, along with the trait anxiety scale (KUAS) were administered to participants in group sessions of 30 to 35 students in their classrooms, during regular school and university hours. The scales were administered to each group in a single session of approximately 10 minutes in duration. Competent assistants carried out the administration of the tests. The university students provided verbal agreement to offer themselves as subjects, after the aims of the study were outlined. There were few refusals. As for the younger pupils, informed consent was obtained. Assurances were made that anonymity would be maintained. The response rate was 93%. The SPSS [27] was used to compute the descriptive statistics, the t rations, and the correlations between nightmares and anxiety.

Results

Regarding the psychometric characteristic of the self-rating scale of nightmares based on a single item, its 1-week test-retest reliability was equal to 0.75 for children, while it was 0.80 for adolescents, and 0.81 for adults, indicating acceptable temporal stability and corroborate the trait (not state)-like of the score. The Cronbach alpha reliability of the anxiety scale (KUAS) ranged between 0.81 and 0.89, indicating acceptable to good internal consistency.

Table 1 sets out the descriptive statistics and the t for the nightmare rating scale among males and females. Reference to this table reveals that the sex-related differences were found only in the ages 15 to 21 in favor of females.

Table 2 presents the descriptive statistics and the t ratio for the trait anxiety scale in males and females. Inspection of this table indicates that the sex differences in anxiety were statistically significant in nine out of the 13 age groups in favor of females, i.e., they were more anxious.

Age	Males			Females			t	p
	N	M	SD	N	M	SD		
12	267	0.94	1.29	231	0.73	1.14	1.89	-
13	261	1.07	1.33	261	0.93	1.24	1.26	-
14	351	0.84	1.11	454	0.96	1.17	1.41	-
15	645	0.82	1.03	606	1.03	1.19	3.4	0.001
16	654	0.79	1.05	570	1.11	1.23	4.85	0.0001
17	502	0.74	0.98	576	1.06	1.18	4.81	0.0001
18	450	0.72	0.93	578	1.06	1.13	5.16	0.0001
19	330	0.8	0.95	265	1.13	1.12	3.82	0.0001
20	219	0.89	1.02	235	1.14	1.13	2.43	0.02
21	144	0.62	0.82	167	0.99	0.95	3.65	0.0001
22	97	0.81	0.89	140	0.89	0.97	0.64	-
23	62	0.85	0.96	69	0.96	0.98	0.6	-
24	41	0.66	0.83	43	0.88	0.96	1.15	-

Table 1: Mean (M), standard deviation (SD), and t ratio for the self-rating scale item to assess nightmares in the past month among males and females in the ages 12-24.

Age	Males			Females			t	p
	N	M	SD	N	M	SD		
12	267	31.65	9.78	231	33.01	10.62	1.48	-
13	261	30.5	9.46	261	33.67	10.7	3.59	0.001
14	351	33.7	9.79	454	34.56	10.63	1.19	-
15	645	34.57	10.03	606	37.81	11.7	5.24	0.0001
16	654	35.28	10.64	570	38.59	11.92	5.08	0.0001
17	502	35.71	10.95	576	39.45	11.49	5.47	0.0001
18	450	37.24	10.3	578	40.39	11.22	4.68	0.0001
19	330	37.83	9.79	265	41.79	12.07	4.32	0.0001
20	219	38.45	9.99	235	40.71	10.93	2.3	0.02
21	144	38.6	11.61	167	40.39	11.34	1.37	-
22	97	36.19	10.3	140	38.93	11.31	1.93	-
23	62	36.6	10.48	69	41.83	12.5	2.6	0.01
24	41	31.5	9.94	43	37.22	10.91	2.51	0.02

Table 2: Mean (M), standard deviation (SD), and t ratio for the anxiety scale among males and females in the ages 12-24.

Table 3 sets out the Pearson correlation coefficients between nightmares and anxiety in the ages 12 to 24. Male and female samples in the same age group were combined because the differences between the correlations were trivial. Reference to this table indicated that all the correlations were statistically significant and positive. These correlations ranged from 0.38 to 0.53 and the median was 0.44.

Age	N	r	p
12	498	0.502	0.001
13	522	0.411	0.001
14	805	0.453	0.001
15	1251	0.426	0.001
16	1224	0.443	0.001
17	1078	0.405	0.001
18	1028	0.394	0.001
19	595	0.446	0.001
20	454	0.527	0.001
21	311	0.412	0.001
22	237	0.384	0.001
23	131	0.435	0.001
24	84	0.462	0.001
Median	8218	0.435	0.001

Table 3: The Pearson correlation (r) coefficients between nightmares and anxiety in the ages 12 to 24.

Discussion

The investigation of the association between nightmares and psychopathology is of great importance for the subjects of etiology, diagnosis, and treatment, as well as for comorbidity. Therefore, increasing attention is being given to this association. Over the last few decades, there has emerged an extensive body of empirical work dealing with this subject. However, a dearth of research with Arab participants exists.

Anxiety disorders and trait anxiety were among the main psychopathologies to study their relation with nightmares, using clinical and non-clinical samples. Unfortunately, the results of these studies have not been consistent. These discrepancies may be related to the sample (large versus small; age; clinical vis- à- vis non-clinical; duration and severity of the disorder; comorbidity, etc.), and the assessment tool (diagnostic criteria of the DSM; psychometric questionnaire; psychological interview, etc.), among other factors. However, it is particularly noteworthy that the positive results on the association between nightmares and anxiety outnumber the negative findings.

The statistically significant correlations found in the present study add to the majority of the existent literature, which suggests that there is a covariation between nightmares and anxiety. However, correlation is, ipso facto, does not mean causality. That is, the present results do not indicate that nightmare is the cause of anxiety or anxiety is the cause of nightmare. In particular, the investigation of causality needs an experimental design.

What is the link between nightmares and anxiety? It has been traditionally thought that the etiology of nightmares was related to a person's daytime anxiety. Recent empirical research strongly supports the view that nightmares are related to psychological problems while awake [4,14].

Comorbidity of nightmares with other psychopathology is an important issue. However, Spoormaker et al. [16] stated that strong relationships and high comorbidities with other mental disorders would not mean that nightmares are not a separate sleep disorder. Comorbidities of nightmares with other mental disorders are high for depressive disorders, anxiety disorders, and psychophysiological insomnia. Because nightmares seem to be persistent, it is more valuable for professionals to diagnose and treat nightmares. Research indicated that nightmares and low well-being are associated [4,28], so treating nightmares would improve the level of well-being of the patient.

The other objectives of the present study have been adequately demonstrated. Consistent with previous studies, the sex-related differences in nightmares were statistically significant [5-7] in some age groups, as well as anxiety [29]. In all the significant differences in the two variables, females obtained the higher mean score than did their male counterparts.

Limitation

Notwithstanding specific strengths of the present investigation, namely using a large sample from an under-represented population in the domain of sleep disorders, from the Arabic context, and the good psychometric characteristics of the psychological tools, specific limitations are acknowledged. Foremost among them is the use of a convenience sample. Moreover, student samples mainly consist of intelligent, young and healthy persons who only represent a small sector of any population. Thus, it would be important to either use a probability sample of students or using older age groups or a clinical Arab sample. Further, it is important to study the association between nightmares and other psychiatric disorders, e.g., depression and insomnia. Further research appears warranted in this endeavor.

Conclusion

As far as the current study on Arab students is concerned, its salient result is the statistically significant and positive correlations between reported nightmares and trait anxiety in all the 13 age groups from 12 to 24 years. That is, participants with high nightmare frequency report themselves as having a higher trait anxiety. By and large, the present results suggest that anxiety level should be considered in participants who experiencing nightmares. Further, treating nightmares would increase the level of subjective well-being of the case.

Acknowledgement

The author would like to thank the participants for their time and good cooperation as well as the reviewers of the manuscript and the editorial board of the journal.

References

1. Silva JAC (2006) Sleep disorders in psychiatry. Metabolism 55: S40-S44.
2. American Academy of Sleep Medicine (2001) International classification of sleep disorders, revised: diagnostic and coding manual. Chicago, Illinois, USA.
3. American Psychiatric Association (2013) Diagnostic and Statistical Manual of Mental Disorders. 5th edn. Arlington, VA, USA.
4. Zadra A, Donderi DC (2000) Nightmares and bad dreams: their prevalence and relationship to well-being. J Abnorm Psychol 109: 273-281.
5. Schredl M, Reinhard I (2011) Gender differences in nightmare frequency: a meta-analysis. Sleep Med Rev 15: 115-121.
6. Abdel-Khalek AM (2010) Prevalence rates of reported nightmares in a cross-sectional sample of Kuwaiti children, adolescents, undergraduates and employees. Sleep Hypn 12: 13-22.
7. Abdel-Khalek AM (2006) Nightmares: prevalence, age and gender differences among Kuwaiti children and adolescents. Sleep Hypn 8: 33-40.
8. Kales A, Soldatos CR, Caldwell AB, Charney DS, Kales JD, et al. (1980) Nightmares: clinical characteristics and personality patterns. Am J Psychiatry 137: 1197-1201.
9. Roberts J, Lennings CL (2006) Peronality, psychopathology and nightmares in young people. Pers Indiv Differ 41: 733-744.
10. Lang R, O' Connor KP (1984) Personality, dream content, and dream coping style. Pers Indiv Differ 5: 211-219.
11. Berquier A, Ashton R (1992) Characteristics of the frequent nightmare sufferer. J Abnorm Psychol 101: 246-250.
12. Ohayon MM, Morselli PL, Guilleminault C (1997) Prevalence of nightmares and their relationship to psychopathology and daytime functioning in insomnia subjects. Sleep 20: 340-348.
13. Köthe M, Pietrowsky R (2001) Behavioral effects of nightmares and their correlations to personality patterns. Dreaming 11: 43-52.
14. Levin R, Fireman G (2002) Nightmare prevalence, nightmare distress, and self-reported psychological disturbance. Sleep 25: 205-212.
15. Schredl M, Landgraf C, Zeiler O (2003) Nightmare frequency, nightmare distress and neuroticism. N Am J Psychol 5: 345-350.
16. Spoormaker VI, Schredl M, van den Bout J (2006) Nightmares: from anxiety symptom to sleep disorder. Sleep Med Rev 10: 19-31.
17. Picchioni D, Goeltzenleucher B, Green DN, Convento MJ, Crittenden R, et al. (2002) Nighmares as a coping mechanism for stress. Dreaming 12: 155-169.
18. Krakow B, Kellner R, Pathak D, Lambert L (1995) Imagery rehearsal treatment for chronic nightmares. Behav Res Ther 33: 837-843.
19. Hartmann E, Russ D, Oldfield M, Sivan I, Cooper S (1987) Who has nightmares? The personality of the lifelong nightmare sufferer. Arch Gen Psychiatry 44: 49-56.
20. Wood JM, Bootzin RR (1990) The prevalence of nightmares and their independence from anxiety. J Abnorm Psychol 99: 64-68.
21. Belicki K (1992) Nightmare frequency versus nightmare distress: relations to psychopathology and cognitive style. J Abnorm Psychol 101: 592-597.
22. Chivers L, Blagrove M (1999) Nightmare frequency, personality and acute psychopathology. Pers Indiv Differ 27: 843-851.
23. Beullens J (1996) Nightmares in psychiatry. Acta Neuropsychiatr 8: 12-16.
24. Lancee J, Spoormaker VI, van den Bout J (2010) Nightmare frequency is associated with subjective sleep quality but not with psychopathology. Sleep Biol Rhythms 8: 187-193.
25. Abdel-Khalek AM (2000) The Kuwait University Anxiety Scale: psychometric properties. Psychological Reports 87: 478-492.
26. Abdel-Khalek AM, Maltby J (2009) Differences in anxiety scores of college students from Germany, Spain, the United Kingdom, and the USA. Psychol Rep 104: 624-626.
27. SPSS, Inc. (2009) SPSS: Statistical data analysis : Base 18.0, Users guide. SPSS: Chicago, Illinois, USA.
28. Blagrove M, Farmer L, Williams E (2004) The relationship of nightmare frequency and nightmare distress to well-being. J Sleep Res 13: 129-136.
29. Abdel-Khalek AM, Alansari BM (2004) Gender differences in anxiety among undergraduates from ten Arab countries. Soc Behav Personal 32: 649-655.

Sleep Abnormalities and Sleep Breathing Disorders in Children with Drug-Resistant Catastrophic Epileptic Encephalopathy

Anna Michela Gaeta[1*], **Anna Annunziata**[1], **Francesca Gaeta**[2], **Gianfranco Scotto Di Frega**[1] **and Giuseppe Fiorentino**[1]

[1]*Division of Respiratory Physiopathology, Monaldi Hospital, Naples, Italy*

[2]*Department of Medicine and Surgery, University of Salerno, Baronissi (Salerno), Italy*

[*]**Corresponding author:** Anna Michela Gaeta, Division of Respiratory Physiopathology, Monaldi Hospital, Naples, Italy, E-mail: annamichelagaeta@hotmail.it

Abstract

Undiagnosed obstructive sleep apnoea is common in patients with medically refractory epilepsy. The aim of this study is to evaluate sleep alterations and the prevalence of Sleep Breathing Disorders (SBD) in a paediatric population with catastrophic epileptic encephalopathy. To diagnose SBD, polysomnography (PSG) was performed in eleven patients (nine males, two females), with ages ranging between 3 and 11 years old, with epileptic encephalopathy characterized by drug-resistant seizures, occurring both in sleeping and waking, mental retardation and cerebral palsy. All the patients presented alterations of the sleep architecture and were positive for SBD. In particular, seven patients presented a severe form of Obstructive Sleep Apnoea Syndrome (OSAS) with apnoea/hypopnea index (AHI) greater than10/hr, two patients presented a moderate form with AHI between 5/hr and 10/hr, two patients presented a mild form with AHI lower than 4/hr. In conclusion, SBD and sleep disruption appeared to be in comorbidity with catastrophic epileptic encephalopathy. Their treatment might also have a positive impact in seizures control and quality of life.

Keywords: SBD: Sleep-Related Breathing Disorders; Epilepsy; PSG: Polysomnography; OSAS: Obstructive Sleep Apnoea Syndrome; Drug-Resistant Seizures, AHI: Apnoea/Hypopnea Index.

Introduction

Recurrent unprovoked seizures occur in 1–2% of children. The incidence of epilepsy plateaus in early childhood and decreases after 10 years of age [1, 2, 3]. Approximately 10–40% of children with epilepsy will continue to have seizures despite optimal medical management with antiepileptic drugs (AEDs) [4, 5, 6]. In 2001, the International League Against Epilepsy (ILAE)Task Force on Classification and Terminology recognized epileptic encephalopathies as a distinct category. The epileptic catastrophic encephalopathies are a rare group of conditions characterized by epileptic seizures that are often, but not always, intractable to treatment and associated with significant neurodevelopmental delay [7, 8]. The relation between epilepsy and sleep disorders is well known and their mutual effects are widely documented [9, 10]. Night seizures significantly reduce sleep efficiency [11]. In particular, Sleep Breathing Disorders (SBD) induce a chronic modification of the sleep architecture and a state of intermittent oxygen desaturation, resulting in poor control of seizures and excessive daytime sleepiness [12]. Obstructive apnoea is common in medically refractory epilepsy adult patients [13].

The comorbidity between SBD and epileptic catastrophic encephalopathies in the paediatric population is very poorly investigated in literature and rarely considered in general practice. This study aims to assess the presence of sleep abnormalities and SBD in a cohort of children with catastrophic epileptic encephalopathy, characterized by seizures refractory to standard antiepileptic drugs.

Materials and Methods

Patients were enrolled in the study according to the following criteria: age less than 12 years; clinical and electroencephalographic diagnosis of partial or generalized crypto-symptomatic catastrophic epileptic encephalopathies characterized by drug-resistant seizures, occurring both in sleeping and waking; mental retardation and cerebral palsy; medication regimens optimized; treatment failure with at least three antiepileptic drugs given alone or in combination.

Exclusion criteria were: seizure secondary to infection, cerebral neoplasia and/or haemorrhage, significant history of medical disease (e.g. liver or kidney failure, metabolic illness) or progressive degenerative disease; non epileptic spells, alone or in combinations with epileptic seizures; another primary sleep disorder requiring medication like sedatives or hypnotics, that could affectthe results of study; poor compliance to the polisomnography (PSG) by parents-care givers and/or children; previous diagnosis of Obstructive Sleep Apnoea Syndrome (OSAS).

Data including age, sex, body mass index (BMI), Mallampati index were collected. Computed tomography-magnetic resonance brain study, chest X-ray study and Electrocardiography (ECG) were performed through all population.

Before the study, each patient underwent a detailed interview about personal history, a general clinical examination and a somatometric data collection. Parents or care-givers were asked about patients sleep characteristic, such as total nocturnal sleep time, history of excessive daytime sleepiness, insomnia, nocturnal snoring, and awakenings during sleep.

Parents or care-givers also completed the Brouillette questionnaire on symptoms of OSAS. According the questionnaire, OSAS was no predicted for scores less than -1, inconclusive from -1 to 3,5 and predicted > 3,5. No change in antiepileptic therapy was performed during the study, or in the four previous months.

Electroencephalographic assessment

Characteristics of epilepsy like frequency of epileptic seizures, circadian rhythm of seizures, previous and current AEDs use were reviewed. The diagnosis of epilepsy was made by an epileptologist based on clinical history of recurrent epileptic seizures and supporting electroencephalographic data. Seizure classification and drug resistant epilepsy definition were based using ILAE criteria [7, 8, 14].

Drug resistant epilepsy was defined as any recurrent complex partial or generalized seizure in the past six months despite adequate use and compliance whit at least two tolerated and appropriately chosen AEDs in the past [14].

Polysomnographic recording

The polysomnographic studies were performed in the sleep laboratory of the A.O. Ospedali dei Colli - A.O.R.N. Monaldi in Naples. Overnight sleep studies were carried out in all subjects using a digital PSG equipment (SOMNOlab V 2.01.0001, Weinmann Medical technology, Germany).

The subject was prepared about 1 h before the recording by attaching electrodes using average 12-18 channels. The recording time ranged from 4 to 8 h, started at the patients' usual bedtime, and continued until spontaneous awakening. Patients have not taken sedative or hypnotic medication before the study. All signals were digitally recorded and were reproduced on paper. At all times, patients were under supervision of a qualified technician and raw data were manually scored by 30-second epoch, according to published standards, before final interpretation (9).

The polisomnographic recording included a pressure transducer for nasal air-flow and a thermistor for nasal-oral air-flow, piezoelectric chest and abdominal belts, pulse oximetry monitoring, a snore microphone, two anterior tibial channels, submental electromyogram, electro-oculogramm, electroencephalogram (C3/A2-C4/A1 O2/A1,O1A2 of the 10-20 International placement electrode system), electrocardiogram (modified V2 lead), a body position sensor and simultaneous video monitoring.

The following sleep architecture parameters were assessed: total sleep time (TST, time from sleep onset to the end of the final sleep epoch minus time awake), time in bed (TIB), sleep latency (SL), sleep efficiency (TST/time in bed*100), percentage of each stage in total sleep time, snoring percentage.

Sleep stages were visually scored following standard criteria. The respiratory parameters evaluated were: oxygen desaturation index (ODI), average oxygen saturation, nadir oxygen saturation, oxygen saturation less than 90% for more than 30% of the registration period (T 90%) and apnoea-hypopnea index (AHI).

The polysomnographic diagnosis of patients was diagnosed according to American Academy of Sleep Medicine guidelines [15].

An event was defined as obstructive apnoea when the duration was more than two breaths, the amplitude reduction in the thermal sensor was 90% or more, and the respiratory effort was continued or increased throughout the entire period of decrease airflow.

An event was defined as hypopnea when the duration was more than two breath, the amplitude reduction in the nasal pressure was 50% or more, and the associated oxygen desaturation was 3% or more, or there was presence of arousal or awakening.

Apnoea- hypopnea index was defined as the number of obstructive apnoeas and hypopneas per hour of the total sleep time. Obstructive sleep apnoea was diagnosed if the obstructive index was more than one on PSG.

The severity of obstructive sleep apnoea increase with increasing obstructive index: apnoea/hypopnea index scores were classified as mild (1-5/hour), moderate (5-10/hour), and severe (> o = 10/hours).

Sleep hypoventilation syndrome (SHVS) was diagnosed in presence of sustained hypoxemia with arterial oxygen saturation <90% for more than 30% of the registration period, during sleep, not related to apnoea or hypopnea episodes.

Primary snoring was diagnosed if there is not polysomnographic evidence of sleep apnoea or hypoventilation in a patient with history of snoring.

Results

Demographic data

The cohort of the patients was composed by eleven Caucasian subjects. Nine of them were males and two were females. There were no obese children (Table 1).

Clinical results

Nine patients presented hypersomnia, morning headaches, nicturia and impaired concentration, (Brouillette questionnaire > 3,5).

Of these, five patients complained awakenings and two patients presented choking during sleep.

Two patients showed only daytime sleepiness. Nine subjects were referred for snoring or sleep-related breathing problems.

The clinical profile of the patients included diagnosis of epileptic syndrome associated neurological symptoms.

All patients had both diurnal and nocturnal complex seizures and were in therapy with a various combination of Lamotrigine, Carbamazepine, Phenobarbital, Phenytoin, Valproate and Levetiracetam.

Electroencephalographic results

The epileptic syndromes included generalized encephalopathy (five), Lennox Gastaut syndrome (LGS) (one), partial secondary generalized epilepsy (PSGE) (three), tuberous sclerosis complex (TSC) (one), Malignant migrating partial seizures (one). (Table 1).

The seizure type, often combined in a given patient, included spasms and tonic seizure (three), polymorphous seizures (four), tonic-clonic seizures (seven), and partial with or without secondary generalization (five).

All patients presented seizures during the recording night. Seizures occurred more frequently during the stage 3 of non-REM sleep.

Patient	Sex	Age (yo)	Mallampati Index	Epileptic syndrome
1	M	7	3	Generalized encephalopathy
2	F	6	3	LGS
3	F	6	4	TSC
4	M	8	2	Generalized encephalopathy
5	M	8	2	Generalized encephalopathy
6	M	3	4	Generalized encephalopathy
7	M	6	4	PSGE
8	M	11	3	Malignant migrating partial seizures
9	M	11	3	PSGE
10	M	7	3	PSGE
11	M	5	4	Generalized encephalopathy

Table 1: Clinical characteristics of the 11 study patients. (M: male; F: Female, LSG: Lennox-Gastaud syndrome; PSGE: partial secondary generalised epilepsy; TSC: tuberous sclerosis complex).

Polysomnographic results

The eleven patients resulted positive for OSAS. In particular, seven patients presented severe OSAS, two presented moderate OSAS and two patients were found to have mild OSAS. SHVS was diagnosed in five patients. Mallampati score has a strong linear correlation with AHI and hence OSAS (Table 2).

Patient	ODI/h	AHI/h	Average SpO2 (%)	Nadir SpO2 (%)	T90 (%)
1	4.1	1.2	95.1	82.3	22.1
2	17.2	28.7	95.2	52.7	16.8
3	4.4	3.9	96.7	82.4	55.3
4	5.0	5.5	93.6	86.1	0.4
5	13.9	14.3	94.8	87.2	8.8
6	14.4	16.3	96.4	75.3	13.3
7	13.9	11.8	95.0	81.2	42.6
8	6.6	26.4	95.7	83.5	40.2
9	31.1	7.7	89.3	80.8	57.4
10	27.5	18.3	92.1	82.1	25.3
11	32.1	26.2	86.4	63.4	60.5

Table 2: The respiratory polysomnographic parameters of the 11 study patients. (AHI: Apnoea-Hypopnea Index; Average SpO2: Average Oxygen Saturation; Nadir SpO2%: Nadir Oxygen Saturation ODI: Oxygen Desaturation Index; Nadir SpO2%: Nadir Oxygen Saturation; T90%: oxygen saturation less than 90% for more than 30% of the registration period).

Very often the episodes of apnoea and hypopnea occurred during the epileptic crisis. Seven patients showed a significant reduction of the total time in bed and of the total sleep time. All patients presented a reduction of REM sleep percentage. Apnoea/hypopnea index and average oxygen saturation are negatively correlated with REM sleep percentage ($p<0.05$). Nadir oxygen saturation negatively correlates with the efficiency of sleep ($p<0.05$). No other significant correlation with polysomnographic data were detected.

Discussion

This pilot study shows that paediatric patients with drug-resistant epilepsy, cerebral palsy and mental retardation often present sleep disruption and are frequently affected by obstructive sleep apnoea. Abnormalities in sleep architecture included reduction of the total time in bed, of the total sleep time and of REM sleep percentage. In our study apnoea/hypopnea index and average oxygen saturation are negatively correlated with REM sleep percentage. Nadir oxygen saturation negatively correlates with the efficiency of sleep. We have also demonstrated that the severity of OSAS strongly influence the quality of sleep.

The limit of the study is that we can't generalize our findings because of the small number of patients analysed. This conclusion of our pilot study should be supported by a larger sample size.

Several studies have reported that epilepsy and OSAS, when coexist, profoundly exacerbate each other's [16]. On the one hand, OSAS has been hypnotized to exacerbate seizure frequency by disrupting REM sleep [17], on the other hand, children with epilepsy report sleep deprivation as a significant seizures-precipitating factor and drug poor control.

In our population, we believe that the epilepsy encephalopathy itself caused the observed abnormalities in sleep architecture. We also argue that the respiratory abnormalities, may have contributed to the results.

In fact, OSAS and sleep deprivation very often coexist with drug-resistant epilepsy in childhood and adult patients [18]. In addition, sleep deprivation in children might be associated with cognitive and behavioural dysfunction, and consequent downgrading of the quality of life [19].

Nevertheless, is very difficult to recognize symptoms associated with sleep breathing disorders in these patients, despite the significant abnormalities of the sleep architecture and the serious impairment of respiratory parameters, characterized by frequent episodes of apnoeas and severe nocturnal oxygen desaturation [20].

Consequently, sleep breathing disorders are underdiagnosed in patients with epilepsy, especially in children with catastrophic epileptic encephalopathy [21]. One possibility is that antiepileptic drugs increases daytime sleepiness with the influence of the sleep architecture, acting as a confounding factor. AEDs can also induce insomnia [22]. Antiepileptic medications may also contribute to sleep disorders. For example, in a patient predisposed to obstructive sleep apnoea (OSAS), barbiturates and benzodiazepines may worsen the frequency of apnoeas and hypopneas by decreasing upper airway resistance or arousal mechanisms [23, 24]. In our population of patients it is possible that AEDs may have contributed to the changes seen in the sleep architecture. As demonstrated in this pilot study, it can be extremely useful to look at the Mallampati index since Mallampati score has been found to have a strong linear correlation with AHI. In fact, in children, a high Mallampati score is more predictive of the presence of OSAS than in adults because the main cause of the obstruction is pharyngeal [25].

Previous studies have also demonstrated that an improvement in seizure frequency in refractory epileptic patients is achieved with the treatment of OSAS [26, 27]. The screening for SBD to recognize an altered nocturnal respiratory function in the medically refractory epilepsy population is particularly outstanding to set up early intervention strategies [28, 29].

This may lead to overall improved night oxygen saturation, seizure control, sleep quality, daytime functioning and quality of life.

Conclusion

Sleep architecture and nocturnal respiratory parameters are abnormal in children with catastrophic refractory epileptic encephalopathy. In this population SBD very often occur. Although the abnormalities could be determined by respiratory events, they could be ascribed to the encephalopathy itself.

The findings of this pilot study offer preliminary data regarding nocturnal respiratory parameters and sleep abnormalities in children with drug resistant epileptic encephalopathy and support the perspective of a prospective study with a larger sample size, with the objective to better design the polysomnographic profile in this paediatric population.

References

1. Camfield CS, Camfield PR, Gordon K, Wirrell E, Dooley JM (1996) Incidence of epilepsy in childhood and adolescence: a population-based study in Nova Scotia from 1977 to 1985. See comment in PubMed Commons below Epilepsia 37: 19-23.
2. Hauser WA, Hesdorffer DC (1990) Epilepsy: frequency, causes and Consequences. Demos 33.
3. Hauser WA, Kurland LT (1975) The epidemiology of epilepsy in Rochester, Minnesota, 1935 through 1967. See comment in PubMed Commons below Epilepsia 16: 1-66.
4. Berg AT, Shinnar S, Levy SR, Testa FM, Smith-Rapaport S, et al. (2001) Early development of intractable epilepsy in children: a prospective study. See comment in PubMed Commons below Neurology 56: 1445-1452.
5. Camfield C, Camfield P, Gordon K, Smith B, Dooley J (1993) Outcome of childhood epilepsy: a population-based study with a simple predictive scoring system for those treated with medication. J Pediatr 122:861–868.
6. Sillanpää M, Jalava M, Kaleva O, Shinnar S (1998) Long-term prognosis of seizures with onset in childhood. N Engl J Med 338: 1715–1722.
7. McTague A , Cross JH (2013)Treatment of Epileptic Encephalopathies. 27: 175-184.
8. Berg AT, Berkovic SF, Brodie MJ, Buchhalter J, et al. (2010) Revised terminology and concepts for organization of seizures and epilepsies: report of the ILAE Commission on Classification and Terminology, 2005-2009. Epilepsia 51:676-85.
9. Mallow B (1996) Sleep and epilepsy Sleep and Epilepsy. Neurol. Clin 14:765-89. Curr Opin Neurol 13:171-5.
10. Méndez M, Radtke RA (2001) Interactions between sleep and epilepsy. See comment in PubMed Commons below J Clin Neurophysiol 18: 106-127.
11. Beth MA (2007) The interaction between sleep and epilepsy. Epilepsia 48: 36–38.
12. Bazil CW, Castro LH, Walczak TS (2000) Reduction of rapid eye movement sleep by diurnal and nocturnal seizures in temporal lobe epilepsy. See comment in PubMed Commons below Arch Neurol 57: 363-368.
13. Malow BA, Levy K, Maturen K, Bowes R (2000) Obstructive sleep apnea is common in medically refractory epilepsy patients. Neurology 55:1002-7.
14. Kwan P, Arzimanoglou A, Berg AT, Brodie MJ et al. (2009) Definition of drug resistant epilepsy: Consensus proposal by the ad hoc Task Force of the ILAE Commission on Therapeutic Strategies. Epilepsia.
15. Iber C, Ancoli-Israel S, Chesson A, Quan SF (2007) The AASM manual for the scoring of sleep and associated events: rules terminology and technical specifications. Westchester, IL: American Accademy of Sleep Medicine.
16. Kaleyias J, Cruz M, et al. (2008) Spectrum of Polysomnographic Abnormalities in Children with Epilepsy. Pediatric Neurology 39: 170–176.
17. Manni R1, Tartara A (2000) Evaluation of sleepiness in epilepsy. See comment in PubMed Commons below Clin Neurophysiol 111 Suppl 2: S111-114.
18. Malow BA, Weatherwax KJ, Chervin RD, Hoban TF, Marzec ML, (2003) Identification and treatment of obstructive sleep apnea in adults and children with epilepsy: a prospective pilot study. Sleep Med 4:509–515.
19. Baglietto MG1, Battaglia FM, Nobili L, Tortorelli S, De Negri E, et al. (2001) Neuropsychological disorders related to interictal epileptic discharges during sleep in benign epilepsy of childhood with centrotemporal or Rolandic spikes. See comment in PubMed Commons below Dev Med Child Neurol 43: 407-412.
20. Boitano JO, Louis J (2013) Pulmonary issues in patients with chronic neuromuscular disease. Am J Respir Crit Care Med 187:1046-55.
21. Décary A, Rouleau I, Montplaisir J (2000) Cognitive deficits associated with sleep apnea syndrome: A proposed neuropsychological test battery. Sleep: Journal of Sleep Research & Sleep Medicine 23:69-381.
22. Vaughn BV1, D'Cruz OF (2004) Sleep and epilepsy. See comment in PubMed Commons below Semin Neurol 24: 301-313.
23. Ettore B, Mascio RD, Sasanelli F (1986) Adverse Reactions to Antiepileptic Drugs: A Multicenter Survey of Clinical Practice. Epilepsia 27:323–330.
24. Malow BA (2007) The interaction between sleep and epilepsy. Epilepsia 48:36–38.
25. Kumar HVM, Schroeder JW (2014) Mallampati Score and Pediatric Obstructive Sleep Apnea. J Clin Sleep Med. 10: 985–990.
26. Segal E, Vendrame M, Gregas M, Loddenkemper T, Kothare SV (2012) Effect of treatment of obstructive sleep apnea on seizure outcomes in children with epilepsy. Pediatr Neurol 46:359-62.
27. Li P, Ghadersohi S, Jafari B, Teter B, Sazgar M (2012) Characteristics of refractory vs. medically controlled epilepsy patients with obstructive sleep apnea and their response to CPAP treatment. Seizure 21:717-21.
28. Koh S, Ward SL, Lin M, Chen LS (2000) Sleep apnea treatment improves seizure control in children with neurodevelopmental disorders. Pediatr Neurol 22:36-9.
29. Segal E, Vendrame M, et al. (2012) Effect of Treatment of Obstructive Sleep Apnea on Seizure Outcomes in Children with Epilepsy. Pediatric Neurology 46: 359–362.

28

Sleep Apnea Management in "Possible IPF" and "Idiopathic NSIP"

Krishna M Sundar[1*], Mary Beth Scholand[1], Alika M Willis[1] and Subhashree Sundar[2]

[1]*Department of Medicine, University of Utah, Salt Lake City, Utah, USA*

[2]*Department of Operations Management & Information Systems, David Eccles School of Business, University of Utah, USA*

***Corresponding author:** Krishna M Sundar, MD, Associate Professor (Clinical), Division of Pulmonary, Critical Care & Occupational Medicine University of Utah, 26N 1900E, Salt Lake City, UT 84132, USA, E-mail: krishna.sundar@hsc.utah.edu

Abstract

Purpose: The clinical course of patients with possible idiopathic pulmonary fibrosis (IPF) and idiopathic non-specific interstitial pneumonia (NSIP) is not well understood. While these patients are clinically followed for disease progression before rendering therapy, the import of sleep-disordered breathing on the disease course is unknown.

Methods: Retrospective analysis of possible IPF and idiopathic NSIP patients seen at a single center with review of clinical data pertinent to therapy for co-morbid sleep-disordered breathing was done.

Results: 7 patients with possible IPF based upon radiologic possible UIP patterns (5 male and 2 female) and 6 patients with idiopathic NSIP (5 female and 1 male) were followed for an average duration of 40 and 30 months respectively. 6/7 patients with possible IPF required continuous positive airway pressure (CPAP) therapy for sleep-disordered breathing and out of this 5/6 were compliant with therapy. Of idiopathic NSIP patients, 2/6 presented with acute exacerbations. All 6 patients required therapy for OSA out of which 5/6 were treated with CPAP and 1 treated with supplemental oxygen. Patients with possible IPF appeared to stabilize their disease following treatment of OSA and none of the study patients experienced any recurrence of acute exacerbations on CPAP therapy.

Conclusions: OSA can be an important problem in patients with possible IPF and idiopathic NSIP. Treatment with nocturnal CPAP therapy in these patients with concomitant OSA may result in stability of underlying interstitial lung disease.

Keywords: Idiopathic interstitial pneumonias; Idiopathic pulmonary fibrosis; Obstructive sleep apnea; Continuous positive airway pressure

Introduction

Idiopathic interstitial pneumonias represent a difficult group of diseases where the disease evolution is unpredictable and there are no good treatment options. Sleep-related hypoxemia is well-described in patients with interstitial lung disease although benefit of treating OSA on the course of fibrotic disease is unknown [1]. Poor sleep quality in patients with fibrotic disorders especially idiopathic pulmonary fibrosis (IPF) contributes to poor daytime functioning [2,3]. Sleep quality is in IPF patients is affected by nocturnal hypoxemia, the severity of which correlates with daytime measures of physical and social functioning [3].

Besides sleep-related hypoxemia, obstructive sleep apnea (OSA) is also being increasingly recognized in patients with interstitial lung disease (ILD) [4]. While initial reports focused on the high prevalence of OSA in IPF patients [5,6], recent reports indicate that OSA is prevalent in ILD from a variety of etiologies [4,7]. The implications of treating the commonly-encountered OSA in ILD patients are unclear. A benefit of treating OSA on progression of IPF has been shown [8], but similar results are unavailable for other types of ILDs. IPF can be a difficult diagnosis especially if radiologic patterns do meet criteria for UIP on high-resolution chest CT (HRCT) [9]. Such patients with radiologic possible usual interstitial pneumonia (UIP) are not always subjected to a definitive surgical lung biopsy and are followed expectantly. Similar to patients with IPF, patients with another idiopathic interstitial pneumonia – non-specific interstitial pneumonia (NSIP) are difficult management problems especially when occurring without a secondary cause such as underlying rheumatologic disease. In order to understand whether OSA is a significant comorbidity in these idiopathic interstitial pneumonias beside definitive UIP, this study was carried out. A retrospective analysis of patients with idiopathic NSIP and possible IPF (possible UIP by radiology) was done to assess the implications of the diagnosis of OSA and potential benefit of CPAP therapy in non-IPF interstitial lung disease.

Methods

Patient records with diagnoses of IPF, UIP and NSIP seen at Utah Valley Pulmonary Clinic between 2006 and 2011 were reviewed. All patients with defined or undifferentiated connective tissue diseases were excluded based on serology testing that included testing for rheumatoid factor, anti-nuclear antibodies, Jo-1 antibody, Scl-70, SS-A/SS-B antibodies, anti-RNP and evaluation for symptomatology consistent with rheumatoid arthritis, scleroderma, Sjogren's syndrome, polymyositis-dermatomyositis, and mixed connective tissue disease.

Of patients with idiopathic interstitial pneumonias, patients with a definite UIP-pattern on HRCT or on surgical lung biopsy (that suggested the diagnosis of IPF) were excluded. Patients with a possible UIP or an NSIP appearance on the CT scans were selected for further review. Clinical history, radiological abnormalities, and pulmonary function abnormalities at baseline and on follow-up were reviewed including acute exacerbations and use of specific immunosuppressive therapy. Acute exacerbations were defined as an acute clinical change with worsening of dyspnea occurring in less than a 4 week period characterized by new chest radiographic opacities that were not felt to be secondary to infection, embolic disease or heart failure [10]. Chest CT scans were reviewed by a radiologist blinded to the clinical data and radiologic diagnoses of possible UIP and NSIP were accorded based upon 2011 IPF consensus guideline criteria [9].

In order to assess the benefit (or lack of) on the course of the underlying interstitial lung disease from treatment of sleep-disordered breathing, only patients with follow-up PFT and CT scan data for more than one year were included.

Results

13 patients were given diagnoses of possible IPF or NSIP based upon clinical and radiological features (Tables 1 and 2) based on extensive review of records of ILD patients going back 5 years. Out of 57 ILD patients reviewed, only 19 patients met criteria for diagnosis of possible IPF or idiopathic NSIP. Out of these 19 patients, only 13 patients had representative CT abnormalities consistent with possible UIP or idiopathic NSIP and had relevant follow-up data for more than 1 year with CT scans and pulmonary function tests. All patients with chronic interstitial lung disease are typically evaluated for sleep-disordered breathing at this center because of either a clinical history of snoring, abnormal nocturnal oximetry or daytime symptoms of fatigue and/or sleepiness. The reasons for polysomnography (PSG) in each of these patients were not fully documented in their medical records and no screening questionnaires such as STOP-BANG or Epworth Sleep questionnaire were consistently admnistered.

Of the 7 patients with possible IPF (Table 1), only one patient underwent a non-diagnostic transbronchial biopsy. Diagnosis of possible IPF was made solely on basis of CT scan findings of possible UIP (9). Of the 6 patients with idiopathic NSIP (Table 2), four had the diagnosis confirmed on surgical lung biopsy while the other two patients underwent transbronchial biopsies that did not reveal abnormalities inconsistent with NSIP.

Characteristic	Patients with OSA n=5 (AHI mean 38.2)	Patient without OSA n=1	Patient with OSA but not on therapy n=1 (AHI 53)
Age (mean ± SD)	74.6 ± 7.2	71	64
BMI (mean ± SD)	27.2 ± 1.8	21	28.4
Sex	3:2 (M:F)	F	M
Duration of dyspnea (years) (mean ± SD)	4 ± 3.7	No reported dyspnea	1
Duration of PFT follow up (months)	28.2 ± 10.7	25	63
FVC (mean) Initial Final	2.65 ± 0.53 2.58 ± 0.52	2.94 2.85	4.11 3.15
DLCO (mean) Initial Final	13.5 ± 1.74 13.04 ± 1.36	14 12.4	23.2 16.6
CT abnormalities Duration of follow up Mean (range) Significant change	24 (12-45) No (one patient had some worsening of traction bronchiectasis)	63 No	25 No
Medication use Opiates Benzodiazepines Proton-pump inhibitors	3/5 None 3/5	No No No	Yes No Yes

Table 1: Characteristics of patients with possible IPF (Abbreviations: IPF – Idiopathic pulmonary fibrosis; OSA – Obstructive sleep apnea; AHI – Apnea-hypopnea index; BMI – Body mass index; PFT – Pulmonary function test; FVC – Forced vital capacity in liters; DLCO – single breath carbon monoxide diffusion capacity in ml/min/mmHg (CO))

All patients were Caucasian. All were non-smokers except patient 4 in idiopathic NSIP group who had a smoking history of 2 pack-years. The mean age in the possible UIP group was 72.6 years with a male to female ratio of 5:2 (Table 1). In comparison, the mean age in the idiopathic NSIP group was 61.2 years with a female to male ratio of 5:1 (Table 2). The mean duration of dyspnea was longer in patients with possible UIP as compared to those with NSIP due to two of the patients in the NSIP group presenting with acute exacerbations (Tables 1 and 2).

Patient	1	2	3	4	5	6
Age (years)	52	68	50	68	51	78
Sex	F	F	F	F	M	F
BMI	44	27.4	30.2	32.7	35.3	27
Duration of dyspnea (years)	0.75	0.5	0.1	1	2	0.5
Acute exacerbation	Yes	Remote	Yes	No	No	No
Duration of PFT follow up (months)	26	33	40	15	38	58
FVC (liters) Initial Final	2.62 2.52	3.19 2.78	0.92 2.21	2.35 2.13	2.26 2.14	1.9 1.69
DLCO Initial Final	17.2 19.3	11.7 10.4	5.0 16.9	16.6 11.8	16.3 15	12.4 6.4
6 MWT Distance (m) Desaturation below 88%	366 yes	480 yes	443 no	420 yes	480 no	322 no
CT findings Duration of follow up(months) Progression	11 Improved	12 Mild worsening	24 Improved	13 No changes	16 Very mild worsening	54 Worsened
Use of daytime oxygen	Yes	Yes	no	no	no	Yes
Medication use Immunosuppression Proton-pump inhibitors	Azathioprine Yes	Prednisone Yes	Azathioprine No	None Yes	None Yes	Mycopheno-late Yes
AHI	51	12	5	7	9.6	4.7

Table 2: Characteristics of patients with idiopathic NSIP (Abbreviations: NSIP – Nonspecific interstitial pneumonia; AHI – Apnea-hypopnea index; BMI – Body mass index; PFT – Pulmonary function test; FVC – Forced vital capacity in liters; DLCO – single breath carbon monoxide diffusion capacity in ml/min/mmHg (CO); 6MWT – 6 minute walk test.)

Patients with possible IPF were followed for a longer duration with only 1/7 patients showing significant disease progression. 5/7 patients with possible IPF and documented sleep apnea received CPAP therapy and on follow up, showed stability in lung function and CT abnormalities. A similar course was noted in the one patient without evidence of OSA on polysomnography (Table 1). The patient with OSA who refused CPAP therapy showed significant decline in both forced vital capacity and diffusion capacity over a five-year period but did not show any significant progression of disease based on CT appearances (Table 1). None of the patients in the possible UIP group experienced acute exacerbations or significant lower respiratory tract infections. None of the patients used supplemental oxygen during daytime even though two patients showed desaturations below 88% on the six-minute walk test.

2/6 patients with idiopathic NSIP presented with acute exacerbations; these patients presenting with acute exacerbations required hospitalization and underwent surgical lung biopsy and treatment with high-dose steroids. Following clinical improvement on steroids, they were maintained on oral azathioprine therapy for nearly two years after which the azathioprine was tapered off. Two other patients in the NSIP group were treated with immunosuppressive therapy for disease progression based on worsening CT scans, dyspnea and pulmonary function tests. Only 2/6 patients in the idiopathic NSIP group were followed without any evidence of disease progression on CT scans or PFTs. 3/6 patients with idiopathic NSIP required supplemental oxygen during day and night. All patients in the idiopathic NSIP group were diagnosed with OSA. All patients had mild OSA except patient 1 that had severe OSA based on an AHI of 51 (Table 2). Except for patient 6 who had an AHI of 4.7, all other patients received CPAP therapy in addition to other treatments. None of the patients experienced any acute exacerbations over the duration of follow-up including the ones that presented with acute NSIP exacerbations at initial contact.

Table 3 details the polysomnographic details of patients with possible IPF and idiopathic NSIP. Patients with possible IPF tended to have more severe degree of obstructive sleep apnea (all of them had apnea-hypopnea indices of 15 or more) and majority of them appeared to tolerate CPAP therapy well. Patients with idiopathic NSIP tended to have mild degree of OSA. Consistent with greater severity of OSA, patients with possible IPF tended to have greater sleep fragmentation, decreased REM and slow sleep time and lesser sleep efficiency as compared to idiopathic NSIP patients (Table 3). Significant oximetric desaturation was noted during these PSG studies in both possible IPF and idiopathic NSIP groups (Table 3). Compliance data available on patients after a year of therapy showed that nearly all patients with possible IPF and idiopathic NSIP used CPAP for more than 4 hours a night for more than 90% of the time of the duration of CPAP data download.

	Possible UIP (n=6)	Idiopathic NSIP (n=6)
AHI mean ± SD	36.2 ± 15.3	14.9 ± 17.9
Arousal index mean ± SD	20.2 ± 12.5	9.5 ± 4.7
PLMS index mean ± SD	17.4 ± 29.7	25.3 ± 52.4
Desaturation index mean ± SD (Percentage time below 89%)	28.6 ± 23.4	10.6 ± 20.4
Sleep efficiency mean ± SD (%)	72.5 ± 17.3	77.3 ± 12.2
Sleep stages (Percentage of TST) Stage II (%) Slow wave sleep stage (%) REM stage (%)	65.2 ± 14.2 15.8 ± 12.1 11.3 ± 7.1	56.5 ± 15.5 24.5 ± 12.5 15.9 ± 7.3

Table 3: Polysomnographic details in patients with possible IPF and idiopathic NSIP (Abbreviations: IPF – Idiopathic pulmonary fibrosis; NSIP – Nonspecific interstitial pneumonia; AHI – Apnea-hypopnea index; PLMS – Periodic limb movement; TST – Total sleep time; REM – Rapid eye movement.)

Discussion

During evaluation for ILD, many patients are rendered diagnoses of UIP and NSIP based on CT findings [9,11,12]. If these patients do not meet definitive CT or pathology criteria for UIP, then a diagnosis of possible IPF is considered [9]. Both possible IPF and idiopathic NSIP are difficult management situations where disease course has to be understood before therapeutic decisions can be confidently made [9,12]. While patients with idiopathic NSIP can behave like NSIP secondary to connective tissue disease [13], patients with possible IPF may not evolve like IPF patients and in those not undergoing definitive surgical lung biopsies, watchful expectancy of disease course is done [14].

Given the unpredictable clinical course of IPF and NSIP, there may be potential benefit in addressing co-morbidities in these disorders. The typical comorbidities that occur in these patients are similar to what is seen in IPF patients and include gastro-esophageal reflux disease (GERD), pulmonary hypertension and OSA [15]. Unlike other comorbidities such as GERD [16] and pulmonary hypertension [17], the impact of OSA on ILD is unclear. Given the high prevalence of obstructive sleep apnea in ILD patients, there may be particular benefit from addressing OSA in patients with ILD. Prevalence rate for OSA in one study that included sarcoidosis and scleroderma patients was 68% [4]. For IPF patients, studies have shown OSA prevalence ranging from 59-88% [5,6].

The association of OSA to non-IPF idiopathic interstitial pneumonias is not known. One study examining the association of OSA and GERD in fibrosing lung diseases included 19 fibrotic NSIP patients [7]. We report the first study examining the association of OSA in patients with idiopathic NSIP and possible IPF. This study does not answer the degree of association of OSA in idiopathic interstitial pneumonias because of the small numbers of patients, the selection bias from study population being drawn from a single site and because of inclusion of patients with only established follow-up visits. This descriptive analysis does however demonstrate that OSA can be an important comorbidity in patients with both possible IPF and idiopathic NSIP. To answer the question of prevalence of OSA in idiopathic interstitial pneumonias, a study of unselected IPF and NSIP patients (with and without symptoms of sleep disordered breathing) needs to be performed. The common finding of OSA in idiopathic interstitial pneumonias may be explained in part by the elderly population in which these fibrotic lung diseases are commonly encountered. The prevalence of OSA increases with age [18] and the average age of patients in idiopathic NSIP is in the 50s and of possible IPF in the 70s [9,12]. Secondly, increasing body-mass index (BMI) can predispose to OSA [19] and 4/6 patients with NSIP had BMI>30 that may have increased their propensity to OSA. While the presence of chest restriction in interstitial lung disease can impose higher inspiratory pressure gradients predisposing to dynamic obstruction following upper airway skeletal muscle relaxation during sleep, studies on IPF patients have not consistently shown a relation between measures of chest restriction and AHI [5,6].

The impact of treating OSA in patients with idiopathic interstitial pneumonias has not received attention until recently [5,6,20]. While there may be preliminary evidence that treating OSA in patients with IPF may improve long-term survival [8], such data does not exist for patients with possible IPF or idiopathic NSIP. Our study suggests that possible IPF patients may benefit from treatment of concomitant OSA. In our treated patients, there was little progression of disease and no acute exacerbations after initiation of CPAP therapy. Moreover, the duration of follow-up of possible IPF patients on CPAP in this study was substantial (Possible IPF patients - 40.2 ± 33.7 months) and no other interventions apart from CPAP and GERD therapy were rendered in these patients. Multiple mechanisms may explain a positive benefit of CPAP on the course of possible IPF. These include a reduction of GERD following CPAP therapy [21] - whether this benefit of CPAP extends to reduction in microaspiration that has been implicated in the injury-fibrosis cascade of IPF is unknown [22]. Secondly, stabilization of the intra-thoracic pressure swings occurring from OSA events may reduce the tractional injury on the peripheral lung lobules that are the seat of IPF progression [23]. Thirdly, positive pressure therapy may exert mechanical effects on the lower lung parenchyma and thereby influence the course of fibrosis. Studies have shown that stiffened lung promotes further contractile fibroblast proliferation that may favor pulmonary fibrosis progression [24]. Fourthly, the effects on chronic intermittent hypoxia or sustained hypoxia on course of lung fibrosis are unknown although there is burgeoning evidence on the effect of hypoxia on allergen-induced airway inflammation in rats [25].

This longitudinal study did not show a significant impact on the progression of idiopathic NSIP from OSA therapy. In our series, out of 6 patients with idiopathic NSIP, 2 presented with acute exacerbations while 2 others exhibited progressive disease and therefore these patients received immunosuppressive for halting disease progression. Idiopathic NSIP patients tend to be younger with a female predominance and excepting for one patient, all the NSIP patients in this study had mild OSA. Unlike possible UIP, idiopathic NSIP may have different pathogenetic mechanisms and this group may tend to behave like NSIP secondary to connective tissue disease [12,13]. While the benefits of treating mild OSA in idiopathic NSIP can be debated, no acute exacerbations were observed in the NSIP patients compliant with CPAP therapy.

Conclusion

This study reveals that OSA has to potential to affect the course of patients with idiopathic interstitial lung disease other than IPF. Patients with the radiologic pattern of possible UIP are a difficult population of patients especially if a surgical biopsy to definitively diagnose IPF cannot be done. Given that possible IPF is a difficult problem in the elderly for which no therapeutic alternatives are available, therapy of comorbid OSA offers the benefit to affect disease course favorably. Larger multicenter studies exploring the complex relationship between fibrotic lung disease and OSA are required to understand the benefits that can be obtained from CPAP therapy in these patients.

Acknowledgment

The authors thank Dr. Howard Mann, Professor, Department of Radiology, University of Utah for review of chest CT scans of patients involved in this study.

References

1. Miyahara Y, Miyahara Y, Naito T, Ikeda S (1995) Monitoring of nocturnal oxygen desaturation using pulse oximeter and apnomonitor in patients with chronic pulmonary disease. Respiration 62: 348-352.
2. Krishnan V, McCormack MC, Mathai SC, Agarwal S, Richardson B, et al. (2008) Sleep quality and health-related quality of life in idiopathic pulmonary fibrosis. Chest 134: 693-698.
3. Mermigkis C, Stagaki E, Amfilochiou A, Polychronopoulos V, Korkonikitas P, et al. (2009) Sleep quality and associated daytime consequences in patients with idiopathic pulmonary fibrosis. Med Princ Pract 18: 10-15.
4. Pihtili A, Bingol Z, Kiyan E, Cuhadaroglu C, Issever H, et al. (2013) Obstructive sleep apnea is common in patients with interstitial lung disease. Sleep Breath 17: 1281-1288.
5. Mermigkis C, Stagaki E, Tryfon S, Schiza S, Amfilochiou A, et al. (2010) How common is sleep-disordered breathing in patients with idiopathic pulmonary fibrosis? Sleep Breath 14: 387-390.
6. Lancaster LH, Mason WR, Parnell JA, Rice TW, Loyd JE, et al. (2009) Obstructive sleep apnea is common in idiopathic pulmonary fibrosis. Chest 136: 772-778.
7. Pillai M, Olson AL, Huie TJ, Solomon JJ, Fernandez-Perez ER, et al. (2012) Obstructive sleep apnea does not promote esophageal reflux in fibrosing interstitial lung disease. Respir Med 106: 1033-1039.
8. Mermigkis C, Bouloukaki I, Antoniou KM, Mermigkis D, Psathakis K, et al. (2013) CPAP therapy in patients with idiopathic pulmonary fibrosis and obstructive sleep apnea: does it offer a better quality of life and sleep? Sleep Breath 17: 1137-1143.
9. Raghu G, Collard HR, Egan JJ, Martinez FJ, Behr J, et al. (2011) An official ATS/ERS/JRS/ALAT statement: idiopathic pulmonary fibrosis: evidence-based guidelines for diagnosis and management. Am J Respir Crit Care Med 183: 788-824.
10. Collard HR, Moore BB, Flaherty KR, Brown KK, Kaner RJ, et al. (2007) Acute exacerbations of idiopathic pulmonary fibrosis. Am J Respir Crit Care Med 176: 636-643.
11. Jawad H, Chung JH, Lynch DA, Newell JD Jr (2012) Radiological approach to interstitial lung disease: a guide for the nonradiologist. Clin Chest Med 33: 11-26.
12. Kligerman SJ1, Groshong S, Brown KK, Lynch DA (2009) Nonspecific interstitial pneumonia: radiologic, clinical, and pathologic considerations. Radiographics 29: 73-87.
13. Kinder BW, Collard HR, Koth L, Daikh DI, Wolters PJ, et al. (2007) Idiopathic nonspecific interstitial pneumonia: lung manifestation of undifferentiated connective tissue disease? Am J Respir Crit Care Med 176: 691-697.
14. Wells AU (2013) The revised ATS/ERS/JRS/ALAT diagnostic criteria for idiopathic pulmonary fibrosis (IPF)--practical implications. Respir Res 14 Suppl 1: S2.
15. King C, Nathan SD (2013) Identification and treatment of comorbidities in idiopathic pulmonary fibrosis and other fibrotic lung diseases. Curr Opin Pulm Med 19: 466-473.
16. Lee JS, Ryu JH, Elicker BM, Lydell CP, Jones KD, et al. (2011) Gastroesophageal reflux therapy is associated with longer survival in patients with idiopathic pulmonary fibrosis. Am J Respir Crit Care Med 184: 1390-1394.
17. Shlobin OA, Nathan SD (2011) Pulmonary hypertension secondary to interstitial lung disease. Expert Rev Respir Med 5: 179-189.
18. Bixler EO1, Vgontzas AN, Ten Have T, Tyson K, Kales A (1998) Effects of age on sleep apnea in men: I. Prevalence and severity. Am J Respir Crit Care Med 157: 144-148.
19. Peppard P, Young T, Palta M, Dempsey J, Skatrud J (2000) Longitudinal study of moderate weight change and sleep-disordered breathing. JAMA 284: 3015-3021.
20. Mermigkis , Bouloukaki I, Antoniou KM, Mermigkis D, Psathakis K, et al. (2013) CPAP therapy in patients with idiopathic pulmonary fibrosis and obstructive sleep apnea: does it offer a better quality of life and sleep? Sleep Breath 17: 1137-1143.

21. Shepherd KL, Holloway RH, Hillman DR, Eastwood PR (2007) The impact of continuous positive airway pressure on the lower esophageal sphincter. Am J Physiol Gastrointest Liver Physiol 292: G1200-1205.
22. Raghu G, Meyer KC (2012) Silent gastro-oesophageal reflux and microaspiration in IPF: mounting evidence for anti-reflux therapy? Eur Respir J 39: 242-245.
23. Leslie KO (2012) Idiopathic pulmonary fibrosis may be a disease of recurrent, tractional injury to the periphery of the aging lung: a unifying hypothesis regarding etiology and pathogenesis. Arch Pathol Lab Med 136: 591-600.
24. Hinz B (2012) Mechanical aspects of lung fibrosis: a spotlight on the myofibroblast. Proc Am Thorac Soc 9: 137-147.
25. Broytman O, Braun RK, Morgan BJ, Pegelow DF, Hsu PN, et al. (2014) Effects of Chronic Intermittent Hypoxia on Allergen-Induced Airway Inflammation in Rats. Am J Respir Cell Mol Biol.

Sleep Medicine Knowledge among Medical Students in Seven Egyptian Medical Faculties

Nevin FW Zaki[1*], Rana Marzouk[2], Osman I[3], Alamah HY[4], Zaied WS[5], Haggag A[2], Hassan A[6], Allam M[7], Saadeldeen O[8], Russell Rosenberg[9], Heidy Reiny[10] and Ahmed S BaHammam[11,12]

[1]*Department of Psychiatry and Manager of Sleep Research Unit, Egypt*

[2]*Faculty of Medicine, Mansoura University, Mansoura, Egypt*

[3]*Faculty of Medicine, Banha University, Banha, Egypt*

[4]*Faculty of Medicine, Tanta University, Tanta, Egypt*

[5]*Faculty of Medicine, Menofia University, Egypt*

[6]*Faculty of Medicine, Zagazig University, Zagazig, Egypt*

[7]*Faculty of Medicine, Alkasr Elainy University, Egypt*

[8]*Faculty of Medicine, Ain Shams University, Egypt*

[9]*Atlanta School of Sleep Medicine, USA*

[10]*Fusion Sleep Atlanta Georgia, USA*

[11]*The University Sleep Disorders Center, Department of Medicine, College of Medicine, King Saud University, Saudi Arabia*

[12]*The Strategic Technologies Program of the National Plan for Sciences and Technology and Innovation in the Kingdom of Saudi Arabia, Riyadh, Saudi Arabia*

***Corresponding author:** Nevin FW Zaki, Faculty of Medicine, Department of Psychiatry, Mansoura University, Gomhoria Street, Elmansoura, Egypt, E-mail: nevinfzaki@yahoo.com

Abstract

Introduction: Egyptian medical education system awards students the bachelor degree of medicine after six academic years and a rotating house-officer year. There are no structured sleep educative programs in Egypt.

Aim of work: This study aimed to assess the knowledge of Egyptian final year medical students and house-officers about normal sleep and sleep disorders.

Subjects and methods: Medical schools distributed throughout Egypt were surveyed asking sixth year medical students (males and females) and house-officers to participate. Seven faculties of medicine were selected. To screen for knowledge on normal sleep and sleep disorders, the Assessment of Sleep Knowledge in Medical Education Survey was used; the participants were classified to low scorers versus high scorers depending upon their ability to answer 60% of the questions correctly.

The participants were separated into comparative groups (males vs. females). 6th year students vs. house officers and according to their faculty location.

Results: A total of 726 participants completed the survey (52.8% males, 78.9% were 6th year medical students and 21.1% were house-officers). There was a statistically significant difference in the scores of the participants with regard to their Faculty location and gender, while no statistically significant difference was found with regards to the study year.

Conclusion and recommendation: Medical students in the screened Egyptian faculties possess poor knowledge about sleep medicine, which reflects the deficient educative processes in this field of medicine. Medical faculties should provide better sleep medicine education through a formal sleep medicine degree-awarding program.

Keywords: Sleep education; Sleep medicine awareness; Medical education; Sleep medicine knowledge

Introduction

Sleep disorders are highly prevalent disorders that affect nearly all age groups, and are associated with decrements in perceived health [1]. The International Classification of Sleep Disorders-3 (ICSD-3) classifies over 80 different sleep disorders, which can be diagnosed and treated [2].

Obstructive sleep apnea (OSA), which is one of the commonest sleep problems affecting approximately 4% of middle-aged males, has been associated with several serious medical co-morbidities such as hypertension, coronary artery disease, stroke and diabetes [3] which can be missed when physicians do not have enough training or education in the field of sleep medicine.

Sleep disorders are common in the Egyptian population. It was reported that the prevalence of sleep paralysis is about 44% [4]. Moreover, Allah et al. [5] reported that insomnia among elderly Egyptians was about 33.6%. A study conducted by Shaheen et al. [6] demonstrated that 42.3% of patients with epilepsy who attended the outpatient neurology clinic at Fayoum University in Egypt had OSA.

Elawady [7] reported that 30.1% of hospital based patients in Egypt have OSA. Thus, a large number of Egyptian patients with sleep complaints remain undiagnosed, which is most probably due to inadequate sleep medicine education and training among healthcare providers [8].

Sleep disorders clinics were established in the USA and some European countries in 1970s. In 1990, 37% of American medical schools offered no formal education in sleep medicine [9].

Egypt requires 6 years of undergraduate study to become a house officer and a 7th year of clinical rotations to become a general practitioner [10]. Given the effect that sleep disorders have on the health and well-being of a significant percentage of the society, it is frustrating to know that little structured time is given to these topics in the medical school curriculum. Physicians-regardless of specialty-will inevitably gets in touch with patients having sleep complaints and should have the knowledge and awareness to diagnose them.

Several studies have assessed the status of sleep medicine knowledge worldwide; however, none has been conducted in Egypt, which is considered one of the influential countries in the Arab world, Africa and the Middle-Eastern region.

Therefore, we conducted a survey to assess the knowledge of sixth year medical students and house officers about sleep and sleep disorders and the current time given for sleep medicine education in Egyptian medical schools and whether the findings will differ from worldwide statistics gathered about the same topic.

Subjects and Methods

Study population

The study was conducted between January 2015 and June 2015. The Ethics Committee of Mansoura Faculty of Medicine approved the study protocol, and informed consent was obtained from all participants. We targeted faculties of medicine distributed throughout the country that have been established over 30 years ago.

Seven medical faculties satisfying this criterion were selected including: Alkasr Elainy University (KAU), Ain Shams University (ASU), Mansoura University (MU), Zagazig University (ZU), Tanta University (TA), Banha University (BU), Menofia University (MeU). Sixth year (final year) medical students and house officers were invited to participate.

Participants were informed that their completion of the survey was purely voluntary and would take 30 min. They were also informed that responses would remain confidential and anonymous. Among the surveyed students and house officers, 726 agreed to participate in the study.

Questionnaire

The questionnaire for medical students comprised demographics, including age, gender, nationality and academic year.

Knowledge in sleep medicine was assessed using the Assessment of Sleep Knowledge in Medical Education (ASKME) Survey, which is a validated tool for the assessment of medical education in sleep [11].

Medical education is offered in English in all the included Egyptian universities; therefore, there was no need to translate the questionnaire into Arabic. The ASKME survey is a validated 30-item questionnaire that includes five separate areas of sleep knowledge: 1) basic sleep principles, 2) circadian sleep/wake control, 3) normal sleep architecture, 4) common sleep disorders and 5) the effects of drugs and alcohol on sleep.

The items were presented in a "true," "false" or "I don't know" format. The questionnaire has a high degree of internal consistency reliability and validity. The total score is determined by simply adding the correct answers.

The ASKME was administered primarily via a dedicated Internet Web site designed by the study team. A hard-copy version of the instrument was available for students who did not have access to the electronic version. For this subcategory of respondents, feedback was provided by hard-copy answer sheets and responses were manually entered into the database.

Participants were divided into two groups: those who scored ≥60% (the "high score group") and those who scored <60% (the "low score group"), since the pass sore in Egyptian universities is 60%.

A total of 726 respondents completed the ASKME. Respondents were divided into two groups: 1) Sixth-year medical students (n = 573); 2) house officers (n = 153).

Statistical analysis

Continuous data are presented as means ± standard deviations (SD), and categorical data are presented in the text and tables as an absolute number (n) and percentage (%). The continuous variables were compared using the independent samples t-test, and the categorical variables were compared using the chi-square (χ^2) test.

A p value ≤0.05 was considered to be significant. Standard statistical software (SPSS: Statistical Package for the Social Sciences, 20, Chicago, Illinois, USA) [12] was used for the data analysis.

Results

The participants had a mean age of 22.69 ± 2.44 years, and males represented 52.8% of the sample. Students from the Capital universities (Ain Shams and Elkasr Elainy were n = 223).

The responses were distributed as follows: Mansoura University (MU) = 103, Tanta university (TU) = 98, Ain shams University (ASU) = 119, Elkasr Elainy (KAU) = 104, Banha university (BU) = 100, Menoufia (MeU) = 105, and Zagazig university (ZU) = 97.

Final year (sixth year) students were 573 (78.9%), and house-officers were 153 (21.1%). Demographic features and sample characteristics are presented in Table 1.

The Mean total score for female students was slightly higher than that of males (12.3 and 11.17, respectively) there was a significant statistic difference among both sexes on the means of total score (p = 0.018) Table 2. On analyzing scores across the university location the range of means for the total score was variable.

The lowest mean was Zagazig University (9.4) while the highest mean was Mansoura university (12.3) and a statistical difference existed between the total score of the students according to their university location (p = 0.006).

On the other hand, there was no obvious difference in the means of the total scores across the study year (p = 0.6). Around 35.1% of the sample obtained a score range 1-10, 61.7% obtained a score range 11-20 and only 2.5% of the sample obtained a score range from 21-30. Means and standard deviations, minimums and maximums and ranges of the total ASKME scores are presented in Table 2.

Age in years	**Mean ±SD**	22.69 (±2.44)	
	Min	20	
	Max	32	
Student's nationality		**Number**	**%**
	Egypt	689	94
	Malaysia	3	0.4
	Palestine	18	2.5
	Sudan	3	0.4
	Saudi Arabia	2	0.3
	Others	11	1.5
Study year	6th year (final)	573	78.9
	House officer	153	21.1
Gender	Males	383	52.8
	Females	343	47.2
Faculty	Mansoura	103	14.18
	Tanta	98	13.22
	Ain-Shams	119	16.39
	Elkasr-Elainy	104	14.32
	Banha	100	13.77
	Menoufia	105	14.46
	Zagazig	97	13.36

Table 1: Demographics & sample characteristics.

		Mean(SD)	**Min**	**Max**	**p**
Gender					
	Male	11.17(4.4)	0	24	0.018
	Female	12.3(4.2)	1	22	
Study year					
	Final year	11.6(4.4)	0	22	0.63
	House-officers	11.8(4)	2	24	
University					
	Mansoura	12.3(4.9)	0	22	0.006

	Tanta	13.7(4)	4	24	
	Ainshams	13(3.4)	5	21	
	Alkasr-alainy	11.6(3.8)	0	22	
	Banha	9.9(3.6)	0	17	
	Menoufia	11.3(4.5)	1	22	
	Zagazig	9.4(4.4)	0	19	
Frequency distribution of score ranges					
Total score(1-10)			256(35.1%)		
Total score(11-20)			451(61.7%)		
Total score(21-30)			18(2.5%)		

Table 2: Means and standard deviations and ranges of total scores on the ASKME according to gender, study year and faculty location.

The participating students were divided into two groups. The low scorers (<60% correct answers) were 663 forming around 91% of the total sample. While high scorers (>60% correct answers) were 63. Table 3 presents the percentage of high scorers versus low scorers rated by their gender, study year and faculty location.

Gender and faculty location had significant differences in the numbers and percentages of high versus low scorers (p = 0.01, p = 0.00 respectively) Table 3, while there was no statistically significant difference between both study year groups (i.e., final year and house officers) as regard their scores on the ASKME (p = 0.46).

	Low scorers	**High scorers**	**p**
	n(%)	**n(%)**	
Male	359(49.4)	24(3.3)	0.01
Female	304(41.9)	39(5.4)	
Final year	524(72.2)	49(6.7)	0.46
House-officers	139(19.1)	14(1.9)	
Mansoura	89(12.3)	14(1.9)	
Tanta	78(10.7)	18(2.5)	
Ainshams	108(14.9)	11(1.5)	
AlkasrAlainy	99(13.6)	5(0.7)	0
Banha	99(13.6)	1(0.1)	
Menoufia	94(12.9)	11(1.5)	
Zagazig	94(12.9)	3(0.4)	
Total	663(91.5)	63(8.5)	

Table 3: The numbers and percentage of high and low scorers across sex, academic level and faculty location.

The Percentage of correct answers obtained on each question in the ASKME survey is summarized in Table 4. A significant difference was observed between males and females in nine out of 30 questions. However, on comparing universities to each other the difference was significant in twenty out of the thirty survey questions. When we compared capital based universities (Ainshams and Alkasr-Elainy) to universities in other districts or governorates away from Cairo, there was no statistically significant difference (p = 0.2) (Table 4).

University /Variable	High scorers >60% correct answers	Low scorers <60% correct answers	Total	p-value
Capital universities (Alkasr ElAiny and Ein Shams)	207	16	223	0.2
Universities outside the capital (Governates)	456	47	503	
Total N	663	63	726	

Table 4: Difference between capitals based universities and governorates universities.

Discussion

This study demonstrates that the knowledge of sleep medicine among Egyptian medical students is limited. Furthermore, the results showed no statistically significant difference in medical students' knowledge in Egyptian medical faculties located in the capital and universities located in smaller cities. We aimed to check whether sleep medicine field is given more attention in capital based universities which attract larger number of students and are more prestigious regarding their ranking over the Egyptian universities and Africa but the results showed equality in student's knowledge.

There is no professional certification program for sleep medicine in Egypt. A limited number of physicians in Egypt have been trained in sleep medicine and the majorities have received their training abroad and through affiliation with international universities worldwide.

According to the geographic location and study year, there was no difference in the knowledge between final year students and house officers. The research team assumed that house-officers might show more knowledge regarding sleep medicine since they are more exposed to the clinical setting during their year of clinical rotations and the possibility of encountering a patient with sleep complaints is higher. Nevertheless, the results showed no significant differences between the two groups.

It is obvious that sleep medicine education is defective and insufficient. Students who scored high, most likely acquired knowledge through self-efforts due to their personal interest in the field. Additionally, some students direct their efforts toward passing the PLAB or the USMLE which makes them more knowledgeable in fields that are not sufficiently covered within the Egyptian curricula. No study has assessed sleep medicine knowledge among medical students in different academic years in Egypt. In the current study, only 8.5% of participants correctly answered ≥60% of the questions. Previous studies reported similar results in different countries. Table 4 summarizes the results obtained from similar studies worldwide. We concentrated on studies involving medical students rather than studies involving physicians of postgraduate or specialty training. In a study that assessed the knowledge of sleep medicine among medical students in Singapore, researchers reported that less than 10% of medical school seniors scored >70% on questions in sleep medicine [13]. In another study only 2% of third and fourth year medical students, when tested, scored >66% in basic sleep medicine knowledge [14]. A third study found that second year medical students and physician specialists recorded an equally poor knowledge of sleep medicine [15]. Other medically related fields reported a similar lack of education in sleep medicine, indicating inadequate sleep medicine acquaintance for physicians during undergraduate education and even in the postgraduate training period [15]. The two remarkable studies to date, which investigated the inclusion of education about sleep and sleep medicine, were conducted in 1979 by Orr [16], and again in 1993 [17]. The latter study found that less than 2 hours of sleep education was typically provided during medical school and approximately 30% of schools provided no formal education. Furthermore, surveys of practicing physicians and pediatricians find greatly limited sleep knowledge, therefore further emphasizing the need for education on sleep and sleep disorders during medical education [18-20].

Findings of this research study are also in concordance with the few studies that have been conducted in countries outside the United States. It was a noticeable finding that inadequate knowledge about sleep and sleep disorders is widespread. For example, 160 physicians attending a pulmonary conference in Pakistan were found to have very limited knowledge of sleep apnea [21]. A group of 215 physicians in Turkey received an average score of 47% on a questionnaire assessing on knowledge about sleep [22]. Another study noted that only 15% of 209 physicians in Saudi Arabia had ever even attended a lecture on sleep [23]. Clearly, there is a great need for advancement of sleep education in medical education in this region of the world. The average amount of time spent on sleep education in Saudi Arabia was just under 2.5 h, with 27% responding that their medical school provides no education regarding sleep. Even more striking were the country-based findings, with three countries (Indonesia, Malaysia and Viet Nam) providing no education, and only Australia and the United States/Canada providing more than 3 h [19].

In Egypt and the Middle East, medical student's exposure to the sleep medicine during medical training remains limited with no professional sleep medicine programs in majority of universities or clinical fellowships. For example, undergraduate medical students in Mansoura and Ain Shams University learn about sleep medicine for the first time in the second year of their education where they attend an hour lecture introducing the basic concepts of normal sleep during included in the curriculum of behavioral science. The second exposure to sleep medicine is during their internal medicine rotation where they have two lectures; one hour for sleep disorders during psychiatry clinical rounds and another hour for sleep-related breathing disorders during pulmonary medicine clinical rotations. However, the average sleep education hours are only 2.5 hrs. At the residency level, sleep medicine is not considered a core educational requirement for several of the primary specialties, such as Internal Medicine, Surgery, and Family Medicine in Egypt this is similar to findings of Simmons [24]. The current organizational structures do not facilitate ideal care for patients with sleep problems. It is not appropriate to restrain clinical training in sleep medicine given the high public health burden of sleep disorders,

Despite brief education, some students could complete the first two years of training without being introduced to the concept that a medical sleep specialist can diagnose and treat conditions that affect sleep and vigilance. This is similar to what has been reported earlier

[25] that the absence of rotations through an integrated sleep medicine experience does not allow students to ratify their solid impression, or obtain a proper idea of what specialization in sleep medicine might be like. Additionally, Teodorescu [26] reported that sleep medicine occupied only <2% of the content in 31 textbooks on four major specialties related to sleep medicine, which included (neurology, psychiatry, pulmonary medicine and geriatrics). During 5 years of undergraduate medical education in Saudi Arabia, Almohaya et al. [8] reported that fewer than 3 hours were assigned to teaching sleep medicine. Simmons [24] found that the average number of educational hours was 3.92 h for the schools with curriculum time in Sleep Medicine, (2.96 h across all 49 responding schools). The same was found in China where Luo [27] revealed that Chinese medical students had little knowledge about sleep disorders. Similar results were reported among Nigerian students as well [28]. The Institute of Medicine (IOM) report suggested that sleep medicine exposure should begin prior to entering into residency and early on as part of the medical school curricula [29].

The suggested solutions as proposed by Quane [30] include incorporating basic sleep science topics into the educational curricula of the preclinical years (such as physiology, neuro-anatomy, neurochemistry and neuroscience), integrating sleep history and physical signs and examination into clinical medicine and integrating sleep disorders into problem-solving and clinical training sessions.

This study clearly suggests that sleep medicine education in Egypt is inadequate. However, there are limitations of this study that need to be acknowledged, and an additional exploration of this topic is necessary in an equal sample of both sexes. An in depth evaluation could have enriched results by screening undergraduates at different years including all six academic years. Moreover, we did not obtain formal reports about sleep medicine curricula in each medical school nor did us interview staff members responsible for teaching sleep medicine. We did not survey for the abilities of medical students and physicians to understand the medical comorbidities and health hazards that can be caused by sleep disorders which should be a goal of future research studies.

Sleep disorders pose a significant burden on individuals and the healthcare system. Enhanced training similar to that available in the US is well needed in our medical school training.

Conclusion and Recommendations

Medical students in the screened Egyptian universities possess poor knowledge about sleep medicine, which reflects the inadequate educational activities in this field of medicine. In order to improve the recognition of sleep disorders among practicing physicians and medical students, universities and medical faculties must provide adequate sleep medicine education through a formal sleep medicine degree-awarding program. Further steps should be taken by the authorities to include sleep medicine as a subspecialty of Egyptian postgraduate clinical training. Medical students should also learn about sleep and sleep loss in order to regulate their own sleep effectively. The challenges of teaching medical students sleep medicine can best be met by actively integrating information about sleep and sleep disorders into the existing medical school curriculum.

Author Contribution

Study conception and design: Nevin Zaki, Rana marzouk.

Acquisition of data: RMI Osman, HY Alamah, WS Zaied, A Haggag, A Hassan, M Allam, O Saadeldeen.

Analysis and interpretation of data: Nevin Zaki, Russel Rosenberg, Heidy Reiny.

Drafting of manuscript: Nevin Zaki, Russel Rosenberg, Heidy Reiny, Ahmad Bahammam.

Critical revision: Nevin Zaki, Russel Rosenberg, Heidy Reiny, Ahmad Bahammam.

Running head: Sleep Education in Egypt.

Financial disclosure: The authors have no financial support related to the published article or any off-label or investigational use. Signed forms are provided with submission.

Conflicts of interest: The authors have no conflicts of interest related to the published article signed forms are provided with submission.

References

1. Roth T, Coulouvrat C, Hajak G, Lakoma MD, Sampson NA, et al. (2011) Prevalence and perceived health associated with insomnia based on DSM-IV-TR; International Statistical Classification of Diseases and Related Health Problems, Tenth Revision; and Research Diagnostic Criteria/International Classification of Sleep Disorders, Second Edition criteria: results from the America Insomnia Survey. Biol Psychiatry 69: 592-600.
2. (2014) International classification of sleep disorders-third edition (ICSD-3). AASM Resource Library.
3. Young T, Finn L, Peppard PE, Szklo-Coxe M, Austin D, et al. (2008) Sleep disordered breathing and mortality: eighteen-year follow-up of the Wisconsin sleep cohort. Sleep 31: 1071-1078.
4. Jalal B, Hinton DE (2013) Rates and characteristics of sleep paralysis in the general population of Denmark and Egypt. Cult Med Psychiatry 37: 534-548.
5. Allah ESA, Abdel-Aziz HR, El-Seoud AR (2014) Insomnia: Prevalence, risk factors, and its effect on quality of life among elderly in Zagazig City, Egypt. J Nursing Education and Practice 4: 52.
6. Shaheen HA, Abd El-Kader AA, Gohary AME, El-Fayoumy NM, Afifi LM (2012) Obstructive sleep apnea in epilepsy: a preliminary Egyptian study. Sleep Breath 16: 765-771.
7. El-Awady ME, Hammouda K, Hassan A, El-Fotouh AS (2014) REM Sleep Behavior Disorder and Excessive Daytime Sleepiness among Egyptians: A Hospital-Based Study. Egyptian Journal of Neurology, Psychiatry & Neurosurgery 51: 421.
8. Almohaya A, Qrmli A, Almagal N, Alamri K, Bahammam S, et al. (2013) Sleep medicine education and knowledge among medical students in selected Saudi Medical Schools. BMC medical education 13: 133.
9. Avidan AY, Vaughn BV, Silber MH (2013) The current state of sleep medicine education in US neurology residency training programs: where do we go from here? Journal of clinical sleep medicine: JCSM: official publication of the American Academy of Sleep Medicine 9: 281.
10. Barnard H (2002) Medical education in Egypt. Ned Tijdschr Geneeskd 146: 1147-1149.
11. Zozula R, Bodow M, Yatcilla D, Cody R, Rosen RC (2001) Development of a brief, self-administered instrument for assessing sleep knowledge in medical education: "the ASKME Survey". Sleep 24: 227-233.
12. Orzechowski KM, Nicholas SS, Baxter JK, Weiner S, Berghella V (2014) Implementation of a universal cervical length screening program for the prevention of preterm birth. Am J Perinatol 31: 1057-1062.
13. Mahendran R, Subramaniam M, Chan YH (2004) Medical students' behaviour, attitudes and knowledge of sleep medicine. Singapore Med J 45: 587-589.

14. kovacić Z, Marendić M, Soljić M, Pecotić R, Kardum G, et al. (2002) Knowledge and attitude regarding sleep medicine of medical students and physicians in Split, Croatia. Croat Med J 43: 71-74.
15. Strohl KP (2011) Sleep medicine training across the spectrum. Chest 139: 1221-1231.
16. Orr WC, Stahl ML, Dement WC, Reddington D (1980) Physician education in sleep disorders. J Med Educ 55: 367-369.
17. Rosen RC, Rosekind M, Rosevear C, Cole WE, Dement WC (1993) Physician education in sleep and sleep disorders: a national survey of U.S. medical schools. Sleep 16: 249-254.
18. Lee KA, Landis C, Chasens ER, Dowling G, Merritt S, et al. (2004) Sleep and chronobiology: recommendations for nursing education. Nurs Outlook 52: 126-133.
19. Mindell JA, Bartle A, Wahab NA, Ahn Y, Ramamurthy MB, et al. (2011) Sleep education in medical school curriculum: a glimpse across countries. Sleep Med 12: 928-931.
20. Salas RE, Gamaldo A, Collop NA, Gulyani S, Hsu M, et al. (2013) A step out of the dark: improving the sleep medicine knowledge of trainees. Sleep Med 14: 105-108.
21. Hussain SF, Zahid S, Haqqee R, Khan JA (2003) General physicians' perspective of sleep apnea from a developing country. Southeast Asian J Trop Med Public Health 34: 420-423.
22. Gelir E, Ardiç S, Izci B (2004) A questionnaire survey among Turkish physicians about sleep disorders. Tuberk Toraks 52: 348-355.
23. BaHammam AS (2000) Knowledge and attitude of primary health care physicians towards sleep disorders. Saudi Med J 21: 1164-1167.
24. Simmons MS, Pullinger A (2012) Education in sleep disorders in US dental schools DDS programs. Sleep Breath 16: 383-392.
25. Pastores SM, O'Connor MF, Kleinpell RM, Napolitano L, Ward N, et al. (2011) The Accreditation Council for Graduate Medical Education resident duty hour new standards: History, changes, and impact on staffing of intensive care units*. Critical care medicine 39: 2540-2549.
26. Teodorescu MC, Avidan AY, Teodorescu M, Harrington JJ, Artar AO, et al. (2007) Sleep medicine content of major medical textbooks continues to be underrepresented. Sleep medicine 8: 271-276.
27. Luo M, Feng Y, Li T (2013) Sleep medicine knowledge, attitudes, and practices among medical students in Guangzhou, China. Sleep Breath 17: 687-693.
28. Ozoh OB, Iwuala SO, Desalu OO, Ojo OO, Okubadejo NU (2015) An Assessment of the Knowledge and Attitudes of Graduating Medical Students in Lagos, Nigeria, Regarding Obstructive Sleep Apnea. Annals of the American Thoracic Society 12: 1358-1363.
29. Chesson JAL, Chervin RD, Benca RM, Greenough GP, O'Hearn DJ, et al. (2013) Organization and Structure for Sleep Medicine Programs at Academic Institutions: Part 2-Goals and Strategies to Optimize Patient Care, Education, and Discovery. Sleep 36: 803.
30. Quan SF, Anderson JL, Hodge GK (2013) Use of a supplementary internet based education program improves sleep literacy in college psychology students. Journal of clinical sleep medicine: JCSM: official publication of the American Academy of Sleep Medicine 9: 155.

30

The Severity of Obstructive Sleep Apnea Syndrome is related to Red Cell Distribution Width and Hematocrit Values

Aida M Yousef[1] **and Wael Alkhiary**[2*]

[1]*Department of Chest Medicine, Mansoura Faculty of Medicine, Mansoura University, Egypt*

[2]*Department of Clinical Pathology, Mansoura Faculty of Medicine, Mansoura University, Egypt*

***Corresponding author:** Dr. Wael Alkhiary MD, MSc, PhD, Department of Clinical Pathology, Mansoura Faculty of Medicine, Mansoura University, Egypt, E-mail: wkhiary@yahoo.com

Abstract

Background: Obstructive sleep apnea syndrome (OSAS) is a common sleep disorder characterized by recurrent upper airway collapse during sleep. Recently, some hematological parameters as red cell distribution width (RDW), mean platelet volume (MPV), and platelet distribution width (PDW) have been emerged as inflammatory biomarkers. Limited, controversial data is available on the association between these hematological parameters and the severity of OSAS. Therefore, we aimed to investigate the levels of these parameters in patients with OSAS and its correlation with the severity of OSAS.

Methods: The clinical data, polysomnography and laboratory results of complete blood pictures of 116 patients with OSAS were retrospectively collected and statistically analyzed.

Results: Obstructive sleep apnea syndrome was associated with increased levels of hematocrit, RDW, MPV, PDW, and platelets count. RDW is positively correlated with Apnea–hypopnea index, oxygen desaturation index, Epworth sleepiness scale, and negatively correlated with minimum oxygen saturation and rapid eye movement sleep.

Conclusion: RDW may be a marker for the severity of OSAS. As RDW is included in a complete blood count, it could provide an easy, inexpensive tool for triaging OSAS patients for polysomnography evaluation.

Keywords: Erythrocyte indices; Mean platelet volume; Polysomnography; Obstructive sleep apnea; Sleep disorders

Introduction

Obstructive sleep apnea syndrome (OSAS) is a common sleep disorder characterized by recurrent upper airway collapse during sleep. This results in a reduction or complete cessation of the airflow that leads to arousals, sleep fragmentation, and oxyhemoglobin desaturation. Patients with OSAS undergo repetitive episodes of hypoxia and reoxygenation that may have systemic effects [1-3], so that, OSAS is considered a systemic inflammatory disease, not a local abnormality [4,5].

Recently, some hematological parameters have emerged as inflammatory biomarker in various diseases. Red cell distribution width (RDW), a laboratory measure of the variability of red blood cell sizes, is the index of the erythrocyte heterogeneity. RDW is calculated by division of standard deviation (SD) of RBC volume by MCV [6]. RDW is widely used to identify the potential cause of anemia. Increased values have however been recently reported in several cardiovascular disorders, such as coronary artery disease [7], heart failure [8,9], and stroke [10]. Moreover, RDW is also associated with all-cause, cardiac and non-cardiac mortality [11].

The mean platelet volume (MPV), that measure platelet size, has been considered as a marker and determinant of platelet function. Increased MPV may reflect either increased platelet activation or increased numbers of large, hyper-aggregated platelets [12], and may represent a link between hypercoagulability and inflammation [13]. Another marker of platelet activation is the platelet distribution width (PDW) [14].

Red cell and platelets indices have been extensively investigated in various diseases. Limited, controversial information is available, however, on the association between red cell [15-19] and platelets [15, 20-25] parameters and the severity of OSAS. Therefore, the aim of this study was to investigate the levels of these parameters in patients with OSAS and to assess whether there is any correlation between the severity of OSAS and any of these parameters.

Material and Methods

Between January 2011 and June 2014 a total of 264 patients admitted to the sleep unit underwent a polysomnographic evaluation and were diagnosed as OSAS patients. 116 out of the 264 met the inclusion and exclusion criteria of this study and were enrolled in this study. Inclusion criteria were patients who are with symptoms of nocturnal snoring and/or excessive daytime sleepiness. Exclusion criteria were any known cardiac disease (congestive heart failure, ischemic vascular disease, or arrhythmias), lung disease (chronic obstructive pulmonary disease, asthma and IPF), diabetes mellitus, hypertension, smoking, and chronic renal or hepatic diseases, a history of recent blood transfusion (three weeks), and known hematologic disease such as leukemia or myelodysplastic syndrome. Patients diagnosed with obesity hypoventilation, overlap syndrome, complex sleep apnea, central sleep apnea, Cheyne-Stokes sleeping disorder, or REM-induced OSAS were excluded from the PSG results. These patients were excluded because these diseases have comorbidities that could cause inflammation.

Detailed medical history, physical examination, routine laboratory investigations, a respiratory function test, electrocardiogram (ECG), and chest X-ray were assessed. Initially, patients were already grouped into three OSAS severity categories: mild (AHI 5 to <15), moderate (AHI 15 to <30), and severe (AHI >30). Further, we combined mild and moderate groups into one group (AHI 5 to <30). As a control group, 62 individuals (ages 44-63) diagnosed with simple snoring (AHI <5) were chosen.

Polysomnograpgic sleep study: In sleep-laboratory, all patients had been assessed regarding their degree of OSAS by subjecting them to basic full night formal PSG sleep study (sleep screen recorder viasys company Germany) in the supine position for definitive diagnosis. PSG was performed and scored according to standard criteria using nasal pressure cannula and tracheal sounds (suprasternal microphone) for airflow measurement. Respiratory events were scored manually. Apnea was defined as cessation of airflow for ≥10 s. Hypopnea was defined as a 30% reduction accompanied by a 4% decrease in capillary oxygen saturation (SpO2) of airflow or a 50% reduction of airflow accompanied by a 3% decrease in SpO2. Classification of a hypopnea as obstructive, central, or mixed performed calibrated respiratory inductance plethysmography. Hypopnea was classified as obstructive in the presence of continued movement in the respiratory inductive plethysmograph (RIP). The oxygen desaturation index (ODI) is the number of times per hour of sleep in which the blood's oxygen level drops by 3 percent or more from baseline. The apnea hypopnea index was taken as the average number of apnea and hypopnea events per hour of sleep. Epworth Sleepiness Scale (ESS) consists of eight questions answered by the patient with regard to daily activities measured on a scale of zero to three and having proportionate values starting from a minimum of zero to a maximum of twenty-four points.

Measurement of laboratory parameters. Fasting (8 hours) venous blood samples were drawn from the antecubital vein, using a sterile 21-gage needle syringe without stasis, between 8 and 9 AM after polysomnography and after 20 min rest. Tripotassium ethylenediaminetetraacetic acid (K3 EDTA) based anticoagulated blood samples were drawn in Vacutainer tubes (Vacutainer, Becton, Dickinson and Company, Franklin Lakes, NJ, USA) and standardized to be assessed within 30 minutes from blood sampling time. Complete blood counts were performed using the Abbott Cell-Dyne 3700 System (Abbott Diagnostics, Santa Clara, CA, USA).

Statistical Analysis. All variables were tested for normality with the Kolmogorov-Smirnov test. Normally distributed continuous variables are expressed as mean ± standard deviation. Non-normally distributed continuous variables are summarized as medians. Categorical variables are expressed as numbers (percentages). Comparisons between independent groups were made using the Mann-Whitney test. Correlations between non-continuous variables and continuous variables with a non-normal distribution were assessed using Spearman's correlation. Correlations between continuous variables were assessed using Pearson's correlation. Univariate and multivariate linear regression analysis were performed to determine the independent correlations of studied parameters. value<0.05 was considered statistically significant. The statistical analysis was performed with SPSS for Windows version 18.0 (SPSS, Chicago, IL, USA).

Results

Patient characteristics

The demographic and clinical characteristics of the patients and controls are shown in Table 1. The patients in this study were subdivided according to AHI into mild, moderate, combined mild and moderate and severe OSAS. We included a total of 116 patients with OSAS [34 patients (29.3%) mild, 20 patients (17.3%) moderate and 62 patients (53.4%) severe] and 62 simple snoring control cases. There were no statistically significant differences between the two groups regarding Age, sex distribution, and BMI. There was no lung disease in both groups.

	Control (n=62)	Total patients (n=116)	Mild to moderate (n=54)	Severe (n=62)	P1	P2	P3	P4	P5
AHI (events/hour)	0.9 (0.2-3.2)	34.5 (5.2-105)	12 (5.2-27.7)	58 (30-105)					
Age (years)	51 (44-63)	51 (39-70)	50 (40-65)	51 (39-70)	0.99	0.523	0.667	0.465	0.521
BMI (kg/m^2)	32.3 (25.5-36.6)	32.8 (23-43.4)	32.5 (23-40)	34.8 (28-43.4)	0.184	<0.001*	0.036*	0.142	<0.001*
Polysomnographic study results									
Oxygen Desaturation Index	1.2 (0.4-3.5)	38 (0.9-105)	12 (0.9-38)	62 (31-105)	<0.001*	<0.001*	<0.001*	<0.001*	<0.001*
Minimum Oxygen Saturation	92 (91-94)	76.5 (42-93)	84 (54-93)	68 (42-88)	<0.001*	<0.001*	<0.001*	<0.001*	<0.001*
Basal Oxygen Saturation	97.3 (96.3-98.5)	93 (79-98)	93 (80-98)	92 (79-95.5)	<0.001*	<0.001*	0.011*	<0.001*	0.084
Epworth Sleepiness Scale	5 (2-8)	11 (4-17)	7 (4-13)	13 (4-17)	<0.001*	<0.001*	<0.001*	<0.001*	<0.001*

Sleep Efficiency	92.9 (88-96.5)	85.7 (37.8-99)	85.9 (37.8-94)	85 (64-99)	<0.001*	0.001*	0.488	<0.001*	0.44
Rapid Eye Movement sleep	23.1 (20.6-25)	11.9 (1.3-36)	13.6 (4.1-36)	11.6 (1.3-20)	<0.001*	<0.001*	0.010*	<0.001*	0.040*
Laboratory variables									
WBC (X109/L)	6.2 (4-9.8)	7.1 (3.9-11)	6.2 (3.9-9.8)	7.4 (4.1-11)	0.183	0.087	0.152	0.606	0.289
RBCs (X106/L)	5.11 (4.5-6.1)	5.14 (3.4-7.1)	5.16 (3.4-7.1)	5.13 (4-5.9)	0.213	0.436	0.521	0.129	0.356
Hemoglobin (g/dL)	13.2 (10.8-15.2)	13.5 (9.9-16.9)	13.8 (9.9-16)	13.5 (10.8-16.9)	0.29	0.394	0.407	0.422	0.956
Hematocrit (%)	45.4 (40-50.1)	45 (39.9-54.3)	43.4 (39.9-49.5)	45.1 (40.1-54.3)	0.701	0.916	0.215	0.193	0.143
MCV	86 (80.1-94.9)	85 (65.3-95.3)	85 (77.9-95.3)	85.4 (65.3-94.3)	0.068	0.113	0.468	0.198	0.714
RDW (%)	12.9 (11.5-14.9)	13.6 (12-19)	13 (12-14.8)	14 (12.4-19)	0.010*	0.001*	0.028*	0.408	0.008*
Platelet count (X109/L)	222 (158-347)	193 (91-384)	198 (121-384)	189 (91-361)	0.040*	0.086	0.588	0.07	0.845
MPV (fl)	8.6 (7.5-9.6)	10.9 (8.2-14.6)	10.9 (8.3-13.8)	11 (8.2-14.6)	<0.001*	<0.001*	0.308	<0.001*	0.634
PDW (fl)	13.4 (9.4-15.1)	14.7 (9.4-21.9)	13.9 (9.8-21.9)	14.9 (9.4-20)	0.014*	0.005*	0.113	0.177	0.888

Table 1: Demographic, clinical and laboratory characteristics of studied groups. (P1: Comparison between total patients versus control group. P2: Comparison between severe versus control group. P3: Comparison between mild, moderate and severe. P4: Comparison between mild+ moderate versus control. P5: Comparison between severe versus mild+ moderate. Categorical variables are expressed in frequency (percentage); numerical variables are expressed in median (range). AHI: Apnea-hypopnea index; BMI: body mass index; WBC: White blood cells; RBCs: Red blood cells; RDW: Red cell distribution width; PDW: Platelets distribution width; MPV: Mean platelet volume, *Significant).

OSAS patients had significantly higher oxygen desaturation index, Epworth sleepiness scale and significantly lower minimal, basal oxygen saturation, sleep efficiency and rapid eye movement sleep when compared to control subjects. In addition, RDW was significantly higher in OSAS, severe OSAS versus control subjects and severe versus mild to moderate OSAS (Table 1 and Figure 1). Moreover, platelets count was significantly higher in OSAS. In addition, MPV was significantly higher in OSAS, mild to moderate and severe OSAS versus control subjects.

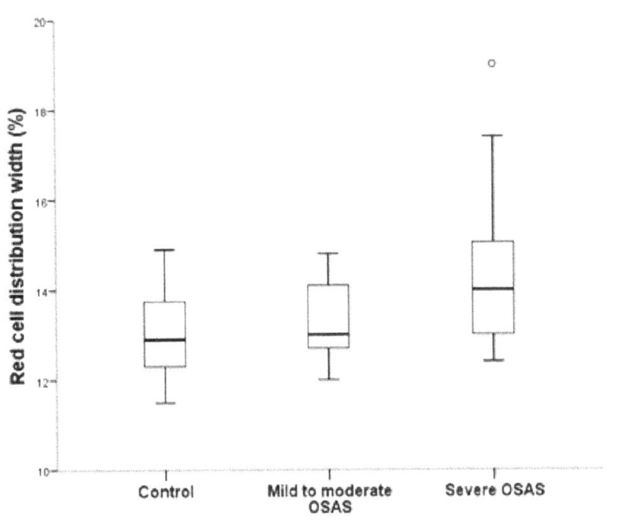

Figure 1: RDW distribution in OSAS patients and control subjects.

Moreover, PDW was significantly higher in OSAS and severe OSAS versus control subjects (Table 1). Furthermore, there was a significant negative correlation between hematocrit and minimal oxygen saturation in mild to moderate OSAS group (r=-0.479, p=0.011, data not shown).

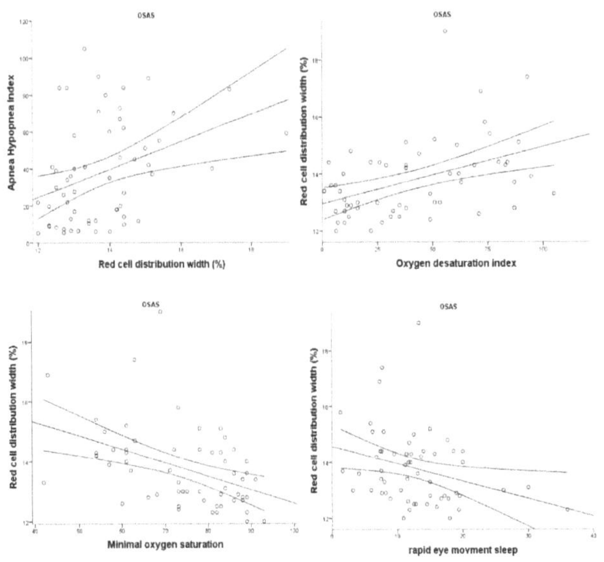

Figure 2: Correlations between RDW and AHI, oxygen saturation index, minimal oxygen saturation and rapid eye movement sleep in total OSAS group.

In the patient population, AHI showed significantly positive correlation with oxygen desaturation index, Epworth sleepiness scale, hematocrit, RDW and significantly negative correlation with minimal oxygen saturation, and basal oxygen saturation in OSAS group (Table 2). Moreover, RDW showed significantly positive correlation with oxygen desaturation index, Epworth sleepiness scale, hematocrit and significantly negative correlation with minimal oxygen saturation and rapid eye movement sleep in OSAS group (Table 2 and Figure 2).

	AHI		RDW		Hematocrit		MPV		PDW	
	r	p	r	p	r	p	r	p	r	p
Oxygen Desaturation index	0.917	<0.001*	0.437	0.001*	0.047	0.020*	0.047	0.726	0.042	0.757
Minimum oxygen saturation	-0.644	<0.001*	-0.456	<0.001*	-0.035	0.052	-0.035	0.793	-0.064	0.631
Basal oxygen saturation	-0.363	0.005*	-0.204	0.125	0.089	0.063	0.089	0.506	-0.129	0.335
Epworth sleepiness scale	0.816	<0.001*	0.365	0.005*	-0.001	0.051	-0.001	0.993	-0.012	0.929
Sleep efficiency	0.098	0.463	-0.084	0.53	0.129	0.749	0.129	0.334	0.223	0.092
Rapid eye movement sleep	-0.183	0.169	-0.321	0.014*	0.018	0.004*	0.018	0.892	0.107	0.423
WBC (X109/L)	0.108	0.42	0.246	0.062	0.204	0.016*	0.204	0.125	-0.114	0.392
RBCs (X106/L)	-0.008	0.955	0.222	0.094	0.375	0.444	0.375	0.004*	0.319	0.015*
Hemoglobin (g/dL)	0.002	0.991	-0.023	0.864	0.214	0.057	0.214	0.106	0.207	0.119
Hematocrit (%)	0.26	0.049*	0.618	<0.001*	-	-	0.162	0.225	0.766	0.074
RDW (%)	0.399	0.002*	-	-	0.618	0.162	0.214	0.107	0.141	0.766
Platelets count (X109/L)	0.081	0.544	-0.08	0.552	-0.36	0.326	-0.36	0.006*	-0.511	<0.001*
PDW (fl)	0.065	0.629	0.141	0.292	0.766	0.074	0.766	<0.001*	-	-
MPV (fl)	0.099	0.458	0.214	0.107	0.162	0.225	-	-	0.766	<0.001*

Table 2: Correlations between different parameters in OSAS patients group (AHI: Apnea-Hypopnea Index; WBC: White Blood Cells; RBCs: Red Blood Cells; RDW: Red Cell Distribution Width; PDW: Platelets Distribution Width; MPV: Mean Platelet Volume, *Significant).

Hematocrit showed significantly positive correlation with oxygen desaturation index, WBCs, MCV and significantly negative correlation with rapid eye movement sleep in OSAS group. Additionally, Hematocrit showed significantly positive correlation with PDW and significantly negative correlation with minimal oxygen saturation in mild to moderate OSAS group (Table 2).

Linear regression analysis

Independent variables including age, body mass index, apnea-hypopnea index, and oxygen desaturation index were applied as covariates in linear analysis. The multivariate analysis including variables which showed $p<0.05$ at univariate analysis (AHI and oxygen desaturation index) was done. Only oxygen desaturation index is an independent predictor of RDW, and higher oxygen desaturation index is a predictor of higher RDW ($\beta=0.035$, $p=0.023$) ($p=0.016$, OR=1.088, 95% CI=1.016-1.165) (Tables 3 and 4). Multiple regression analysis was done on all other outcomes, namely hematocrit, MPV, and PDW. However all results were non-significant (data are not shown).

	β coefficient	SE	p
Age (years)	0.014	0.020	0.470
Body mass index	0.011	0.019	0.568
Apnea-hypopnea index	-0.019	0.016	0.246

Oxygen Desaturation Index	0.035	0.015	0.023

Table 3: Predictors of red cell distribution width by linear regression analysis.

	Univariate			**Multivariate**				
	p	**OR**	**95% C.I.**		**p**	**OR**	**95% C.I.**	
Age	0.287	1.041	0.967	1.121				
Body Mass Index	0.759	1.011	0.943	1.085				
Apnea-Hypopnea Index	0.007*	1.031	1.009	1.054	0.141	0.95	0.888	1.017
Oxygen Desaturation Index	0.001*	1.038	1.015	1.062	0.016*	1.088	1.016	1.165
Hemoglobin.	0.968	1.008	0.696	1.46				

Table 4: Independent predictors of red cell distribution width by multivariate logistic regression analysis (*Significant).

Discussion

This study is a comprehensive one of only a few controversial studies examining the relationship between almost-single-hematological parameter and AHI in OSAS. We have shown that RDW, MPV, and PDW are higher in OSAS. Additionally, hematocrit and RDW are positively correlated with AHI. These findings reveal the importance of full blood count and indices in OSAS patients, and suggest that hematocrit and RDW might be a related marker of OSAS severity.

Recently, the concept of OSAS as a simple respiratory abnormality during sleep has been diverted to a systemic response due to multiple pathogenetic mechanisms of oxidative stress [26-30], increased sympathetic **overactivity** [31], coagulation fibrinolysis imbalance, and platelets activation [32]. All these factors lead to a state of systemic inflammation [4, 33-35], endothelial dysfunction [3], metabolic dysregulation [36], and hypercoagulability [32].

Red cell distribution width indicates the variability in the size of blood erythrocytes. RDW is measured by automated hematology analyzers as part of a complete blood count [37]. The exact mechanism of a high RDW level in patients with OSAS and its association with AHI is not clear. However, this may be related to oxidative stress and chronic inflammation in OSAS, both playing major roles in the pathogenesis of OSAS. Oxidative stress has been shown to be associated with RDW and antioxidants were shown to be significantly associated with a decrease in RDW [38]. Additionally, A state of chronic inflammation exists in OSAS and lead to increased secretion of interleukin-6 (IL-6) and other pro-inflammatory cytokines [39,40]. RDW may reflect the bone marrow's response to systemic, ongoing inflammation [41]. Inflammation may influence erythropoiesis, erythrocyte circulatory half-life and erythrocyte deformability, promoting anisocytosis and thus increasing RDW levels [40]. Recently, it was demonstrated that greater RDW levels were independently associated with greater high-sensitivity CRP levels, a well-established marker of inflammation [39,41]. Further, high RDW levels may be related to increased neurohormonal activity in OSAS [42].

Our results may appear similar to previous two studies in literature [16,17], regarding the elevation and correlation of RDW to the severity of AHI. However, there is a major difference in the study design between these two studies and ours. We have designed the current study cautiously, to avoid confounding diseases; that may affect RDW results, so that no difference between patients and controls regarding comorbidity diseases. In contrast, these previous studies [16,17], that have not excluded or equalize the effect of comorbidity as coronary artery disease [7,11], diabetes mellitus [43], and hypertension [44], which could lead to elevation of RDW.

In addition to its positive correlation with the severity of OSAS, RDW was also associated with most of the sleep parameters in patients with OSAS. More specifically, RDW was positively correlated with oxygen desaturation index, Epworth sleepiness scale (EES), an established marker of daily sleepiness [45], and negatively correlated with both of minimum oxygen saturation rapid eye movement (REM) sleep. This supports our proposed role of RDW as a simple surrogate marker for the severity of OSAS. To the best of our knowledge, these all associations have not been reported before.

Blood viscosity is defined as the internal resistance of the blood to shear forces. Blood viscosity is determined by plasma viscosity, hematocrit (volume fraction of erythrocytes, which constitute 99.9 % of the cellular elements), and the mechanical behavior of erythrocytes [46]. Thus, hematocrit plays an important role in blood coagulability, as it affects blood viscosity and platelet aggregation, and hypoxic individuals often have increased hematocrit [47]. Increased blood clotting, caused by changes in the rheological properties (flow properties) of blood and plasma, seems to be an important factor linking OSAS and CV complications [48]. In this study, although hematocrit levels were not increased in patients with OSAS, hematocrit was positively correlated with AHI, the severity of index of OSAS. In literature, few studies have determined that patients with OSAS have increased hematocrit levels [49-54], and only one study revealed that the hematocrit correlate positively with OSAS severity [49], similar to this study. However, Reinhart et al. [54] found no relation between hematocrit and the severity of OSAS. Both short-term, and long-term CPAP therapy were found to decrease hematocrit levels in OSAS patients [52,55].

Patients with OSAS have a complex array of factors that may result in a state of hypercoagulability [32]. Hypoxemia experienced by patients during apnea triggers the release of inflammatory factors that alter the micromilieu of the blood, resulting in hypercoagulability [56]. Regarding platelets, the major finding of this study was that, compared to the control, MPV and PDW were increased in total group subjects with OSAS, and in patients with severe OSAS. Additionally, platelets count was increased in total group subjects with OSAS. This may support the evidence for platelet activation in OSAS, which may contribute to the increased incidence of cardiovascular events in patients with OSAS [57,58]. Moreover, this study is the first to demonstrate elevated platelets count in patients with OSAS. However, no correlations were found between any of these platelets indices and severity of OSAS or the sleep parameters, contrary to our results of RDW, and hematocrit. In this study, we excluded the possible confounding effects of several factors/diseases on the studied hematological parameters, as hypertension, cardiovascular diseases, smoking, and diabetes mellitus. There were no statistical differences regarding these factors between OSAS patients and controls.

There is controversy about MPV and PDW levels in patients with OSAS. Varol et al. [19] found that MPV was significantly higher in patients with severe OSAS when compared with control subjects and MPV was correlated with AHI. Alternatively, the results of the study of Kurt et al. [15] revealed that PDW, but not MPV, was higher in severe OSAS. In accordance with our results, Nena et al. [20] reported that both of MPV and PDW levels were significantly higher in severe OSAS patients than in control and mild to moderate OSAS. However, their study did not exclude cardiac or lung disease, chronic renal or hepatic disease, hypertension, or smoking.

The exact mechanism of platelet activation in patients with OSAS is unclear and may be complex, Three main pathways may be implicated; sympathetic overactivity [59], hypoxia [60], and inflammation [61,62], all being well-known features of OSAS [3-5].

There are potential limitations of this study. First, as it is a retrospective study, we did not include a marker of inflammation, neurohormonal activation, or oxidative stress to evaluate its correlation with these CBC parameters. Second, this study cannot discriminate causality from association with regard to the link between RDW and OSAS in relation to inflammation and oxidative stress. Third, this is not a follow-up study, so we do not have the prognostic outcome results of OSAS patients with high RDW values, including the influence of CPAP therapy on these patients. Fourth, we did not measure nutritional status of vitamin B and folate levels, which are one of the potential causes of increased levels of RDW. However, our study population is not anemic, and the possible effect of these vitamins deficiencies can be neglected.

Conclusions

In conclusion, our study has established that RDW, MPV, PDW, and platelets count all are increased in OSAS. RDW is positively correlated with AHI, oxygen desaturation index, EES, and negatively correlated with minimum oxygen saturation and REM sleep. Thus, RDW may be a marker for the severity of OSAS. As RDW is included in a complete blood count, it could provide an easy, inexpensive tool for triaging OSAS patients for polysomnography evaluation. It is highly possible that RDW will become one of the items of the standard evaluation test panel for OSAS patients and patients with severe OSAS could be identified based on RDW at the first examination and given priority for testing and treatment.

References

1. Zamarron C, García Paz V, Riveiro A (2008) Obstructive sleep apnea syndrome is a systemic disease. Current evidence. See comment in PubMed Commons below Eur J Intern Med 19: 390-398.
2. Lavie L (2015) Oxidative stress in obstructive sleep apnea and intermittent hypoxia - Revisited - The bad ugly and good: Implications to the heart and brain. See comment in PubMed Commons below Sleep Med Rev 20C: 27-45.
3. Hoyos CM, Melehan KL, Liu PY, Grunstein RR, Phillips CL (2015) Does obstructive sleep apnea cause endothelial dysfunction? A critical review of the literature. See comment in PubMed Commons below Sleep Med Rev 20C: 15-26.
4. Zamarrón C, Morete E, del Campo Matias F (2012) Obstructive Sleep Apnoea Syndrome as a Systemic Low-Grade Inflammatory Disorder. In Cardiovascular Risk Factors, Armen Gasparyan (Ed.); ISBN: 978-953-51-0240-3, InTech.
5. Gileles-Hillel A, Alonso-Álvarez ML, Kheirandish-Gozal L, Peris E, Cordero-Guevara JA, et al. (2014) Inflammatory Markers and Obstructive Sleep Apnea in Obese Children: The NANOS Study. Mediators of Inflammation ID 605280: 1-9.
6. Evans TC, Jehle D (1991) The red blood cell distribution width. See comment in PubMed Commons below J Emerg Med 9 Suppl 1: 71-74.
7. Su C, Liao LZ, Song Y, Xu ZW, Mei WY (2014) The role of red blood cell distribution width in mortality and cardiovascular risk among patients with coronary artery diseases: a systematic review and meta-analysis. See comment in PubMed Commons below J Thorac Dis 6: 1429-1440.
8. van Kimmenade RR, Mohammed AA, Uthamalingam S, van der Meer P, Felker GM, et al. (2010) Red blood cell distribution width and 1-year mortality in acute heart failure. See comment in PubMed Commons below Eur J Heart Fail 12: 129-136.
9. Allen LA, Felker GM, Mehra MR, Chiong JR, Dunlap SH, et al. (2010) Validation and potential mechanisms of red cell distribution width as a prognostic marker in heart failure. See comment in PubMed Commons below J Card Fail 16: 230-238.
10. Ani C, Ovbiagele B (2009) Elevated red blood cell distribution width predicts mortality in persons with known stroke. See comment in PubMed Commons below J Neurol Sci 277: 103-108.
11. Montagnana M, Cervellin G, Meschi T, Lippi G (2011) The role of red blood cell distribution width in cardiovascular and thrombotic disorders. See comment in PubMed Commons below Clin Chem Lab Med 50: 635-641.
12. Park Y, Schoene N, Harris W (2002) Mean platelet volume as an indicator of platelet activation: methodological issues. See comment in PubMed Commons below Platelets 13: 301-306.
13. Gasparyan AY, Ayvazyan L, Mikhailidis DP, Kitas GD (2011) Mean platelet volume: a link between thrombosis and inflammation? Curr Pharm Des 17: 47-58.
14. Vagdatli E, Gounari E, Lazaridou E, Katsibourlia E, Tsikopoulou F, et al. (2010) Platelet distribution width: a simple, practical and specific marker of activation of coagulation. See comment in PubMed Commons below Hippokratia 14: 28-32.
15. Kurt OK, Yildiz N (2013) The importance of laboratory parameters in patients with obstructive sleep apnea syndrome. See comment in PubMed Commons below Blood Coagul Fibrinolysis 24: 371-374.
16. Ozsu S, Abul Y, Gulsoy A, Bulbul Y, Yaman S, et al. (2012) Red cell distribution width in patients with obstructive sleep apnea syndrome. See comment in PubMed Commons below Lung 190: 319-326.
17. **Sökücü SN, Karasulu L, Dalar L, Seyhan EC, Altın S (2012) Can red blood cell distribution width predict severity of obstructive sleep apnea syndrome? See comment in PubMed Commons below J Clin Sleep Med 8: 521-525.**
18. Karakas MS, Er A, Gülcan AR, Altekin RE, Yalçinkaya S, et al. (2013) Assesment of red cell distribution width (RDW) in patients with obstructive sleep apnea syndrome. Journal Of Turgut Ozal Medical Center 20: 208-214.

19. Gunbatar H, Sertogullarindan B, Ekin S, Akdag S, Arisoy A, et al. (2014) The correlation between red blood cell distribution width levels with the severity of obstructive sleep apnea and carotid intima media thickness. See comment in PubMed Commons below Med Sci Monit 20: 2199-2204.

20. Varol E, Ozturk O, Gonca T, Has M, Ozaydin M, et al. (2010) Mean platelet volume is increased in patients with severe obstructive sleep apnea. See comment in PubMed Commons below Scand J Clin Lab Invest 70: 497-502.

21. Nena E, Papanas N, Steiropoulos P, Zikidou P, Zarogoulidis P, et al. (2012) Mean Platelet Volume and Platelet Distribution Width in non-diabetic subjects with obstructive sleep apnoea syndrome: new indices of severity? See comment in PubMed Commons below Platelets 23: 447-454.

22. Kanbay A, Tutar N, Kaya E, Buyukoglan H, Ozdogan N, et al. (2013) Mean platelet volume in patients with obstructive sleep apnea syndrome and its relationship with cardiovascular diseases. See comment in PubMed Commons below Blood Coagul Fibrinolysis 24: 532-536.

23. Karakaş MS, Altekin RE, Baktır AO, Küçük M, Cilli A, et al. (2013) Association between mean platelet volume and severity of disease in patients with obstructive sleep apnea syndrome without risk factors for cardiovascular disease. See comment in PubMed Commons below Turk Kardiyol Dern Ars 41: 14-20.

24. Sökücü SN, Ozdemir C, Dalar L, Karasulu L, Aydın S, et al. (2014) Is mean platelet volume really a severity marker for obstructive sleep apnea syndrome without comorbidities? See comment in PubMed Commons below Pulm Med 2014: 754839.

25. Akyüz A, Akkoyun DÇ, Oran M, Değirmenci H, Alp R (2014) Mean platelet volume in patients with obstructive sleep apnea and its relationship with simpler heart rate derivatives. See comment in PubMed Commons below Cardiol Res Pract 2014: 454701.

26. Ayas NT, Hirsch AA, Laher I, Bradley TD, Malhotra A, et al. (2014) New frontiers in obstructive sleep apnoea. See comment in PubMed Commons below Clin Sci (Lond) 127: 209-216.

27. Sánchez-Armengol A, Villalobos-López P, Caballero-Eraso C, Carmona-Bernal C, Asensio-Cruz M, Barbé F, et al. (2015) Gamma glutamyl transferase and oxidative stress in obstructive sleep apnea: a study in 1744 patients. Sleep Breath.

28. Andaku D, D Almeida V, Carneiro G, Hix S, Tufik S, et al. (2015) Sleepiness, inflammation and oxidative stress markers in middle-aged males with obstructive sleep apnea without metabolic syndrome: a cross-sectional study. Respir Res; 16:3.

29. Hopps E, Canino B, Calandrino V, Montana M, Lo Presti R, et al. (2014) Lipid peroxidation and protein oxidation are related to the severity of OSAS. See comment in PubMed Commons below Eur Rev Med Pharmacol Sci 18: 3773-3778.

30. Li J, Wang L, Jiang M, Mao Y, Pan X (2014) Relationship between serum homocysteine level and oxidative stress in patients with obstructive sleep apnea-hypopnea syndrome. Zhonghua Yi Xue Za Zhi; 94: 2510-2513.

31. Tauman R, Lavie L, Greenfeld M, Sivan Y (2014) Oxidative stress in children with obstructive sleep apnea syndrome. See comment in PubMed Commons below J Clin Sleep Med 10: 677-681.

32. Abboud F, Kumar R (2014) Obstructive sleep apnea and insight into mechanisms of sympathetic overactivity. See comment in PubMed Commons below J Clin Invest 124: 1454-1457.

33. Liak C, Fitzpatrick M (2011) Coagulability in obstructive sleep apnea. See comment in PubMed Commons below Can Respir J 18: 338-348.

34. Htoo AK, Greenberg H, Tongia S, Chen G, Henderson T, et al. (2006) Activation of nuclear factor kappaB in obstructive sleep apnea: a pathway leading to systemic inflammation. See comment in PubMed Commons below Sleep Breath 10: 43-50.

35. Burioka N, Koyanagi S, Fukuoka Y, Okazaki F, Fujioka T, et al. (2009) Influence of intermittent hypoxia on the signal transduction pathways to inflammatory response and circadian clock regulation. See comment in PubMed Commons below Life Sci 85: 372-378.

36. May AM, Mehra R (2014) Obstructive sleep apnea: role of intermittent hypoxia and inflammation. See comment in PubMed Commons below Semin Respir Crit Care Med 35: 531-544.

37. Lam JC, Mak JC, Ip MS (2012) Obesity, obstructive sleep apnoea and metabolic syndrome. See comment in PubMed Commons below Respirology 17: 223-236.

38. Perkins SL (2003) Examination of blood and bone marrow. In: Greer JP, Foerster J, Lukens JN, Rodgers GM, Paraksevas F, Glader BE, eds. Wintrobe's Clinical Hematology. 11th ed. Salt Lake City, UT: Lippincott Williams & Wilkins: 5-25.

39. Semba RD, Patel KV, Ferrucci L, Sun K, Roy CN, et al. (2010) Serum antioxidants and inflammation predict red cell distribution width in older women: the Women's Health and Aging Study I. See comment in PubMed Commons below Clin Nutr 29: 600-604.

40. Yokoe T, Minoguchi K, Matsuo H (2003) Elevated levels of C- reactive protein and interleukin-6 in patients with obstructive sleep apnea syndrome are decreased by nasal continuous positive airway pressure. Circulation 107: 1129-1134.

41. Weiss G, Goodnough LT (2005) Anemia of chronic disease. See comment in PubMed Commons below N Engl J Med 352: 1011-1023.

42. Lippi G, Targher G, Montagnana M, Salvagno GL, Zoppini G, et al. (2009) Relation between red blood cell distribution width and inflammatory biomarkers in a large cohort of unselected outpatients. See comment in PubMed Commons below Arch Pathol Lab Med 133: 628-632.

43. Celik A, Koc F, Kadi H, Ceyhan K, Erkorkmaz U, et al. (2012) Relationship between red cell distribution width and echocardiographic parameters in patients with diastolic heart failure. See comment in PubMed Commons below Kaohsiung J Med Sci 28: 165-172.

44. Malandrino N, Wu WC, Taveira TH, Whitlatch HB, Smith RJ (2012) Association between red blood cell distribution width and macrovascular and microvascular complications in diabetes. See comment in PubMed Commons below Diabetologia 55: 226-235.

45. Tanindi A, Topal FE, Topal F, Celik B (2012) Red cell distribution width in patients with prehypertension and hypertension. See comment in PubMed Commons below Blood Press 21: 177-181.

46. Johns MW (1991) A new method for measuring daytime sleepiness: the Epworth sleepiness scale. See comment in PubMed Commons below Sleep 14: 540-545.

47. Dikmenoglu N, Ciftçi B, Ileri E, Güven SF, Seringeç N, et al. (2006) Erythrocyte deformability, plasma viscosity and oxidative status in patients with severe obstructive sleep apnea syndrome. Sleep Med 7: 255–261.

48. Zubieta-Calleja GR, Paulev PE, Zubieta-Calleja L, Zubieta-Castillo G (2007) Altitude adaptation through hematocrit changes. See comment in PubMed Commons below J Physiol Pharmacol 58 Suppl 5: 811-818.

49. Somers VK, White DP, Amin R, Abraham WT, Costa F, Culebras A, et al. (2008) Sleep apnea and cardiovascular disease: an American Heart Association/American College of Cardiology Foundation Scienti?c Statement from the American Heart Association Council for High Blood Pressure Research Professional Education Committee, Council on Clinical Cardiology, Stroke Council, and Council On Cardiovascular Nursing. In collaboration with the National Heart, Lung, and Blood Institute National Centeron Sleep Disorders Research (National Institutes of Health). Circulation 118: 1080–1111.

50. Choi JB, Loredo JS, Norman D, Mills PJ, Ancoli-Israel S, et al. (2006) Does obstructive sleep apnea increase hematocrit? See comment in PubMed Commons below Sleep Breath 10: 155-160.

51. Hoffstein V, Herridge M, Mateika S, Redline S, Strohl KP (1994) Hematocrit levels in sleep apnea. See comment in PubMed Commons below Chest 106: 787-791.

52. Krieger J, Sforza E, Delanoe C, Petiau C (1992) Decrease in haematocrit with continuous positive airway pressure treatment in obstructive sleep apnoea patients. See comment in PubMed Commons below Eur Respir J 5: 228-233.

53. Chin K, Ohi M, Kita H, Noguchi T, Otsuka N, et al. (1996) Effects of NCPAP therapy on fibrinogen levels in obstructive sleep apnea syndrome. See comment in PubMed Commons below Am J Respir Crit Care Med 153: 1972-1976.
54. Nobili L, Schiavi G, Bozano E, De Carli F, Ferrillo F, et al. (2000) Morning increase of whole blood viscosity in obstructive sleep apnea syndrome. See comment in PubMed Commons below Clin Hemorheol Microcirc 22: 21-27.
55. Reinhart WH, Oswald J, Walter R, Kuhn M (2002) Blood viscosity and platelet function in patients with obstructive sleep apnea syndrome treated with nasal continuous positive airway pressure. Clin Hemorheol Microcirc 27: 201-207.
56. Zhang X, Yin K, Wang H, Su M, Yang Y (2003) Effect of continuous positive airway pressure treatment on elderly Chinese patients with obstructive sleep apnea in the prethrombotic state. See comment in PubMed Commons below Chin Med J (Engl) 116: 1426-1428.
57. Phillips CL, McEwen BJ, Morel-Kopp MC, Yee BJ, Sullivan DR, et al. (2012) Effects of continuous positive airway pressure on coagulability in obstructive sleep apnoea: a randomized, placebo-controlled crossover study. Thorax 67: 639-644.
58. Shimizu M, Kamio K, Haida M, Ono Y, Miyachi H, et al. (2002) Platelet activation in patients with obstructive sleep apnea syndrome and effects of nasal-continuous positive airway pressure. See comment in PubMed Commons below Tokai J Exp Clin Med 27: 107-112.
59. Geiser T, Buck F, Meyer BJ, Bassetti C, Haeberli A, et al. (2002) In vivo platelet activation is increased during sleep in patients with obstructive sleep apnea syndrome. See comment in PubMed Commons below Respiration 69: 229-234.
60. Feres MC, Cintra FD, Rizzi CF, Mello-Fujita L, Lino de Souza AA, et al. (2014) Evaluation and validation of a method for determining platelet catecholamine in patients with obstructive sleep apnea and arterial hypertension. See comment in PubMed Commons below PLoS One 9: e98407.
61. Tyagi T, Ahmad S, Gupta N, Sahu A, Ahmad Y, et al. (2014) Altered expression of platelet proteins and calpain activity mediate hypoxia-induced prothrombotic phenotype. See comment in PubMed Commons below Blood 123: 1250-1260.
62. Ghoshal K, Bhattacharyya M (2014) Overview of platelet physiology: its hemostatic and nonhemostatic role in disease pathogenesis. See comment in PubMed Commons below ScientificWorldJournal 2014: 781857.
63. Tsiara S, Elisaf M, Jagroop IA, Mikhailidis DP (2003) Platelets as predictors of vascular risk: is there a practical index of platelet activity? See comment in PubMed Commons below Clin Appl Thromb Hemost 9: 177-190.

Application of Cognitive-behavioral Therapy in Obstructive Sleep Apnea: Comparison of CPAP Therapy and CBT on the Executive Functions of the Brain

Maryam Talebi[1]*, Kazem Rasoolzadeh Tabatabaye[1] and Ensiye Vahedi[2]

[1]*Tarbiat Modares University, Tehran, Iran*
[2]*School of Medical Sciences, Baqiyatallah University of Medical Sciences, Tehran, Iran*

Abstract

Purpose: Sleep apnea disorder brings about negative effects to the quality of life of the people involved. Debilitation of cognitive functioning is one of the consequences of this condition. Scant researches have been carried out to explore the efficacy of cognitive therapy on mitigating clinical symptoms and cognitive functions of the brain. The novelty of the present study is in combining cognitive method and medical treatment. This research aims to compare the effectiveness of continuous positive air pressure (CPAP) therapy and cognitive-behavioral treatment (CBT) on improving mental cognitive functions in patients with sleep apnea.

Methods: The study population included all patients referred to the Bahar Sleep Disorders Clinic in Tehran, Iran. The sample consisted of 45 people who were randomly placed into three groups of 15 people (CPAP therapy, cognitive behavioral therapy, and control groups). All three groups were psychologically assessed prior to the intervention. Next, individuals in the cognitive-behavioral group underwent 12 sessions of cognitive training, progressive muscle relaxation, mental visualization, and sleep hygiene. The other group went through CPAP therapy. After the intervention, both groups were assessed psychologically. Data collection instruments included Wisconsin cognitive software, simple Stroop, complex Stroop, continuous performance, polysomnography device, and CPAP devices.

Results: The results indicated that both types of intervention can enhance cognitive functioning; however, a greater efficacy is obtained by combining the two methods compared with the exclusive application of medical treatment.

Conclusion: The authors propose cognitive-behavioral therapy OSA as a complement to medical treatment.

Keywords: Obstructive sleep apnea; CPAP therapy; Cognitive-behavioral therapy; Cognitive functions

Introduction

Sleep is one of the most important natural biological cycles and is featured by a complex pattern. One normally applies the concept of sleep to refer to the effects associated with two circadian (24 hours) and balancing processes such as the adequacy of nocturnal sleep, sleep quantity, and daytime sleepiness.

Sleep is important for two reasons: First, sleep-related complaints are very common among people; second, low sleep quality is considered as an indicator of many psychological diseases [1].

Good quality sleep can lead to mental and physical regeneration of individuals since cellular repair and mental health are dependent on sleep.

The quality and quantity of sleep also affect one's health, and they are always regarded as important factors influencing the quality of life People with sleep disorder are not only characterized by fatigue, but also suffer from a range of complications like those related to cellular repair, defects in learning and memory, increased stress and anxiety, and reduced quality of daily life. Hence, sleep disorder can have detrimental effects on a person›s health and improvement.

According to some researchers, the first damage caused by poor sleep emerges in the ability of brain to plan and organize cognitive functions [2]. Sleep apnea is a common disorder with far-reaching implications for health and it is one of the major consequences of cognitive impairment. Apnea leads to a negative effect on inductive and deductive reasoning, attention, alertness, learning [3] poor performance on the revised version of Wechsler Adult Intelligence Scale [4] psychomotor vigilance task [5,6] repetitive finger-tapping test [7] as well as impaired concentration, problem-solving, and verbal and spatial short-term memory [8]. The prevalence of sleep apnea in adult men is about 3% to 7% and nearly 2% to 5% for adult women [9].

In addition to physical factors underlying sleep disorder, one can point to some psychological roots of this condition including emotional factors, dysfunctional beliefs and attitudes concerning sleep [10,11] as well as behavioral factors such as inadequate sleep hygiene.

People with sleep apnea, due to frequent waking, are unable to enter the phase of rapid eye movement (REM) which is necessary for a good sleep [12] therefore; they experience mental health problems such as anxiety and memory complications. This is because dreams are an opportunity for processing everyday events and a means of memory retention [13]. Dreams provide a ground for, long-term goals, everyday interactions and discharge of anxious emotions.

***Corresponding author:** Maryam Talebi, Student of Psychology, Department of Psychology, Faculty of Humanities, Tarbiat Modares University, Tehran, Iran, E-mail: m.taleby@modares.ac.ir

A cohort study on 4 million American soldiers, revealed that 118 thousand individuals had gone through sleep apnea along with other disorders such as depression (21/8%) post-traumatic stress (11/9%) anxiety (16/7%) psychosis (5/1%) and bipolar disorder (3.3%) [14,15].

Bardwell et al. reported that after they controlled severe sleep apneas, the subjects showed symptoms of depression and fatigue. Hence, they suggested that in addition to controlling this disorder, one has to take psychological symptoms and mood complications into account as well [16]. It is worth noting that depression has caused the most prevalent conditions in subjects with sleep apnea [17].

It is also shown that anxiety and depression decrease as a result of continuous positive air pressure (CPAP), but fatigue might be still there and the treatment may not improve it. In fact, intense apnea disorder is associated with the increase of anxiety and depression

Aloia et al. in their research on the cognitive effects of apnea and treatment with continuous positive air pressure demonstrated that consciousness increases after treatment, but there still remains a weakness in terms of cognitive abilities and mental performance. It is clear that many cognitive deficiencies cannot be compensated by medical care alone [18].

In their follow-up study, Bourke et al. observed a decrease in the level of anxiety, depression, and psychological distress after treatment; nevertheless, not that much improvement was found in cognitive function tests. The authors suggested that such improvement requires a longer treatment period [19]. Bourke reported that some cognitive symptoms can be treated but this will not lead to improvement in mood and affection symptoms. The use of ECT after the treatment by CPAP is evidence indicating that some of the cognitive functions and symptoms (e.g. depression) cannot completely be improved through CPAP. After treatment with continuous positive air pressure (CPAP), the symptoms of mental weakness (psychasthenia), evaluated by MMPI-2 test, remained unchanged [20].

In their samples that were treated with CPAP and were mentally trained, Golay et al. observed a considerable progress in improving quality of life compared to the group without education [20]. The faith-based model of health, which emphasizes patients' mental experience of health and their beliefs, produces more stable treatment effects [21]. Therefore, due to the severity of cognitive side effects and considering the important role of cognitive disabilities in the course of this condition, we employed, in addition to medical treatment, cognitive-behavioral approach as a combination therapy to improve executive functions of patients.

Materials and Methods

This study is a quasi-experimental research with pretest and post-test design and a control group. The research population consisted of all individuals who referred to Bahar sleep disorders clinic. To conduct the study, 45 patients with sleep apnea were chosen using purposive sampling and assigned to the control and experimental groups. The criteria for inclusion were: maximum age of 60 years, no psychotic and personality disorder, no substance abuse, lack of sleep medications, observing ethical principles, and willingness to cooperate. Under the supervision of a psychiatrist and assistance of the clinical psychologist, the researcher applied, using Wisconsin Card Sorting Test, simple and complex Stroop, together with continuous performance task, the relevant components of executive functions to clients whose apnea had been diagnosed using polysomnography device. Also, CPAP therapy was conducted for two consecutive months on the patients and cognitive-behavioral therapy was performed in 12 sessions (90 minutes each) on the experimental group. During this period, subjects in the control group did not receive any intervention and were kept in the waiting list so that in case the effectiveness of treatment was proved they might be treated provided they were inclined to. The sessions included the following: one session dealing with mental training and providing information about the disorder, explaining the objectives of education and getting familiar with the members, agreeing on the time and place, stressing the importance of therapy assignments, assessing sleep problems, evaluating beliefs, relaxation training, and constructive worry worksheet; two sessions for training time management strategies; two sessions of training organization and planning, sleep hygiene and scheduling a new sleep program, sleep restriction, refraining from daily naps, food health; two sessions of training prevention techniques; one session given to enhancing patients' motivation and problem solving skills, summing up ideas, explaining the reality of sleep, introducing the cycle of thinking and feeling and behavior, training thought blocking, mental visualization, and not trying in vain to fall asleep (paradoxical intention) as well as applying all previous instructions; several sessions devoted to teaching the techniques of emotional self-regulation; and eventually, some training sessions meant to increase cognitive flexibility, control and coordinate as well as organize behaviors.

Results

Table 1 provides the average pretest and post-test scores in the experimental and control groups. As can be seen, compared with the control group, the post-test scores of the experimental groups have been improved in all indices.

To examine the differences in the linear combination of dependent variables in the experimental and control groups, we drew on Wilks' Lambda [a probability distribution used in multivariate hypothesis testing, especially with regard to the likelihood-ratio test and multivariate analysis of variance (MANOVA)]multivariate test (Table 2). The results of all four tests show that after controlling the pretest factor, there was a significant difference in the linear combination of dependent variables; hence, the group factor had a significant impact.

Table 3 illustrates the results of intergroup effect test which can be used to examine the differences between each dependent variable. The results of Table 3 show that the mean scores of post-test have been significantly changed in all of the dependent variables except for the index of "correct responses (phase 2)."

Having observed that F value has been significant in all of the related indices except for that of "correct answers (phase 2)," we next used Bonferroni (one of several methods used to counteract the problem of multiple comparisons) post hoc test for the other 17 indices whose F value were significant in order to determine those post-test scores of the groups that have gone through significant changes. In other words, Bonferroni test was employed so as to make a mutual comparison between the experimental and control groups.

Discussion

Regarding the two indices of "correct answers (phase 1)" and "correct answers (phase 2)," it was found that the mean of polytherapy group was significantly higher than that of control group; however, there was no significant difference between the medical treatment and control group. Therefore, it can be said that compared to medical treatment, polytherapy was more effective on the indices of "correct answers (phase 1)" and "correct answers (phase 2). Nevertheless, it has to be noted that there was no significant difference between the mean

Variables	Components	Combination Group		Medical Group		Control Group	
Stroop Test		Pre-test	Post-test	Pre-test	Post-test	Pre-test	Post-test
	Correct answers (phase 1)	(74/0) 13/9	(64/0) 53/9	(59/0) 26/9	(63/0) 40/9	(67/0) 20/9	(64/0) 13/9
	Correct answers (phase 2)	(53/0) 9	(63/0) 40/9	(59/0) 06/9	(60/0) 26/9	(59/0) 07/9	(53/0) 01/9
	Correct answers (phase 3)	(41/0) 80/8	(50/0) 41/9	(51/0) 86/8	(59/0) 07/9	(59/0) 73/8	(56/0) 80/8
	Reaction time (phase 1)	(18/0) 98/0	(16/0) 87/0	(19/0) 97/0	(17/0) 93/0	(18/0) 00/1	(16/0) 00/1
	Reaction time (phase 2)	(14/0) 90/0	(13/0) 80/0	(17/0) 91/0	(14/0) 85/0	(16/0) 94/0	(15/0) 92/0
	Reaction time (phase 3)	(19/0) 02/1	(16/0) 90/0	(18/0) 03/1	(16/0) 97/0	(17/0) 03/1	(13/0) 02/1
	Correct answers (list of related words)	32	66/35	32	40/33	66/31	60/31
		(65/2)	(95/1)	(97/2)	(09/2)	(74/2)	(38/2)
	Correct answers (list of unrelated words)	93/30	40/34	73/30	80/32	80/30	00/31
		(57/2)	(29/1)	(63/2)	(11/2)	(30/2)	(77/1)
Emotional Stroop test	Reaction time (list of related words)	(11/0) 89/0	(08/0) 83/0	(14/0) 89/0	(11/0) 86/0	(12/0) 91/0	(10/0) 90/0
	Reaction time (list of unrelated words)	(08/0) 90/0	(06/0) 83/0	(11/0) 88/0	(09/0) 85/0	(12/0) 89/0	(11/0) 88/0
	Average reaction time	(08/0) 85/0	(06/0) 72/0	(07/0) 84/0	(05/0) 78/0	(09/0) 85/0	(06/0) 84/0
	Error of commission	(68/0) 80/4	(77/0) 20/3	(27/1) 73/4	(74/0) 86/3	(97/0) 66/4	(64/0) 46/4
Performance Test	Error of omission	(64/0) 86/3	(74/0) 46/2	(70/0) 06/4	(63/0) 40/3	(70/0) 93/3	(91/0) 86/3
	Completed classes	(09/1) 06/4	(12/1) 46/5	(03/1) 26/4	(26/1) 20/5	(72/0) 33/4	(59/0) 26/4
	Preservation error	20Dec	40/10	13Dec	20Nov	00/13	00/13
		(43/3)	(09/2)	(27/3)	(30/2)	(72/2)	(92/1)
Wisconsin Classification Test	Other errors	Jun-13	20Aug	80/12	13Oct	86/12	73/12
		(36/4)	(21/2)	(69/4)	(54/3)	(55/3)	(25/2)
	Failure to maintain a sequence	(12/0) 79/0	(09/0) 55/0	(13/0) 81/0	(12/0) 68/0	(12/0) 81/0	(07/0) 80/0
	Attempt to complete the first pattern	33/18	66/14	73/17	53/15	Jun-19	46/18
		(79/7)	(88/5)	(18/6)	(40/4)	(94/5)	(74/4)

Table 1: Mean and SD of research variables in three groups in the pretest and post-test.

Test	Value	F	DF	Sig	Eta
Stroop	0.133	8.996	12	0	0.635
Emotional Stroop	0.105	18.21	8	0	0.675
Performance	0.122	22.94	6	0	0.65
Wisconsin Classification	0.11	13.27	10	0	0.668

Table 2: Multivariate tests (Wilks' lambda statistics).

of post-tests in the polytherapy and medical treatment groups. As for the indices of "reaction time (phase 1)," "reaction time (phase 2)," and "reaction time (phase 3)," it was indicated that both polytherapy and medical treatment had a significant impact, compared to the control group, and they led to the improvement of the subjects' performance. Specifically, polytherapy showed a significantly better effect than medical treatment. Regarding the four indices of "correct answers (list of related words)," "correct answers (list of unrelated words), "reaction time (list of related words)," and "reaction time (list of unrelated words)," we observed that both polytherapy and medical treatment displayed a significant effect, compared to the control group, and they clearly improved subjects' performance. Moreover, it wasremarkable that polytherapy had a significantly better effect than medical treatment. Based on the indices of "average reaction time," "commission error," and "omission error," subjects' performance was better in both experimental groups than that in the control group. Besides, polytherapy revealed a significantly greater performance than medical treatment. With respect to the indices of "completed classes" and "preservation error," we found that subjects' performance was significantly better in both experimental groups, compared to the control group. Even so, although the performance of polytherapy group was slightly better than the medical treatment group, this did not reveal a significant difference. With regard to the three indices of "other errors," "failure to maintain a sequence," and "attempt to complete the first pattern," it was demonstrated that both polytherapy and medical treatment had a significant effect,

Variables	Dependent Variable	SS	DF	F	Sig.	Eta
Stroop Test	Correct answers (phase 1)	1.574	2	3.586	0.038	0.166
	Correct answers (phase 2)	1.485	2	2.745	0.078	0.132
	Correct answers (phase 3)	2.669	2	4.963	0.012	0.216
	Reaction time (phase 1)	273.46	2	21.672	0	0.546
	Reaction time (phase 2)	229.32	2	27.528	0	0.605
	Reaction time (phase 3)	303.67	2	52.08	0	0.743
	Correct answers (list of related words)	111.48	2	54.602	0	0.742
	Correct answers (list of unrelated words)	83.941	2	32.107	0	0.628
	Reaction time (list of related words)	106.7	2	25.907	0	0.577
Emotional Stroop test	Reaction time (list of unrelated words)	106.83	2	28.547	0	0.6
	Average reaction time	406.85	2	74.16	0	0.792
	Error of commission	13.348	2	23.476	0	0.546
Performance test	Error of omission	14.441	2	11.719	0	0.375
	Completed classes	12.58	2	7.773	0	0.296
	Preservation error	36.877	2	14.226	0	0.435
	Other errors	159.16	2	57.396	0	0.756
	Failure to maintain a sequence	0.408	2	56.619	0	0.754
Wisconsin Classification test	Attempt to complete the first pattern	79.667	2	24.189	0	0.567

Table 3: Intergroup effect test.

compared to the control group, and enhanced subjects' performance. Polytherapy had a significantly better impact than medical treatment in this regard as well.

This study aimed to compare two types of interventions including medical treatment and medical cognitive-behavioral polytherapy in terms of improving mental executive functions of patients who had referred to a sleep disorder clinic.

The study results indicated that both the medical approach and the polytherapy method were effective in treating apnea symptoms. However, upon comparison, it was observed that the efficacy of polytherapy was significantly greater than medical treatment. This finding is consistent with the studies by [22-29].

According to the results of this study, it seems that, in explaining the effectiveness of cognitive-behavioral therapy, training the skills of cognitive-behavioral therapy is helpful in terms of some executive functions such as attention, reaction time, problem-solving strategies, and control of impulsive behaviors; an objective that can be attained through improving cognitive functioning or increasing cognitive abilities of individuals involved [30]. Given that cognitive functions can be seriously impaired due to apnea disorder, one may compensate for the defects resulting from the disease by properly taking advantage of cognitive-behavioral treatment as a regular therapeutic activity built upon cognitive principles.

This seems an important suggestion because frequent sleep apneas might damage the performance of central neural system and the implementation of many cognitive tasks. It is proposed that if one effectively learn cognitive control skills and sleep hygiene strategies, we can expect that the neural system and cognitive performance will be improved. This is due to the fact that one of the goals of cognitive-behavioral treatment is to make lifestyle interventions so as to enhance recovery and increase cognitive performance. As mentioned in the introduction, although the basis of treatment is to emphasize changing the content of thought and cognitive processes, practically the major focus of treatment is on a number of central issues related to patients' daily life such as sleep hygiene, emotional self-regulation, increasing cognitive flexibility, and controlling as well as coordinating behavior.

Indeed, despite the many benefits of cognitive-behavioral therapy in improving sleep quality, sleep disorders are often addressed by physicians, and psychologists have only occasionally dealt with them. Notwithstanding the psychological complications of this disorder, seldom are sleep medicine specialists familiar with its methods of treatment. Thus, it appears that increasing the knowledge of specialists with regard to the efficacy of cognitive-behavioral methods and encouraging psychologists to cooperate with physicians at sleep clinics will lead to obtaining better results in treating sleep disorders. Besides, one may use this method in sleep clinics as a complement to medical treatment.

Compliance with Ethical Standards

Funding: The authors declared that this study received no financial support

Conflict of interest: The authors declare that they have no conflict of interest.

Ethical approval: The whole procedures on the human participants were approved by the Board of Ethics of the hospital and university.

Informed consent: Oral informed consent was obtained from all the participants of the study.

References

1. Ağargün MY, Kara H, Anlar Ö (1996) The validity and reliability of the Pittsburgh Sleep Quality Index. Turk Psikiyatri Derg 7: 107-115.
2. Alhola P, Polo-Kantola P (2007) Sleep deprivation: Impact on cognitive performance. Neuropsychiatr Dis Treat 3: 553.
3. Incalzi RA, Marra C, Salvigni BL, Petrone A, Gemma A, et al. (2004) Does cognitive dysfunction conform to a distinctive pattern in obstructive sleep apnea syndrome? J Sleep Res 13: 79-86.
4. Lal C, Strange C, Bachman D (2012) Neurocognitive impairment in obstructive sleep apnea. CHEST 141: 1601-1610.
5. Dorrian J, Rogers NL, Dinges DF (2005) Psychomotor vigilance performance: Neurocognitive assay sensitive to sleep loss. Marcel Dekker New York.
6. Gagnon K, Baril AA, Gagnon JF, Fortin M, Decary A, et al. (2014) Cognitive impairment in obstructive sleep apnea. Pathol Biol 62: 233-240.
7. Lojander J, Kajaste S, Maasilta P, Partinen M (1999) Cognitive function and treatment of obstructive sleep apnea syndrome. J Sleep Res 8: 71-76.
8. Findley LJ, Barth JT, Powers DC, Wilhoit SC, Boyd DG, et al. (1986) Cognitive impairment in patients with obstructive sleep apnea and associated hypoxemia. CHEST 90: 686-690.
9. Lindberg E (2010) Epidemiology of OSA.
10. Morin C, Blais F, Savard J (2002) Are changes in beliefs and attitudes about sleep related to sleep improvements in the treatment of insomnia? Behav Res Ther 40: 741-752.
11. Saunamäki T, Jehkonen M (2007) Depression and anxiety in obstructive sleep apnea syndrome: A review. Acta Neurologica Scandinavica 116: 277-288.
12. Iranzo A, Santamaria J (2005) Severe obstructive sleep apnea/hypopnea mimicking REM sleep behavior disorder. Sleep 28: 203-206.
13. Meyer JS, Sakai F, Karacan I, Derman S, Yamamoto M (1980) Sleep apnea, narcolepsy, and dreaming: Regional cerebral hemodynamics. Ann Neurol 7: 479-485.
14. Sharafkhaneh A, Richardson P, Hirshkowitz M (2004) Sleep apnea in a high risk population: A study of Veterans Health Administration beneficiaries. Sleep Med 5: 345-350.
15. Sharafkhaneh A, Giray N, Richardson P, Young T, Hirshkowitz M (2005) Association of psychiatric disorders and sleep apnea in a large cohort. Sleep 28: 1405.
16. Bardwell WA, Moore P, Ancoli-Israel S, Dimsdale JE (2003) Fatigue in obstructive sleep apnea: Driven by depressive symptoms instead of apnea severity? Am J Psychiatry 160: 350-355.
17. Baran AS, Richert AC (2003) Obstructive sleep apnea and depression. CNS Spectr 8: 128-134.
18. Aloia M, Arnedt J, Stepnowsky C, Hecht J, Borrelli B (2005) Predicting treatment adherence in obstructive sleep apnea using principles of behavior change. J Clin Sleep Med 1: 346-353.
19. Bourke R, Anderson V, Yang JS, Jackman AR, Killedar A, Nixon GM, Davey MJ, Walker AM, Trinder J, Horne RS (2011) Cognitive and academic functions are impaired in children with all severities of sleep-disordered breathing. Sleep medicine 12:489-496
20. Golay A, Girard A, Grandin S, Métrailler JC, Victorion M, et al. (2006) A new educational program for patients suffering from sleep apnea syndrome. Patient Educ Couns 60: 220-227.
21. Tyrrell J, Poulet C, Pe JL, Veale D (2006) A preliminary study of psychological factors affecting patients' acceptance of CPAP therapy for sleep apnoea syndrome. Sleep med 7: 375-379.
22. Sivertsen B, Omvik S, Pallesen S, Bjorvatn B, Havik OE, et al. (2006) Cognitive behavioral therapy vs. zopiclone for treatment of chronic primary insomnia in older adults: A randomized controlled trial. Jama 295: 2851-2858.
23. Goodkind MS, Gallagher-Thompson D, Thompson LW, Kesler SR, Anker L, et al. (2015) The impact of executive function on response to cognitive behavioral therapy in late-life depression. Int J Geriatr Psychiatry 31: 334-339.

24. Espie CA, Inglis SJ, Tessier S, Harvey L (2001) The clinical effectiveness of cognitive behaviour therapy for chronic insomnia: Implementation and evaluation of a sleep clinic in general medical practice. Behav Res Ther 39: 45-60.

25. Quesnel C, Savard J, Simard S, Ivers H, Morin CM (2003) Efficacy of cognitive-behavioral therapy for insomnia in women treated for nonmetastic breast cancer. J Consult Clin Psychol 71: 189.

26. Vincent N, Lewycky S (2009) Logging on for better sleep: RCT of the effectiveness of online treatment for insomnia. Sleep 32: 807-815.

27. Beebe DW, Gozal D (2002) Obstructive sleep apnea and the prefrontal cortex: towards a comprehensive model linking nocturnal upper airway obstruction to daytime cognitive and behavioral deficits. J Sleep Res 11: 1-16.

28. Manber R, Edinger J, Gress J, Kuo T, Kalista T, et al. (2008) Cognitive behavioral therapy for insomnia enhances depression outcome in patients with comorbid major depressive disor-der and insomnia. Sleep 31: 489-495.

29. Harvey AG, Tang NK (2003) Cognitive behaviour therapy for primary insomnia: can we rest yet? Sleep Med Rev 7: 237-263.

30. Hofmann SG (2006) The importance of culture in cognitive and behavioral practice. Cogni Behav Prac 13: 243-245.

A Global Perspective to Falling Asleep

Renata Pendle[1], **Kathy Sexton-Radek**[2*] **and Fatema Marvi**[2]

[1]*Concordia University, Canada*

[2]*Elmhurst College, USA*

[*]**Corresponding author:** Kathy Sexton-Radek, Professor of Psychology, Elmhurst College, Illinois, USA, E-mail: ksrsleep@aol.com

Abstract

Large scale epidemiological studies along with World Health Organization sponsored studies using the International Classification of Functioning, Disability and Health system, have categorized patient complaints about their sleep The current study was designed as a qualitative investigation of an aspect of a common patient sleep complaint—difficulty falling asleep. The aim of the study was to identify some of the sleep onset practices which may or may not include a treatment for sleep onset. A social media approach was used to capture the qualitative comments about sleep from individuals responding to a Facebook questionnaire.

Keywords: Sleep; Patients; Sleep disturbance; Natural remedies; Sleep quality

Introduction

The scope of sleep medicine has been examined worldwide [1-3]. Results from studies of sleep medicine describe the incidence and prevalence of sleep disorders by population by country [2,4]. With these tabulations, the severity and treatment needs of sleep disorders have been identified [5,6]. In an effort to determine factors precipitate to sleep disorders, a survey asking about sleep disturbance and sleep related behaviors was administered to a worldwide audience. The questionnaire was in English and Portuguese (per the first author). A graphical and tabular summary of the individual responses across 26 countries to the questions about their pre-sleep and sleep onset behaviors will be given. Additionally, the clinical implications will be provided for the conclusions.

Method

Greater than 90% of the world's countries have an English speaking population. Study participants are often patients or undergraduates (i.e., homogeneous groups by demographic and medical diagnosis/symptom). Participants were gathered from invitations posted on sleep related blogs and social media. Additionally, a Facebook page was generated with a description of the aim of the research. Consent was gathered by agreement represented in completed questionnaires which was in line with Helsinki guidelines that specifically requests informed consent be given.

A five-item survey asking about sleep difficulty, natural remedies, strategies to fall asleep and other treatments used when sleep is disrupted. The questions were designed with 4-15 choices per item – in a checklist fashion. Each question was treated as a separate variable, coded and entered into an Excel spreadsheet. Survey statistics were used to represent the tabulations among the items by participant. The aim of the study was to identify personal, qualitative factors related to sleep and sleep disturbance.

Findings

A response rate of 181 surveys was collected. 24 male and 157 females in an age range of 18 to 65 years. The responses were collected during the period of August to November of 2014. Individuals responded from 13 countries: Albania, United States, Canada, Brazil, England, Ireland, China, Norway, Sweden, Jamaica, Mexico, Philippines and Italy.

49.7% of the respondents stated they had difficulty falling asleep; of this grouping initiating sleep was the most problematic (35%). Fragmented sleep resulting from frequent wake ups was the second most common reason for poor sleep. 48.9% of the participants that indicated trouble falling asleep had had this problem for ten years or greater. 28% of the respondents indicated that they take a supplement to fall asleep. Melatonin, chamomile and mineral/vitamin supplements were the most popularly used by the respondents. Table 1 lists the types of natural remedy by use in the subgroup of respondents that stated they take them. Table 2 represents alternative medicine practices that 28% of the respondents have tried as a method to fall asleep. Regulation of caffeine intake, co-sleeping and rest & digest (i.e., colloquial phrase for relaxing, sedentary behavior).

Which of the following natural remedies have you tried and regularly use to fall asleep?				
Natural Remedy	**Never tried**	**Have tried**	**Regularly use**	**Response Count**
Amino acids	45	0	1	46

California poppy (Eschscholzia California)	46	0	0	46
Camphor odor	45	1	0	46
Chamomile	26	17	4	47
Feverfew	46	0	0	46
Homeopathic supplement	38	7	1	46
Kava kava	45	1	0	46
Lavender	33	12	2	47
Melatonin	23	18	7	48
Mineral supplements	39	4	3	46
Passion flower	41	4	1	46
Quinoa	44	1	1	46
Soy products	43	1	1	45
Spirulina	44	2	0	46
St John's wort	40	6	0	46
Sulfur	46	0	0	46
Tryptophan	43	2	0	45
Valerian	41	3	2	46
Vitamin supplements	32	11	5	48
Wild lettuce (Lactuca Virosa)	45	0	0	45
Other (please specify)				2
Answered question				**50**
Skipped question				**131**

Table 1: Responses to Facebook Question, "How Do You Fall Asleep?"

Which of the following techniques have you tried and/or regularly use to fall asleep?				
	Never tried	**Have tried**	**Regularly use**	**Response Count**
Acupuncture	39	8	0	47
Alter sleep arrangements (e.g., arrange bed away from window)	25	21	2	48
Co-sleeping	22	18	7	47
Guided imagery	32	13	2	47
Massage	32	15	2	49
Mindfulness	26	21	1	48
Regulate amounts of caffeine and/or energy drinks	11	23	15	49
Rest & digest	27	16	5	48
Savoring day's events	31	13	2	46

Tai chi chuan	42	4	0	46
Tapping (Emotional freedom technique)	45	2	1	48
Other (please specify)				8
Answered question				**50**
Skipped question				**131**

Table 2: Responses to Facebook Question, "How do you fall asleep?"

Discussion

Sleep disturbances have been considered as a worldwide agenda item to address when considering the health of an individual. Of the types of sleep disturbances, insomnia is the most prevalent [7-10]. Respondents posted their responses to a Facebook page about their sleep disturbance and importantly the ways in which they managed it. 50 of the 181 participants utilized alternative medicine and self-management strategies. We feel that the social media approach provided immediate information not commonly communicated in the formal health care system intake interview. The extensive listing of natural remedies and non-pharmaceutical approaches reflects an advantage, we feel, to this social media methodology. The impact of social media on the individual may provide an ease to being more forthcoming and detailed about self-behaviors given the anomy of the online encounter. We think further research with this social media method specific to alternative medicine/non-pharmaceutical approaches usage patterns and sleep quality measures would be useful in more fully understanding what individuals do, globally, to help themselves fall asleep. We think this implicitly implies how individuals consider their sleep quality, importance of sleep in their lives and behaviors, accordingly, that they will do to enhance their sleep. Additionally, the effectiveness of the strategies as well as the role of health care professionals to assist in this area needs exploration.

References

1. Gillian JC, Roehrs T, Roth T (2013) Sleep aids and insomnia. National Sleep Foundation.
2. Glass J, Lanctôt KL, Herrmann N, Sproule BA, Busto UE (2005) Sedative hypnotics in older people with insomnia: meta-analysis of risks and benefits. BMJ 331: 1169.
3. Gradinger F, Boldt C, Hogl B, Cieza A (2011) Identification of problems in functioning of persons with sleep disorder from the health professional perspective using the International Classification of Functionality, Disability and Health (ICF) as a reference: A worldwide expert survey. Sleep Med 12: 97-101.
4. Gradisar M, Gardner G, Dohnt H (2011) Recent worldwide sleep patterns and problems during adolescence: a review and meta-analysis of age, region, and sleep. Sleep Med 12: 110-118.
5. Joya FL, Kripke DF, Loving RT, Dawson A, Kline LE (2009) Meta-analyses of hypnotics and infections: eszopiclone, ramelteon, zaleplon, and zolpidem. J Clin Sleep Med 5: 377-383.
6. Lombardi DA, Folkard S, Willetts JL, Smith GS (2010) Daily sleep, weekly working hours, and risk of work-related injury: US National Health Interview Survey (2004-2008). Chronobiol Int 27: 1013-1030.
7. Sexton-Radek K (2013) A Look at Worldwide Sleep Disturbance. J Sleep Disorders Ther 2: 115.
8. Radek KS (2013) Insomnia Symptom Presentation and Sleep Aids. J Sleep Disorders Ther 2: e122.
9. Walsh JK, Krystal AD, Amato DA, Rubens R, Caron J, et al. (2007) Nightly treatment of primary insomnia with eszopiclone for six months: effect on sleep, quality of life, and work limitations. Sleep 30: 959-968.
10. Zammit G, Erman M, Wang-Weigand S, Sainati S, Zhang J, et al. (2007) Evaluation of the efficacy and safety of ramelteon in subjects with chronic insomnia. J Clin Sleep Med 3: 495-504.

33

An Insight into Mechanisms underlying Sleep Deprivation Induced Cognitive Dysfunction

Priyanka Chanana and Anil Kumar*

Pharmacology Division, University Institute of Pharmaceutical Sciences, UGC Centre of Advanced Study, Panjab University, Chandigarh, India

Abstract

Introduction: Sleep has been found to influence both acquisition and consolidation of memory; therefore, sleep deprivation is often linked to multiple anomalies in cognitive paradigms giving rise cognitive dysfunctions.

Objective: The present study has been designed with an aim to decipher plausible mechanistic interplays involved in the induction of cognitive dysfunction as a direct consequence of sleep deprivation.

Methods: Male *laca* mice were sleep deprived for 24-hours using grid suspended over water method on alternate days extended over the total protocol duration of 21 days. Various neurobehavioral memory evaluating parameters followed by biochemical, acetylcholinesterase (AChE) activity, mitochondrial respiratory enzyme complex activities (I-IV) and histopathological examinations of the mice brain were monitored.

Results: Sleep deprivation of 24-hours on alternate days for 21 days significantly impaired cognitive performance in both memory evaluating paradigms (Morris water maze test and elevated plus maze test) as compared to naïve animals. Additionally animals subjected to sleep deprivation also demonstrated conditions of elevated oxidative stress, impaired mitochondrial enzyme complex activities, increased aceytlcholineestaerase activity, as well as histopathological alterations pertaining to hippocampal and thalamo-cortical regions of mice brain as compared to naïve animals. However, chronic piracetam (100 mg/kg) treatment showed significant protective effect against sleep deprivation induced cognitive dysfunction, oxidative damage, mitochondrial respiratory enzyme complex insuffeciencies, increased acetylcholinesterase activity as well as neuromorphological alterations.

Conclusion: The present study suggests mechanistic interplay between oxidative stresses; mitochondrial impairment as well as acetylcholineesterase activity may influence hippocampal and cortical neuronal survival and thus lead to precipitation of sleep deprivation induced cognitive deficits.

Keywords: Cognition; Hippocampus; Mitochondrial insufficiency; Oxidative stress; Sleep deprivation

Introduction

Extensive research has portrayed the role played by sleep dynamics in nurturing of cognitive profiles via influencing both acquisitions as well as consolidation paradigms of memory formation [1-5]. It has been validated that sleep affects almost every individual component of cognition such as stimulus detection, information encoding, working memory, etc. Against this background, sleep deprivation [SD] is entitled to cause cognitive deficits. The direct effect of SD over cognitive paradigms may be manifested either via decreased alertness and attention lapses as well as slowed responses owing to sleep debt. SD has also led to deleterious structural and functional instabilities of selective encephalic structures controlling cognitive processes which may partially explain the cognitive impairments precipitated by SD [6,7]. The same has been investigated by using potent non-invasive neurophysiological techniques such as Transcranial Magnetic Stimulation (TMS) which specifically evaluates primary motor cortex (M1) and cortico spinal tract excitability in vivo. The significant alterations observed in key characteristics of single and paired TMS techniques (as a consequence of SD) clearly demonstrate significant variations in cortical excitability as well as functionality of inter-neuronal circuitry in the primary motor cortex brought and thus aptly explain pathophysiological substrates of SD induced cognitive impairments [8-10].

Though all this has been well researched but still, there remain several lacunae in the molecular mechanistic interplays that may facilitate SD mediated phenotypes of cognitive deficits. The present study is an endeavor towards the same.

Several plausible mechanisms may be purported for the SD induced cognitive lapses. SD has been directly linked to precipitating situations of elevated oxidative stress [11-13]. SD has been found to be linked to not only elevated generation of free radicals but also depletion in the activity of endogenous antioxidant enzymes [12]. Also, nitric oxide (NO) is thought to be involved in memory consolidation processes in the hippocampus during sleep [14]. Additionally, SD has also been found to be associated with mitochondrial respiratory enzyme complex insufficiencies as well as *Bax* activation [15], directly leading to situations of energy deficits as well as indirect activation of apoptotic responses. This suggests that both conditions of oxidative damage and energy deficits may influence neuromorphological changes as well survival of neurons specifically in areas of the brain responsible for memory encoding and consolidation, particularly the hippocampus [16], which may be partially held responsible for cognitive deficits precipitated as a direct consequence of SD. Furthermore, SD has also demonstrated to increase acetylcholinesterase (AChE) activity, which may probably lead to deficits in memory tasks [17,18].

***Corresponding author:** Anil Kumar, Pharmacology Division, University Institute of Pharmaceutical Sciences, UGC Centre of Advanced Study, Panjab University, Chandigarh, India, E-mail: kumaruips@yahoo.com

Based on this background, the present study was designed with an aim to evaluate the possible crosstalks and mechanistic interplays between pivotal molecular cascades of oxidative damage, mitochondrial enzyme complex insuffeciencies, acetylcholineesterase activity as well as neuromorphological changes in memory controlling encephalic regions to be put forward as cardinal etiological links between SD and induction of cognitive dysfunction.

Material and Method

Animals

Male *laca* mice (22 g to 30 g) bred in Central Animal House (CAH) facility of the Panjab University, Chandigarh, India were used. The animals were housed under standard laboratory conditions and maintained under natural light-dark cycles. The experimental protocol was approved by Institutional Animal Ethics Committee (PU/IAEC/S/14/99) of Panjab University and carried out in accordance with the guidelines of Committee for the Purpose of Control and Supervision of Experimentation on Animals (CPCSEA), Government of India and Indian National Science Academy.

Sleep Deprivation and protocol design

Animals were sleep-deprived for 24-hours (every alternate day) across the 21 days protocol by using modified grid suspended over water method developed by Shinomiya et al. [19]. Briefly, animals in a group of six to eight were sleep deprived by placing on a grid floor (29 × 15 × 7 cm) inside the polyacrylic cages (38 × 23 × 10 cm), filled with water upto 1 cm below the grid surface for 24-hours (every alternate day for 21 days, to comply with clinical situations). The stainless steel rods of the grid (3 mm wide) were set 2-cm apart from each other. Food and water were provided ad libitum. As soon as the animal tried to sleep, it lost its muscle tone and thereby grip over the grid which made it fall in water and thus awakened the animal. The process was continued for total of 21 days. During the course of the protocol behavioral estimations like locomotor activity was ascertained on day 0, 7, 14 and 21; elevated plus maze performance was evaluated on day 15, 16 and 21 as well as morris water maze test performance was evaluated from day 17th to day 21st.

S.No.	Group name	Treatment (mg/kg)
1	Naïve	Animals not subjected sleep deprivation [vehicle treated]
2	SD	Sleep deprived animals [subjected to sleep deprivation of 24 hours on alternate days for 21 days and vehicle treated]
3	Pira (100)	Piracetam (100 mg/kg) administered in sleep deprived animals for 21 days

Table 1: Treatment groups.

Drugs and Treatment Schedule

Animals were randomly divided into different treatment groups (n=10 to 12) as described in (Table 1). The entire study has been performed as per the schematic plan given in the protocol as described in (Figure 1). Across the total protocol duration of 21 days animals were exposed to standardized treatments once daily, based on their treatment groups. While animals in the naive and sleep deprived control groups were treated with vehicle i.e. normal saline i.p; the animals in the standard group were treated with Piracetam (100 mg/kg i.p; prepared in normal saline). Piracetam (Pira) was purchased from CDH, India. The treatments (vehicle as well as standard) were administered to animals in volume of 1 ml/100 g of bodyweight.

Behavioral assessments

Measurement of locomotor activity: To rule out the interference of change in motor activity in the parameters of learning and memory, locomotor activity of animals was evaluated on weekly basis (i.e. day 0, 7, 14 and 21). The locomotor activity was recorded by using an actophotometer (IMCORP, Ambala, India). The instrument consisted of a closed arena or activity chamber in which each animal was placed for total of 8 minutes (3 minutes for habituation and exploration as well as 5 minutes for evaluation of actual locomotor activity). Animals's total activity (ambulation + rearing counts) was recorded and expressed in terms of total photo beam counts cut for 5 min per animal [20].

Assessment of cognitive performance (Morris Water Maze Task): Individual animals were tested for spatial memory using the Morris water maze (MWM) test paradigm [21,22]. The apparatus consisted of

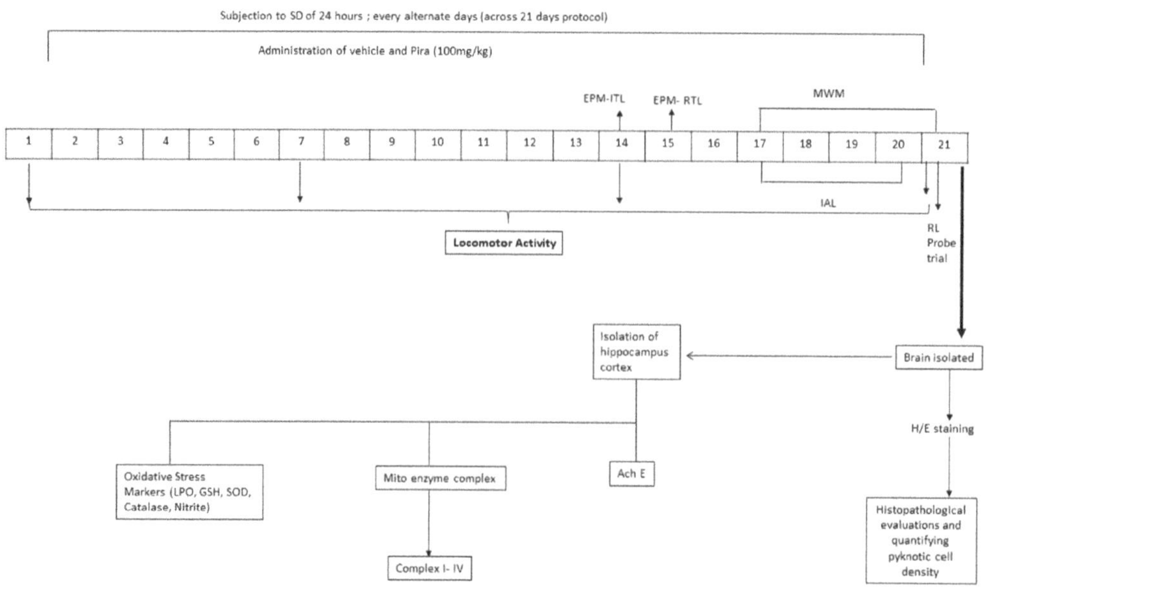

Figure 1: Protocol design.

a circular water tank (120 cm diameter, 30 cm high, filled to a depth of 20 cm with water at 28 ± 1°C). The tank was divided into four equal quadrants (Q1 to Q4) and water in the tank was made opaque with a nontoxic white dye. A platform (4.5 cm in diameter) was placed in one quadrant of the pool (Q4), 1 cm above the water level during the acquisition phase and position of the platform was kept unaltered all through the acquisition phase. The tank was located in a large room with presence of several brightly colored visible clues external to the maze which could be easily used by the mice for spatial orientation and further for memory consolidation. The task was carried out for five consecutive days (17th to 21th day, four days of acquisition and one day of retention trial). During each trial, the position of the clues remained unchanged and animal was subjected to four such consecutive trials (corresponding to each quadrant).

Acquisition phase (training): For each trial, individual mice was smoothly put into the water at one of the four starting positions (corresponding to each quadrant) to locate the submerged platform (maintained at Q4) and allowed to stay on the platform for next 20 seconds. If animal failed to find the platform within 90 seconds, same was gently guided onto the platform. Latency time to locate the hidden platform (known as initial acquisition latency (IAL) also known as escape latency time (ELT) was noted as parameter of acquisition or learning using a video-graphed computer tracking system maintained by EthoVision software (Noldus Information Technology, Wageningen, Netherlands).

Retention phase (Probe Trial): To assess the extent of memory consolidation after learning, retention trial was performed [23] on day 21 wherein the animal was placed into the pool for a total duration of 90 seconds as in the training trial, with the absence of hidden platform from the Q4 quadrant of the pool. Various parameters such as time spent in target quadrant [TSTQ] and number of crossings across the platform area were measured using above mentioned computer tracking system [24].

Elevated Plus Maze Task: The elevated plus maze (EPM) consisted of two opposite black open arms (16 x 9 x 5 cm), crossed with two closed walls of the same dimensions of 12 cm height. The arms were connected with a central square of dimensions 5 × 9 × 5 cm. The entire maze was elevated to a height of 25 cm from the floor. Both acquisition and retention of memory processes were assessed as previously described. Acquisition of memory was tested on day 15 of study protocol. Animal was placed individually at one end of the open arm facing away from the central square. The time taken by the animal to move from the open arm to the closed arm was recorded as the initial transfer latency (ITL; noted on day 15). Cut off time was set to be 90 seconds and if the animal could not enter closed arm within 90 seconds, same was guided to the closed arm and the ITL recording was noted as 90 seconds. Animal was allowed to explore the maze for 30 seconds after recording the ITL and then returned to the home cage. Retention of memory was assessed on day 16th (1st RTL) and 21st (2nd RTL) by placing the mouse again in an open arm and ascertaining the time taken to cross over to the closed arm [25].

Biochemical estimations

Dissection and homogenization: Thereupon, after the last behavioral test, animals were randomized into distinct sets; the first set was used for the biochemical assays (n=5/group). For biochemical analysis, animals were sacrificed by decapitation. Whole brain from each animal was put over ice and dissected into hippocampus and cerebral cortex sections. For antioxidant enzyme activity estimation, a 10% (w/v) tissue homogenates were prepared in 0.1 M phosphate buffer (pH 7.4). The homogenates were centrifuged at 10,000 × g at 4°C for 15 min. Aliquots of supernatants were separated and used for biochemical estimations.

Lipid peroxidation assay: The quantitative measurement of lipid peroxidation in the whole brain was measured in accordance with the method of Wills [26]. The amount of malondialdehyde (MDA) concentration formed was measured by reaction with thiobarbituric acid at 532 nm using Perkin Elmer lambda 20 UV-vis spectrophotometer (Norwalk, CT, USA). The results were expressed as nano moles of MDA per milligram protein using the molar extinction coefficient of chromophore (1.56 × 10 M/cm) and represented as percentage of naive.

Estimation of nitrite levels: The nitrite accumulation in the homogenate supernatant (an indicator of the production of nitric oxide (NO load), was determined via a colorimetric assay using Greiss reagent (0.1% N-(1-napthyl) ethylene diaminedihydrochloride, 1% sulfanilamide and 2.5% phosphoric acid) as per the method reported by Green and co-workers [27]. Equal volumes of supernatant and Greiss reagent were mixed, incubated for 10 min at room temperature; consequently the absorbance of reaction mixture was read at 540 nm using a spectrophotometer (Perkin Elmer lambda 20 UV-Visible spectrophotometer, Norwalk, CT, USA). The concentration of nitrite in the supernatant was determined from a standard curve. The results were expressed as mg/ml and represented as percentage of naïve.

Estimation off reduced glutathione: Reduced glutathione (GSH) was estimated according to the method described by Ellman [28]. 1.0 ml of homogenate was precipitated using 1.0 ml of 4% sulfosalicylic acid by keeping the mixture at 4°C for 1 hour and the samples were immediately centrifuged at 1200 g for 15 min at 4°C. The assay mixture contained 0.1 ml of supernatant, 2.7 ml of phosphate buffer (pH 8.0) and 0.2 ml of 0.01 mL M-dithiobisnitrobenzoic acid. The yellow colour developed was read immediately at 412 nm using spectrophotometer (Perkin Elmer lambda 20 UV-Vis spectrophotometer (Norwalk, CT, USA). The results were expressed as nano moles of GSH per milligram of protein and represented as percentage of naive.

Estimation off catalase: Catalase activity was assayed by the method reported by Luck [29], wherein the breakdown of hydrogen peroxide (H_2O_2) was measured at 240 nm. Briefly, the assay mixture consisted of 3 ml of H_2O_2 phosphate buffer (1.25 × 10^{-2} M H_2O_2) and 0.05 mL of supernatant of tissue homogenate (10%). The change in absorbance was recorded at 240 nm using UV-Vis spectrophotometer (Perkin Elmer lambda 20 spectrophotometer (Norwalk, CT, USA). The results were expressed as micromole H_2O_2 decomposed per milligram of protein/min and represented as percentage of naive.

Superoxide Dismutase activity: Superoxide dismutase (SOD) activity was assayed by the method of Kono [30]. According to the method, reduction of nitro blue tetrazolium (NBT) was inhibited by the SOD and the change in absorbance was recorded for 2 minutes at 30 seconds intervals by measuring absorbance at 560 nm using Perkin Elmer Lambda 20 spectrophotometer. The results were expressed as units/mg protein and represented as percentage of naive.

Protein estimation: The total protein content was measured according to Biuret method described by Lowry and his team [31]. The amount was calculated using a standard curve wherein bovine serum albumin was used as the protein standard.

Mitochondrial enzyme complex estimations: The brain samples of second set of animals were used for evaluation of mitochondrial respiratory enzyme complex activities as described by Berman and Hastings [32]. The whole brain was sectioned into hippocampi and cortical regions and individual sections were then homogenized in isolation buffer (215 mM mannitol, 75 mM sucrose, 0.1% BSA, 20 mM HEPES, 1 mM EGTA, and pH 7.2). Homogenates were centrifuged at 13,000 g for 5 minutes at 4°C. Pellets were re-suspended in isolation buffer with ethylene glycol tetra acetic acid (EGTA) and spun again at 13,000 g at 4°C for 5 min. The resulting supernatants were transferred to new tubes and topped off with isolation buffer with EGTA and again spun at 13,000 g at 4°C for 10 min. Pellets containing pure mitochondria were re-suspended in isolation buffer without EGTA.

Nicotinamide Adenine Dinucleotide (NADH) Dehydrogenase activity: The quantitative analysis of Complex-I was done spectrophotometrically by the method mentioned by King and Howard [33]. The method involved catalytic oxidation of NADH to NAD^+ with subsequent reduction in cytochrome c. The reaction mixture contained 0.2 M glycyl glycine buffer pH 8.5, 6 mM NADH in 2 mM glycyl glycine buffer and 10.5 mM cytochrome c. After addition of requisite amount of solubilised mitochondrial sample to reaction mixture, absorbance change was recorded at 550 nm for 2 minutes and the results were expressed as nano moles of NADH oxidized per minute per milligram protein and represented as percentage of naïve.

Succinate Dehydrogenase (SDH) activity: The spectrophotometric quantification of Complex-II/ SDH was done according to method reported by King [34]. The reaction mixture contained 0.2 M phosphate buffer (pH 7.8), 1% BSA, 0.6 M succinic acid, and 0.03 M potassium ferricyanide. The reaction was initiated by the addition of mitochondrial sample and recording absorbance change at 420 nm for 2 minutes. The results were expressed as nano moles of SDH per milligram of protein and represented as percentage of naïve.

3-(4,5-dimethylthiazol-2-yl)-2,5-diphenyltetrazolium (MTT or mitochondrial redox activity) assay: This method is used to evaluate the mitochondrial redox activity via the conversion of MTT tetrazolium salt to formazan crystals by mitochondrial respiratory chain reactions in isolated mitochondria by the method of Liu et al. [35]. The blue formazan crystals so formed were then further solubilised with dimethylsulphoxide and corresponding absorbance was measured by an ELISA reader at 580 nm filter. The results were expressed number of viable cells per well and represented as percentage of naïve.

Cytochrome Oxidase activity: Cytochrome oxidase activity was assayed in brain mitochondria according to the method developed by Sottocasa et al. [36]. The assay mixture contained 0.3 mM reduced cytochrome C in 75 mM phosphate buffer. The reaction was started by the addition of solubilized mitochondrial sample and the changes in absorbance were recorded at 550 nm for 2 minutes (at intervals of 30 seconds each) and the results represented as percentage of naive.

Acetyl Cholinesterase (AChE) activity assay: AChE activity (marker of cholinergic activity in the brain) was assessed in the hippocampal and cortical regions by the method of Ellman et al. [37]. The assay mixture contained 0.05 ml of supernatant, 3 ml of sodium phosphate buffer (pH 8), 0.1 ml of acetylthiocholine iodide and 0.1 ml of DTNB (Ellman reagent). The change in absorbance was measured for 2 min at 30 seconds interval at 412 nm using a Perkin Elmer UV-Vis spectrophotometer. Results were expressed as micromoles of acetylthiocholine iodide hydrolyzed per minute per mg protein.

Histopathological Analysis by Hematoxylin and Eosin Staining (H&E) Staining

Tissue sections preparation: Third set of animals were scarified immediately after last behavioural test and perfused transcardially with cold phosphate buffered saline (0.1 M, pH 7.4) via the ascending aorta. The whole brain was dissected out and fixed overnight in the same buffer containing 10% (v/v) paraformaldehyde. The brain was then washed with 0.1 M PBS (pH 7.4) for 1 hour, dehydrated in alcohol, and consecutively embedded in paraffin wax to form blocks. Freezing microtome was used to obtain serial coronal sections (5 μm to 10 μm thickness) of whole brain.

Haematoxylin and Eosin (H&E) staining: The brain sections (5 μm to 10 μm) thick were de-waxed and stained with haematoxylin and eosin. Briefly, sections were immersed in the filtered haematoxylin solution for 1 min followed by rinsing with tap water. Then, the sections were immersed in eosin stain for 1 min to 2 min and rinsed thoroughly with tap water followed by dehydration in ascending alcohol solutions (50%, 70%, 80%, 95%, 97% and 100% alcoholic solutions). Now the sections were mounted on labelled slides. The stained sections were viewed under a binocular microscope (Nikon Eclipse 80i, Nikon Instruments Inc., USA) at 40× targeting the thalamo-cortical and hippocampal regions of the brain for the presence of morphological changes and thereby photographed. The thalamo-cortical encephalic area was specifically analyzed for the presence and density of pyknotic nuclei. The number of such pyknotic nuclei per square pixel were then quantified using computer based image processing and analysis (Image J 1.42q, NIH, USA).

Statistical Analysis

The behavioral assessment data was analyzed using two-way analysis of variance (ANOVA) followed by Bonferroni's test. The time spent in target quadrant, number of platform crossings, biochemical estimations, mitochondrial activity estimations, AchE activity as well as pyknotic cell density in the thalamo-cortical encephalic regions were separately analyzed by one way ANOVA followed by Tukey's post hoc test. In all the tests, criterion for statistical significance was considered to be $p<0.05$. All statistical procedures were carried out using sigma stat Graph Pad Prism (Graph Pad prism Software, version 5, San Diego, CA).

Results

Effect of SD on locomotor activity

As observed on day 0, 7, 14 and 21, the mean scores of locomotor activity (ambulation+rearing count per 5 minutes) did not differ significantly between naïve; sleep deprived and piracetam treated groups of animals depicting a rather stable locomotor activity on each day. However, a trend of gradual decrease in locomotor activity across the duration of entire protocol (day 7th, 14th, and 21st) was observed (Figure 2).

Effect of SD on performance in Morris Water Maze (MWM) test paradigm: Maze acquisition trial (Day 17 to 20)

The cognitive performance was assessed using the MWM performance. Mean escape latency/ initial transfer latency (IAL) (to find the submerged platform) was found to be invariable amongst all the groups on the first day of training (i.e. day 17). However, mean escape/transfer latency gradually decreased in all groups on subsequent days of training period from day 18 to day 20 in MWM test. Further, animals exposed to SD of 24 hours on alternate days for 21 days exhibited a significantly poor cognitive performance (depicted by increased mean escape latency) from day 17 to 20 as compared to the naive group (Figure 3). However, treatment with piracetam (100 mg/

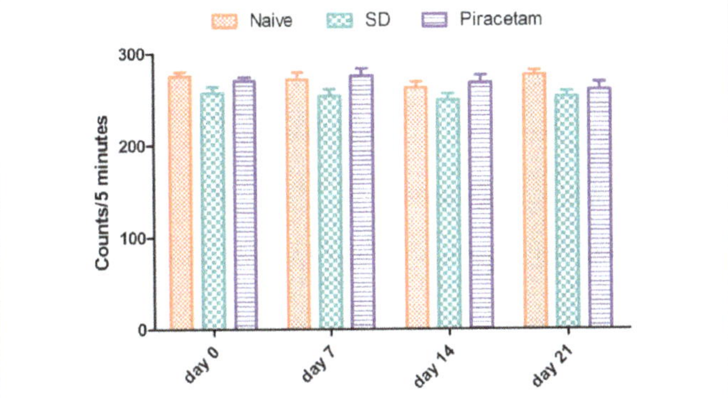

Figure 2: Effect of SD on locomotor activity. Values expressed as mean ± SEM. SD: Sleep deprived for 24-hours every alternate day for 21 days; Pira: Piracetam.

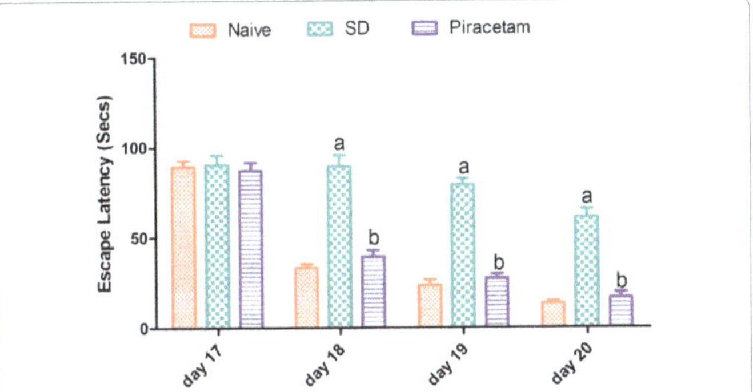

Figure 3: Effect of SD on mean escape latency in morris water maze (MWM) test paradigm. Values are expressed as mean ± SEM. [a]p<0.05 as compared with naive, [b]p< 0.05 as compared with SD, (Two-way ANOVA followed by Bonferroni's test). SD: Sleep deprived for 24 hours every alternate day for 21 days; Pira: Piracetam.

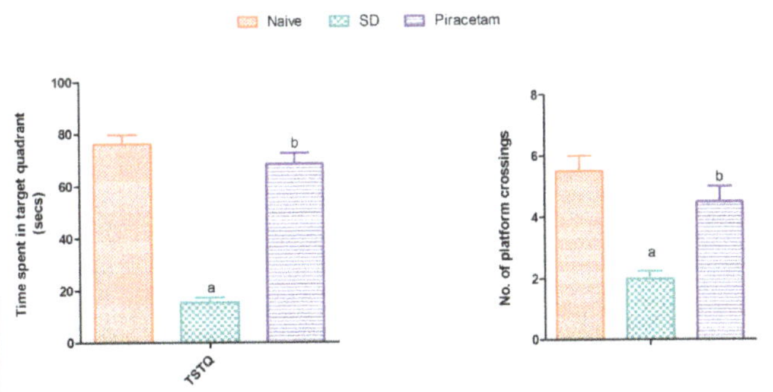

Figure 4: Effect of SD on time spent in target quadrant [TSTQ] and number of crossings across the platform area in morris water maze test. Values are expressed as mean ± SEM. [a]p<0.05 as compared with naive, [b]p<0.05 as compared with SD, (One-way ANOVA followed by Tukey's test). SD: Sleep deprived for 24-hours every alternate day for 21 days; Pira: Piracetam.

kg) significantly improved the cognitive performance (decreased mean escape latency) from second day of the task (day 18) uptil last day of training (day 20) as compared to the SD control group.

Maze retention trial (Day 21)

The probe or retention trial, performed after removal of the hidden platform from the MWM tank was used to evaluate the degree of memory consolidation attained by the animals after four days of training in the acquisition phase of MWM task and whether SD has any effect on degree of memory consolidation. Animals subjected to 24 hours SD on alternate days across the 21 day protocol significantly failed to recall the initial location of the hidden platform in Q4 as evident from lesser time spent in the target quadrant (TSTQ) quadrant and decreased number of crossings across the platform area as compared to naïve group on the day of probe trial (day 21) (Figure 4). Additionally treatment with piracetam (100 mg/kg) for 21 days significantly improved the cognitive performance and intensified memory consolidation (as evidenced by increased TSTQ and increase number of platform area crossings) as compared to control SD group.

Effect of SD on Elevated Plus Maze (EPM) task performance

The present study depicted no significant difference in mean initial transfer latency (ITL; day 15) between naïve, SD and piracetam treated groups. Further, SD of 24 hours on alternate day basis resulted in significant increase in first and second retention transfer latencies (1st and 2nd RTL; day 16 and 21 respectively) as compared to naive group, demonstrating SD induced memory impairment (Table 2). However, treatment with piracetam (100 mg/kg) for 21 days significantly improved the cognitive performance and depicted a decrease in both first and second retention latencies as compared to the control SD animals.

Effect of SD on oxidative stress parameters

As depicted in Table 3, exposing animals to SD of 24-hours on alternate days for a total period of 21 days significantly elevated levels of oxidative stress markers (increase in lipid peroxidation and nitrite levels) as well as depleted endogenous antioxidant activities (decreased reduced glutathione and catalase as well as superoxide dismutase (SOD) activity) in both hippocampi and cortical encephalic regions. Therefore, chronic SD may precipitate conditions of oxidative damage. Additionally, treatment with piracetam (100 mg/kg) for 21 days led to significant antioxidant like property and demonstrated depletion in lipid peroxidation and nitrite levels as well as increase in reduced glutathione, catalase as well as SOD activity (Table 3).

Effect of SD on mitochondrial respiratory enzyme complex activities

As depicted in Figure 5, SD of 24 hours on alternate days extended over a duration of 21 days, significantly depleted the mitochondrial respiratory enzyme complex activities (NADH dehydrogenase, succinate dehydrogenase, cytochrome oxidase activities as well as cell viabilities) in hippocampus and cortex regions of brain in comparison to the naïve group. Nevertheless, chronic treatment with piracetam (100 mg/kg) for 21 days significantly refurbished mitochondrial enzymes complex activities and increased cell viability as compared to SD control animals (Figure 5).

Effect of SD on acetylcholineesterase (AChE) activity

Sleep debt generated as a consequence of SD of 24 hours on alternate days within the 21 days protocol significantly increased AChE activity in hippocampus and cortex regions as compared to the naive group (without SD). However, upon treatment with piracetam (100 mg/kg) for 21 days, a significant attenuation in AChE activity was observed, which was found to be significant as compared to control (SD) vehicle treated animals (Figure 6).

Effect of SD on neuronal morphology and pyknotic cell density as depicted by histopathological sections of mice brains

Histopathological evaluation of hippocampi and thalamocortical

S.No.	Group name	ITL (Day 1)	RTL1 (Day 16)	RTL2 (Day 21)	% deficit in 1st and 2nd RTL
1	Naïve	78.21 ± 4.11	23.32 ± 1.00	27.15 ± 1.72	14.10 ± 2.51
2	SD	79.32 ± 3.61	39.57 ± 4.00[a]	77.36 ± 4.85[a]	48.84 ± 3.01
3	Pira (100)	76.14 ± 4.17	25.16 ± 0.85[b]	32.00 ± 1.50[b]	21.37 ± 2.65

Values are expressed as mean ± SEM. [a]p< 0.05 as compared with naive, [b]p< 0.05 as compared with SD, (Two-way ANOVA followed by Bonferroni's test). Pira: piracetam; SD: Sleep deprived for 24-hours every alternate day for 21 days.

Table 2: Effect of SD on cognitive performance in Elevated Plus Maze task.

Treatment group (mg/kg)	Brain Region	LPO (nmol MDA/mg of protein) (% of Naive)	Nitrite (µmol/ml) (% of Naive)	GSH (nmol of GSH/mg Pr) (% of Naive)	Catalase (µM of H_2O_2/min/ mgpr) (% of Naive)	SOD (Units/mg of protein) (% of Naive)
Naïve	Cortex	0.0179 ± 0.002 (100)	257.51 ± 3.52 (100)	0.802 ± 0.01 (100)	0.670 ± 0.043 (100)	67.58 ± 1.67 (100)
	Hippocampus	0.0231 ± 0.001 (100)	230.62 ± 2.79 (100)	0.896 ± 0.02 (100)	0.619 ± 0.016 (100)	78.32 ± 2.67 (100)
SD	Cortex	0.0949 ± 0.002a (530.16)	689.32 ± 5.62a (267.68)	0.139 ± 0.01a (17.33)	0.127 ± 0.029a (22.52)	25.63 ± 1.27a (37.92)
	Hippocampus	0.1243 ± 0.003a (538.09)	764.65 ± 6.61a (3331.54)	0.176 ± 0.01a (19.64)	0.159 ± 0.014a (27.59)	31.86 ± 1.01a (40.67)
Pira (100)	Cortex	0.0218 ± 0.001b (121.78)	300.65 ± 3.62b (116.75)	0.718 ± 0.02b (89.56)	0.626 ± 0.012b (90.07)	63.52 ± 2.16b (93.99)
	Hippocampus	0.0316 ± 0.002b (136.79)	361.81 ± 3.51b (156.89)	0.817 ± 0.03b (91.25)	0.592 ± 0.036b (95.87)	70.52 ± 3.11b (90.04)

Values are expressed as mean ± SEM. [a]p<0.05 as compared with naive, [b]p<0.05 as compared with SD, (One-way ANOVA followed by Tukey's test). Pira: piracetam; SD: Sleep deprived for 24 hours every alternate day for 21 days.

Table 3: Effect of SD on oxidative stress parameters.

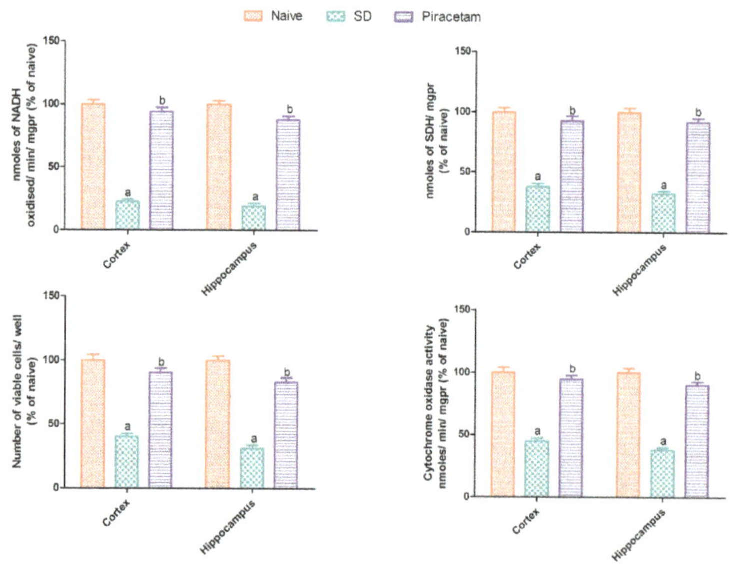

Figure 5: Effect of SD on mitochondrial respiratory enzyme complex activities. Complex-I (NADH dehydrogenase activity); Complex-II (Succinate dehydrogenase activity); Complex-III (MTT/ mitochondrial redox activity); Complex IV (cytochrome c oxidase activity). Values are expressed as mean ± SEM. [a]p<0.05 as compared with naive, [b]p<0.05 as compared with SD, (Two-way ANOVA followed by Bonferroni's test). SD: Sleep deprived for 24 hours every alternate day for 21 days; Pira: Piracetam.

regions of mice brain was conducted under light microscopy. Representative images of brain sections from different groups of animals have been shown in Figure 7A. Brains of naïve animals showed comparatively undamaged and optimum sized neuronal cells as compared to sleep deprived animals. However, disorganization of various cell layers, increased level of cellular spongiosis and increased density of pyknotic cells per 128800 square pixels (signifying activation of neuroinflammatory and apoptotic responses), was observed specifically in hippocampi and thalamo-cortical regions of the brains of sleep deprived animals. However, continued treatment with piracetam (100 mg/kg) significantly attenuated these neuroinflammatory alterations as well as reduced number of pyknotic cells, per 128800 square pixels of area compared to the control SD group, signifying the protective effect of piracetam against neuromorphological alterations in discrete brain areas precipitated as a direct outcome of chronic SD (Figures 7 and 8).

Discussion

The link between SD and other neuropsychiatric disorders like anxiety like behaviour, depression, psychosis and cognitive dysfunction have been suggested to be bidirectional. Both acute and chronic SD has been found to be intricately associated with change in sleep patterns and cognitive deficits both in preclinical as well clinical studies [16,38-41]. Furthermore, single paired and repetitive TMS studies have put forward effect of SD on neurophysiological patterns of cortical excitability which prove to be another etiological target in SD induced cognitive deficits. However, the absence of complex reproducibility of results may be due to heterogeneity in the design

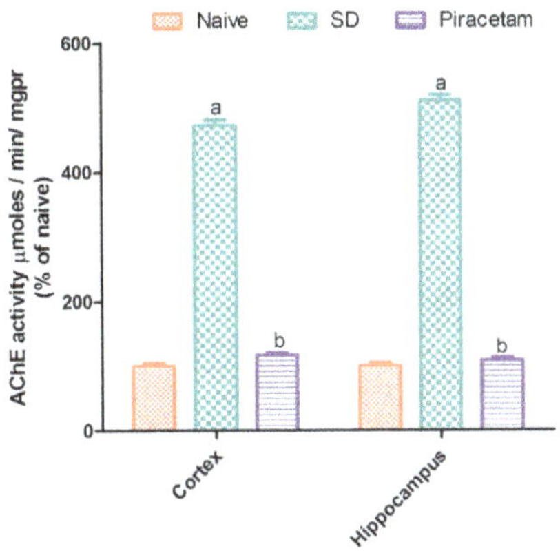

Figure 6: Effect of SD on acetylcholineesterase activity. Values are expressed as mean ± SEM. [a]p<0.05 as compared with naive, [b]p<0.05 as compared with SD, (Two-way ANOVA followed by Bonferroni's test). SD: Sleep deprived for 24 hours every alternate day for 21 days; Pira: Piracetam.

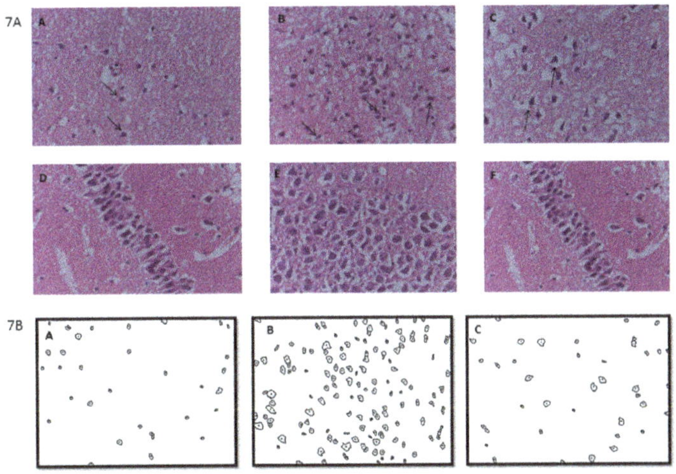

Figure 7A and 7B: Effect of SD on neuronal morphology as depicted by histopathological sections of sleep deprived mice brains. A-C: Thalamocortical regions; D-F: hippocampal regions. A: Naive; B: Sleep deprived (control); C: Piracetam (100); D: Naive; E: Sleep deprived (control); F: Piracetam (100); The pictographs of histopathological sections as modified by software for processing; showing outliners of pyknotic cells; A: Naive; B: Sleep deprived (control); C: Piracetam (100).

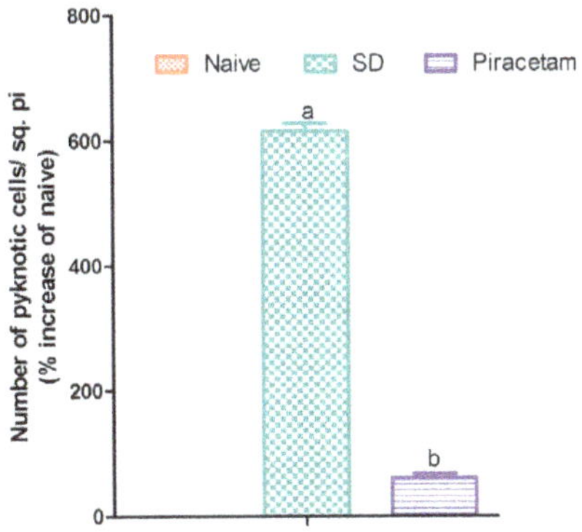

Figure 8: Effect of SD on pyknotic cell expression per 1228800 square pixels of area in thalamo-cortical regions of mice brains; Values are expressed as mean ± SEM. [a]p<0.05 as compared with naive, bp<0.05 as compared with SD, (One-way ANOVA followed by Tukey's test). SD: Sleep deprived for 24-hours every alternate day for 21 days; Pira: Piracetam.

of experimental protocols and number of subjects in each study. Studies have demonstrated that while single TMS characteristics like MEP latency or MEP size are found to be least affected by conditions of SD (clearly suggesting that SD least affects the structural integrity of cortico-spinal pathway), the characteristics of paired TMS are subjectively altered by SD (signifying pathophysiological correlates of cortical intraneuronal excitability) [10]. SD has shown to bring about a decrease in short latency intracortical inhibition (SICI), Short latency Afferent Inhibition (SAI), decrease in intra cortical facilitation (ICF), as well as cortical silent period (CSP), which may signify altered cortical excitability and thus precipitate memory deficits [8,9,42-45]. Besides, alterations in most of the above mentioned TMS characteristics as a

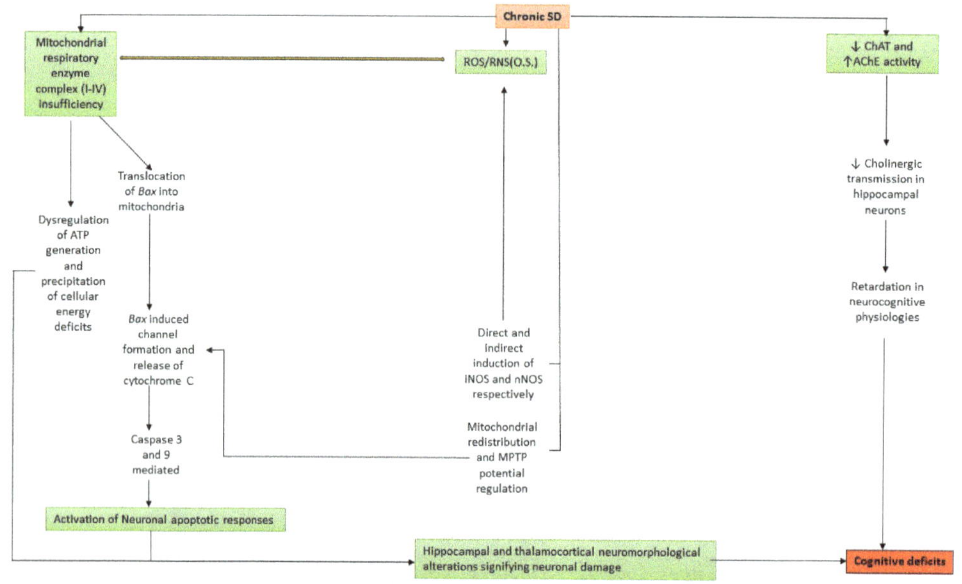

Figure 9: Figure tries to delineate the plausible etiological pathways involved in SD induced cognitive dysfunction. AChE: Acetylcholineesterase; ATP: Adenosine triphosphate; Bax: Bcl-2 associated X protein; ChAT: Choline acetyltranferase; iNOS: inducible nitric oxide synthase; nNOS: Neuronal nitric oxide synthase.

consequence of SD, have also been found to be significantly correlated with deficits in parameters of episodic verbal memory and executive functions in SD subjects, clearly signifying that SD may influence both encoding and consolidation of memory paradigms via alteration of cortical excitability profiles [8,9].

But the exact behavioral and biochemical mechanistic interplays exacerbated by SD that may consequently lead to cognitive deficits are largely unknown. In concordance with the previously mentioned reports, in the present study as well, SD created a sleep debt and induced significant alterations in cognitive functions. The study witnessed marked deviations in escape, transfer latencies as well as retention latencies in neurobehavioral memory evaluating paradigms like EPM as well as MWM. This clearly purports that SD interferes with complex physiologies involved in both acquisition as well as consolidation of cognitive paradigms. Additionally, the study utilized a differential protocol of SD wherein animals were exposed to 24 hours SD on every alternate day to be in line with the clinical situations of sleep management wherein acute and chronic SD behaviors are not witnessed.

Earlier reports have demonstrated acute SD of 72 or 96 hours to be intricately linked with depleted antioxidant enzymes profile as well as elevated production of oxidative free radicals precipitating conditions of oxidative damage [11,13,46]. In line with the acute SD conditions, in the present study as well exposure to alternate days SD over a total period of 21 days not only depicted increased lipid peroxidation, and nitrite production but also diminished glutathione reduction and antioxidant enzymes activities of SOD as well as catalase in discrete encephalic areas of hippocamapus as well as cortex. Additionally present study also depicted that SD led to significant depletions in activities of mitochondrial respiratory enzyme complexes and cellular viabilities in both hippocampus and cortex which may manifest situation of not only cellular energy deficits but also increased production of oxidative free radicals as well as activation of caspase dependent apoptotic responses. Therefore, the present study purports that vicious bidirectional crosstalks between oxidative stress and mitochondrial insufficiencies may hamper neuronal survival in specific encephalic areas controlling memory encoding and consolidation.

Acetylcholine is one of the major neurotransmitters that cardinally modulates memory formation and consolidation which is justified on grounds of earlier reports wherein decrease in the levels of acetylcholine has often led to decline in cognitive performances and and AChE inhibitors serve as targeted therapies for the treatment of dementia [47]. In the current study, the elevated levels of AChE in specific brain sections of hippocampus and cortex clearly put forward that the decrease in the levels of acetylcholine might serve as another etiological link behind the cognitive decline as a direct consequence of 24 hours SD every alternate day for 21 days. This observation has been in line with previous reports wherein acute SD has been found to be associated with increased AChE activity [17,48].

In order to reassure the above mentioned hypothesis that vicious interplays between oxidative damage, mitochondrial insufficiencies and consequent activation of apoptotic responses may serve as pivotal etiological links behind SD induced cognitive deficits, histopathological correlates pertaining to thalamo-cortical and hippocampal regions were evaluated. The results consolidified the fact that SD led to neuromorphological alterations as well as increased pyknotic cell density (via above mentioned cascades) signifying detrimental effects on neuronal survival in thalamo-cortical and hippocamapal regions, thereby leading to alterations in cognitive physiologies. Therefore, it can be purported that vicious and complex mechanistic interplays between oxidative free radicals, mitochondrial respiratory enzyme complex insufficiencies, AChE activity as well as activation of apoptotic responses may serve as cardinal interactive molecular cascades in SD induced cognitive dysfunction. But still confirmative molecular and sub cellular studies may be required to validate the above mentioned set of results. However, Figure 9 tries to elaborate the plausible molecular mechanistic interplays which may play cardinal role apart from other neuropathologies in SD induced cognitive deficits (Figure 9).

Conclusion

The present study suggests that chronic SD may directly head to substantial depletions in cognitive performances. Additionally, it was also suggested that oxidative stress, depleted mitochondrial respiratory enzyme complex activities and cellular survival, increased

AChE activity may bring out neuromorphological alterations in specific encephalic regions which may manifest alterations in cognitive physiologies and thereby serve as cardinal etiologies in SD induced cognitive dysfunction.

Acknowledgments

Authors would like to thank the University Grants Commission, New Delhi for providing financial support under the UGC- RFSMS [Research Fellowship in Sciences for Meritorious Students; award file number: F.5-94/2007(BSR)] scheme.

References

1. Stickgold R, Walker MP (2013) Sleep-dependent memory triage: evolving generalization through selective processing. Nat Neurosci 16: 139-145.
2. Walker MP, Stickgold R (2004) Sleep-dependent learning and memory consolidation. Neuron 44: 121-133.
3. Walker MP (2009) The role of sleep in cognition and emotion. Ann NY Acad Sci 1156: 168-197.
4. Havekes R, Vecsey CG, Abel T (2012) The impact of sleep deprivation on neuronal and glial signaling pathways important for memory and synaptic plasticity. Cell Signal 24: 1251-1260.
5. Abel T, Havekes R, Saletin JM, Walker MP (2013) Sleep, plasticity and memory from molecules to whole-brain networks. Curr Boil 23: R774-788.
6. Dorrian J, Rogers NL, Dinges DF (2005) Psychomotor vigilance performance: Neurocognitive assay sensitive to sleep loss (Doctoral dissertation, Marcel Dekker).
7. Durmer JS, Dinges DF (2005) Neurocognitive consequences of sleep deprivation. Semin Neurol 25: 117-129).
8. Nardone R, Bergmann J, Kunz A, Christova M, Brigo F, et al. (2012) Cortical afferent inhibition is reduced in patients with idiopathic REM sleep behavior disorder and cognitive impairment: a TMS study. Sleep Med 13: 919-925.
9. Chee MW, Chuah LY (2008) Functional neuroimaging insights into how sleep and sleep deprivation affect memory and cognition. Curr Opin Neurol 21: 417-423.
10. Lanza G, Cantone M, Lanuzza B, Pennisi M, Bella R, et al. (2015) Distinctive patterns of cortical excitability to transcranial magnetic stimulation in obstructive sleep apnea syndrome, restless legs syndrome, insomnia, and sleep deprivation. Sleep Med Rev 19: 39-50.
11. Gopalakrishnan A, Ji LL, Cirelli C (2004) Sleep deprivation and cellular responses to oxidative stress. Sleep 27: 27-35.
12. Singh R, Kiloung J, Singh S, Sharma D (2008) Effect of paradoxical sleep deprivation on oxidative stress parameters in brain regions of adult and old rats. Biogerontology 9: 153-162.
13. Khadrawy YA, Nour NA, Ezz HS (2011) Effect of oxidative stress induced by paradoxical sleep deprivation on the activities of Na+, K+-ATPase and acetylcholinesterase in the cortex and hippocampus of rat. Trans Res 157: 100-107.
14. Kalinchuk AV, Lu Y, Stenberg D, Rosenberg PA, Porkka-Heiskanen T (2006) Nitric oxide production in the basal forebrain is required for recovery sleep. J Neurochem 99: 483-498.
15. Andreazza AC, Andersen ML, Alvarenga TA, de-Oliveira MR, Armani F, et al. (2010) Impairment of the mitochondrial electron transport chain due to SD in mice. J Psychiatr Res 44: 775-780.
16. Silva RH, Abilio VC, Takatsu AL, Kameda SR, Grassl C, et al. (2004) Role of hippocampal oxidative stress in memory deficits induced by sleep deprivation in mice. Neuropharmacology 46: 895-903.
17. Benedito MA, Camarini R (2001) Rapid eye movement sleep deprivation induces an increase in acetylcholinesterase activity in discrete rat brain regions. Braz J Med Biol Res 34: 103-109.
18. Camarini R, Benedito MA (1997) Rapid eye movement (REM) sleep deprivation reduces rat frontal cortex acetylcholinesterase (EC 3.1.1.7) activity. Braz J Med Biol Res 30: 641-647.
19. Shinomiya K, Shigemoto Y, Okuma C, Mio M, Kamei C (2003) Effects of short-acting hypnotics on sleep latency in rats placed on grid suspended over water. Eur J Pharmacol 460: 139-144.
20. Kumar A, Kalonia H (2007) Protective effect of *Withania somnifera Dunal* on the behavioural and biochemical alterations in sleep-disturbed mice (grid over water suspended method). Indian J Experimental Biol 45: 524-528.
21. Morris R (1984) Developments of a water-maze procedure for studying spatial learning in the rat. J Neurosci Methods 11: 47-60.
22. Kumar A, Prakash A, Dogra S (2011) Centella asiatica attenuates D-Galactose-Induced Cognitive Impairment, Oxidative and Mitochondrial Dysfunction in Mice. Int J Alzheimer Dis 2011: 347569.
23. Tuzcu M, Baydas G (2006) Effect of melatonin and vitamin E on diabetes-induced learning and memory impairment in rats. Eur J Pharmacol 537: 106-110.
24. Mishra J, Chaudhary T, Kumar A (2014) Rosiglitazone synergizes the neuroprotective effects of valproic acid against quinolinic acid-induced neurotoxicity in rats: Targeting PPARγ and HDAC pathways. Neurotox Res 26: 130-151.
25. Misra S, Tiwari V, Kuhad A, Chopra K (2011) Modulation of nitrergic pathway by sesamol prevents cognitive deficits and associated biochemical alterations in intracerebroventricular streptozotocin administered rats. Eur J Pharmacol 659: 177-186.
26. Wills ED (1966) Mechanism of lipid peroxide formation in animal tissues. Biochem J 99: 667-676.
27. Green LC, Wagner DA, Glagowski J (1982) Analysis of nitrate, nitrite and [15N] nitrate in biological fluids. Anal Biochem 126: 131-138.
28. Ellman GL (1959) Tissue sulfhydryl groups. Arch Biochem Biophys 82: 48670-48677.
29. Luck H (1965) Catalase. Method of Enzymatic Analysis 885-894.
30. Kono Y (1978) Generation of superoxide radical during autoxidation of hydroxylamine and an assay for superoxide dismutase. Arch Biochem Biophys186: 189-195.
31. Lowry OH, Rosenberg NJ, Farr AL, Randall RJ (1951) Protein measurement with the Folin-phenol reagent. J Biol Chem 193: 265-275.
32. Berman SB, and Hastings TG (1999) Dopamine oxidation alters mitochondrial respiration and induces permeability transition in brain mitochondria. J. Neurochem 73: 1127-1137.
33. King TE, Howard RL (1967) Preparations and properties of soluble NADH dehydrogenases from cardiac muscle. Methods Enzymol 10: 275-294.
34. King TE (1967) Preparation of succinate dehydrogenase and reconstitution of succinate oxidase. Methods Enzymol 10: 322-331.
35. Liu Y, Peterson DA, Kimura H, Schubert D (1997) Mechanisms of cellular 3-(4,5-dimethylthiazol-2-yl)-2,5-diphenyltetrazoliniumbromide (MTT) reduction. J Neurochem 9: 581-593.
36. Sottocasa GL, Kuylenstierna B, Ernster L, Berqstrand A (1967) An electron-transport system associated with the outer membrane of liver mitochondria. J Cell Biol 32: 415-438.
37. Ellman GL, Courtney KD, Featherstone RM (1961) A new and rapid colorimetric determination of acetylcholinesterase activity. Biochem Pharmacol 7: 88-95.
38. Mueller AD, Meerlo P, McGinty D, Mistlberger RE (2013) Sleep and adult neurogenesis: implications for cognition and mood. Curr Top Beh Neurosci 25: 151-181.
39. Graves LA, Heller EA, Pack AI, Abel T (2003) Sleep deprivation selectively impairs memory consolidation for contextual fear conditioning. Learn Mem 10(3): 168-176.

40. Smith ME, McEvoy LK, Gevins A (2002) The impact of moderate sleep loss on neurophysiologic signals during working-memory task performance. Sleep 25(7): 784.

41. Xu ZQ, Gao CY, Fang CQ, Zhou HD, Jiang XJ (2010) The mechanism and characterization of learning and memory impairment in sleep-deprived mice. Cell Biochem Biophys 58: 137-140.

42. Kreuzer P, Langguth B, Popp R, Raster R, Busch V, et al. (2011) Reduced intra-cortical inhibition after sleep deprivation: a transcranial magnetic stimulation study. Neurosci Lett 493: 63-66.

43. Civardi C, Boccagni C, Vicentini R, Bolamperti L, Tarletti R, et al. (2001) Cortical excitability and sleep deprivation: a transcranial magnetic stimulation study. J Neurol Neurosurg Psychiatry 71: 809-812.

44. Scalise A, Desiato MT, Gigli GL, Romigi A, Tombini M, et al. (2006) Increasing cortical excitability: a possible explanation for the proconvulsant role of sleep deprivation. Sleep 29: 1595-1598.

45. Placidi F, Zannino S, Albanese M, Romigi A, Izzi F, et al. (2013) Increased cortical excitability after selective REM sleep deprivation in healthyhumans: a transcranial magnetic stimulation study. Sleep Med 14: 288-292.

46. Ramanathan L, Gulyani S, Nienhuis R, Siegel JM (2002) Sleep deprivation decreases superoxide dismutase activity in rat hip-pocampus and brainstem. Neuroreport 13: 1387-1390.

47. Thakkar M, Mallick BN (1991) Effect of REM sleep deprivation on rat brain acetylcholinesterase. Pharmacol Biochem Behav 39: 211-214.

48. Roman V, Hagewoud R, Luiten PG, Meerlo P (2006) Differential effects of chronic partial sleep deprivation and stress on serotonin-1A and muscarinic acetylcholine receptor sensitivity. J Sleep Res 15: 386-394.

Accuracy of the Oxford Sleep Resistance Test versus Simultaneous Electroencephalography to Detect Sleep Onset

Vincent Jobin[1*], Annie Mathieu[1], Pierre Rompré[2], Mélanie Perraton-Brillon[3], Geneviève Rondeau[1] and Pierre Mayer[1]

[1]Department of Medicine, Centre hospitalier de l'Université de Montréal (CHUM),Canada

[2]Faculty of Dental Medicine, Université de Montréal, Canada

[3]Department of Pneumology, Hôpital Maisonneuve-Rosemont, Canada

*Corresponding author: Dr Vincent Jobin, Centre hospitalier de l'Université de Montréal (CHUM)-3840, St-Urbain Street, Montreal, QC, Canada, E-mail: vincent.jobin@umontreal.ca

Abstract

Background: The Oxford Sleep Resistance test (OSLER) is a useful tool to assess daytime vigilance. However, it has not been validated against simultaneous electroencephalography (EEG) recordings in large populations. The main objective of the study was to compare the OSLER values versus EEG-determined Sleep Onset latency (EEG-SOL).

Methods: Patients referred for assessment of daytime vigilance were recruited from a tertiary sleep clinic. Patients underwent the OSLER (4 x 40 minutes trials; if 7 consecutive stimuli are missed, the trial is terminated and sleep onset is concluded to have occurred) with simultaneous EEG recordings. Determination of EEG-SOL using American Academy of sleep Medicine (AASM) criteria to score sleep during daytime testing was compared to OSLER values.

Results: 65 OSLER were performed in 65 subjects for a total of 260 trials (65X4 trials/OSLER). In 136 out of the 260 trials (52.3%), subjects remained awake according to the OSLER, while EEG-SOL was scored in 5 of the 136 trials (3.7%). Of the 124 trials (47.7%) with sleep onset, (i.e. 7 consecutive missed stimuli) the mean sleep onset value was 14.5 ± 10.9 min and EEG-SOL was recorded before the end of the trial in 37 trials (29.8%) (Mean difference EEG-SOL *vs.* OSLER 4.1 ± 5.8 min).

Conclusion: Using current AASM criteria for daytime testing, EEG-determined sleep onset latency is unlikely to occur in subjects with no sleep onset in the OSLER. However, the presence of sleep onset in the OSLER cannot be used as a precise surrogate to detect EEG sleep onset.

Keywords: Sleep; Sleep apnea; Wakefulness; Continuous positive airway pressure; Electroencephalography; Polysomnography

Abbreviations: AASM: American Academy of Sleep Medicine; AHI: Apnea-Hypopnea Index; APAP: Automatically-adjusting Positive Airway Pressure; AUC: Area Under the Curve; BiPAP: Bilevel Positive Airway Pressure; BMI: Body Mass Index; CI: Confidence Interval; CPAP: Continuous Positive Airway Pressure; EEG: Electroencephalography; EEG-SOL: EEG-determined Sleep Onset Latency; EMG: Chin Electromyogram; EOG: Bilateral Electrooculogram; ESS: Epworth Sleepiness Score; LED: Light Emitting Diode; MSLT: Multiple Sleep Latency Test; MWT: Maintenance of Wakefulness Test; ODI: Oxygen Desaturation Index; OSA: Obstructive Sleep Apnea; OSLER: Oxford Sleep Resistance Test; PSG: Polysomnography; RDI: Respiratory Disturbance Index; ROC: Receiver Operating Characteristic; SOL: Sleep Onset Latency

Introduction

The current gold standard to measure the ability to stay awake is the Maintenance of Wakefulness Test (MWT) [1,2]; which requires electroencephalography (EEG) monitoring and is costly. The Oxford Sleep Resistance test (OSLER) is a useful alternative [3]. It is a performance test where the subject is asked to respond to a Light Emitting Diode (LED), a monotonous visual stimulus occurring every three seconds. The OSLER test is not based on EEG and estimates the Sleep Onset Latency (SOL) by the time taken by the subject to fail to respond to seven consecutive visual stimuli. Compared to the MWT, this test is viewed as a simple and inexpensive; not requiring any specialized staff.

The OSLER was first used with 4 x 40 min trials and was first validated to determine sleep onset during daytime studies with non-simultaneous EEG monitoring [3]. The OSLER discriminates well untreated sleepy patients with obstructive sleep apnea (OSA) from normal controls [3]. Using different protocols (1 to 4 trials of 20 to 40 min in length), the OSLER test has subsequently proved to be a useful test, especially in OSA patients, to differentiate normality from hypersomnia as well as to demonstrate an effect of therapy [4-10]. However, little is known about its accuracy when compared to simultaneous EEG measurements of sleep onset in a large cohort of patients using current AASM 2005 definition of sleep onset in daytime studies (MWT, MSLT) versus the previous definition used when the test was first described [2,3,11]. Also, there is debate in the literature in order to determine if an OSLER test consisting of less than 4 trials can be done with similar accuracy in order to simplify the test procedure [3,4].

We hypothesize that in a cohort of patients referred for assessment of daytime vigilance in a tertiary care university hospital: i) the OSLER test is not accurate to detect sleep onset using current AASM criteria defining sleep onset after one epoch of any stage of sleep and ii) the results of the four-trial OSLER test can be estimated by less than four trials. Therefore, the objectives of our study are to compare a SOL obtained using the OSLER *vs.* one obtained by simultaneous EEG monitoring and, to compare the mean OSLER value using 1, 2 or 3 trials with the mean value of the standard four-trial OSLER performed during the day.

Methods

Patients

Patients were recruited after an evaluation at our sleep clinic. We included all consecutive patients who were underwent a MWT after being referred for the test by a sleep specialist, including patients who were referred for a second evaluation/opinion. Exclusion criteria included poor comprehension of French or English and the presence of a physical disability that would make the OSLER test unreliable. Research Ethics Board approved the study protocol. All patients gave a written informed consent.

Experimental protocol

Some patients underwent either a full in-lab polysomnography (PSG) or a home recording, with or without treatment to control their condition (medications or positive pressure therapy). Charts were reviewed in order to obtain an Apnea-Hypopnea Index (AHI) from PSG (level 1 to 3 studies) or an Oxygen Desaturation Index (ODI level 4 study) according to the AASM classification [12]. Since some PSG studies were not done at our laboratory, scoring criteria for respiratory events could differ between studies and are here after referred to as a respiratory disturbance index.

Before the study, some patients answered a standardized questionnaire including the Epworth Sleepiness Score (ESS). They were asked to list all medication, caffeine and alcohol consumption, comorbidities, and sleep hygiene.

Measurements

OSLER trials: OSLER trials (Stowood Scientific Instruments, Oxford, UK) were set at 8:00 am, 10:00 am, 12:00 pm and 2:00 pm through 4 x 40 min duration trials. Patients were seated in a comfortable supportive armchair in a quiet sleep-recording room with low-level illumination.

Patients were instructed to touch the switch of a box, set on their thigh, with the index of their dominant hand, each time they saw a LED; which was delivered for 1 second every 3 seconds at eye's height and 2 meters from the head. Each time the patient missed a LED, a noise was emitted to the technician (seated in a different room) and a visual marker was also seen on a computer screen adjacent to EEG tracings. When 7 consecutive stimuli were missed, a different sound was heard and the trial was terminated. Each trial ended at a maximum of 40 min or when 7 consecutive omissions occurred. Patients were asked to remain in the chair and resist sleep without using extraordinary measures. They were also informed that if the LED stopped, they should put the response box away, remain seated and try to stay awake until the technician comes in the room. Between trials, patients were asked to take a walk in order to minimize fatigue and sleepiness and maintain motivation. The same team of respiratory therapist conducted all tests.

EEG measurement: EEG was monitored simultaneously during OSLER trials using C3/A2, C4/A1, O1/A2, O2/A1 along with chin electromyogram (EMG) and bilateral electrooculogram (EOG) using a Sandman Software recording system.

Data analysis

OSLER: To determine the sleep latency for one 40 min trial, we measured the time before the occurrence of 7 consecutive diodes without response (21 seconds) [3]. This criterion was chosen because it approximates the sleep duration generally used to score one epoch of sleep with Rechtschaffen and Kales scoring rules for an overnight PSG and was the criterion used when the test was first described [3,13]. A session lasting less than 40 min is classified as presence of sleep and SOL is measured [3].

EEG-determined Sleep Onset latency (EEG-SOL): EEG-SOL was defined as single 30 seconds epochs of stage 1, 2 or 3. If no sleep occurred during the OSLER trial, no EEG-SOL was noted. To determine the number and timing of OSLER trials required to best estimate the results of four-trial OSLER; we compared mean results of all possibilities: 1, 2, 3 or 4 trials done at 8:00 am, 10:00 am, 12:00 pm and 2:00 pm comparing each trials independently and with any combination of them.

Statistical analysis

In addition to the behavioral measurement of the sleep latency obtained by the OSLER test, EEG-SOL was calculated for each patient and each trial. Values were not normally distributed and Spearman's rank correlation was used for correlation. The mean bias and variability between methods for trials in which EEG-SOL was measured were compared and displayed as a Bland-Altman plot. Lastly, to determine the number of OSLER trials needed to accurately estimate the mean value of four-trial OSLER test, we analyzed the variance between the trials by using the Wilcoxon signed-rank test and to expressed results for all possibilities (1, 2 or 3 trials); we used Bland-Altman plots and receiver operating characteristic (ROC) curves analysis. Statistical analyses were performed using the SPSS 17.0 statistical software package (SPSS Inc. Released 2007; SPSS for Windows, version 16.0, Chicago, USA). Values are expressed as means ± SD or 95% confidence interval (CI) and medians (interquartile range). A threshold of $p<0.05$ was used for statistical significance.

Results

Patients

Sixty-five consecutive patients (57 men and 8 women, 50.5 years ± 10.8 years) with sleep disorders were included in the study. Clinical diagnoses of patients were: sleep disordered breathing (n=63), idiopathic hypersomnolence concomitant with sleep apnea (n=4), restless leg syndrome (n=2) and narcolepsy (n=1). For one patient, we were not able to retrieve the initial diagnosis. Five patients had more than one sleep disorder. (Figure 1).

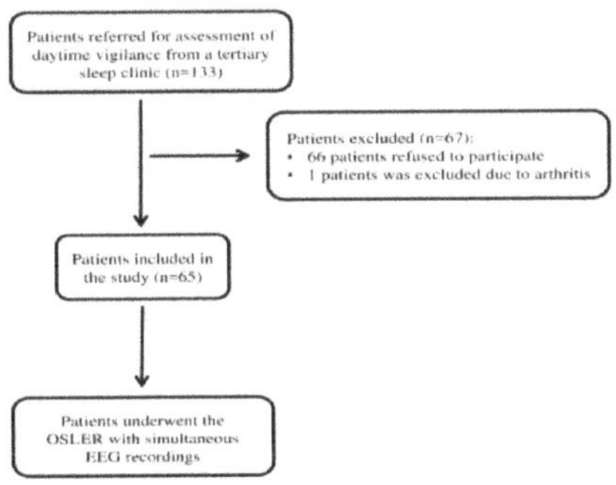

Figure 1: A flowchart of the screening process for included patients. A total of sixty-five patients with sleep disorders were included in the study.

Seven patients were taking stimulants on a regular basis and 62 patients used positive pressure therapy regularly (Continuous Positive Airway Pressure (CPAP), Automatically-adjusting Positive Airway Pressure (APAP) or Bilevel Positive Airway Pressure (BPAP)). For OSA patients, the mean Respiratory Disturbance Index (RDI) was 38.9 ± 26.9 events/hour (n=59). Baseline characteristics of the patients are presented in Table 1 (data were not available for all patients)

Measures of agreement between OSLER and simultaneous EEG

Analysis of OSLER: A total of 65 OSLER were done. The overall mean value for the OSLER was 27.8 ± 12 min. In 19 OSLER (29.2%), patients remained awake (four 40 min trials). In these 19 OSLER, simultaneous EEG-determined sleep was not scored in any but one test (5.2%).

Analysis of individual OSLER trials: In 136 (52.3%) of the 260 OSLER trials performed, while no sleep onset was detected on the OSLER trials, EEG-SOL was recorded using AASM 2005 criteria in 5 trials (3.7%) (Mean difference EEG-SOL *vs.* OSLER 23.8 min ± 12.3 min). Of the 124 OSLER trials (Mean value 14.5 min ± 10.9 min) where sleep onset occurred as defined by failure of the patient to respond to 7 consecutive stimuli, sleep onset by EEG monitoring was found in 37 trials (29.8%) (Mean difference EEG-SOL *vs.* OSLER 4.1 min ± 5.8 min).

Figure 2 shows the results of OSLER trials in which EEG-determined sleep was scored. Note that sleep was scored before the OSLER trial was terminated in a significant proportion of patients.

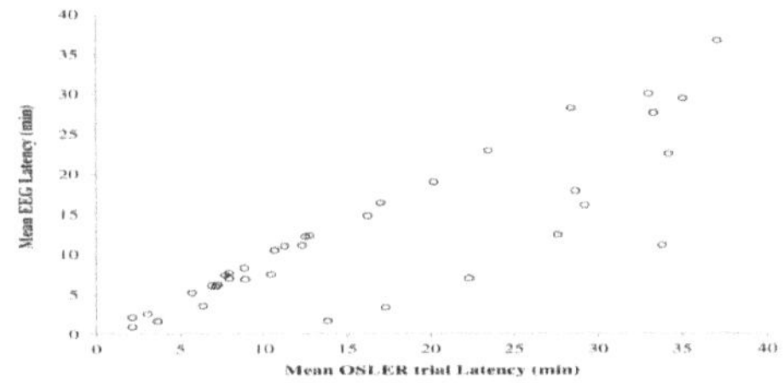

Figure 2: Comparison of sleep latencies between OSLER trials and simultaneous EEG. Data shown for OSLER trials in which EEG-sleep was scored.

In order to compare EEG-SOL with OSLER, a Bland-Altman plot was used in OSLER trials in which EEG sleep was scored (Figure 3).

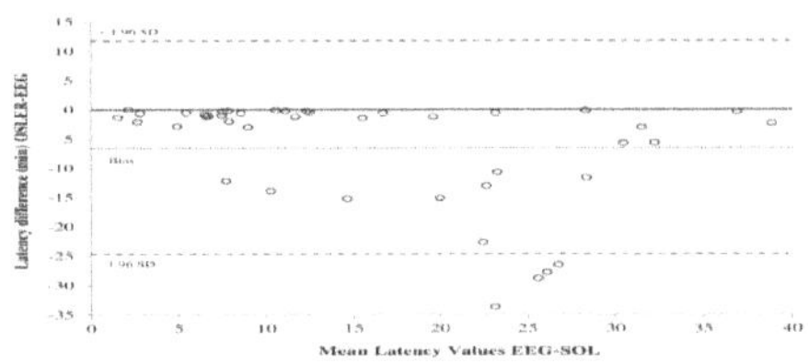

Figure 3: Comparison of sleep latency difference between EEG-SOL and OSLER trials. Bland-Altman plot showing the distribution of the differences between EEG-SOL and OSLER trials in which EEG-sleep was scored (each open circle represents one trial). The line of identity (OSLER and EEG sleep latency is equal) is shown (solid line). The broken lines represent 1.96 ± SD of the observed differences and the dotted line systematic bias.

The bias towards lower values were 6.5 min for EEG-SOL [SD 9.3 95% CI (24.7, 11.7) min].

Assessment of the accurate number of OSLER trials to estimate the four-trial

OSLER test: The median OSLER value for each trial was 40.0 min with inter-quartile range 40.0 (14.8 to 40.0), 40.0 (13.9 to 40.0), 34.2 (8.6 to 40.0) and 37.1 (12.5 to 40.0) at 8:00 am, 10:00 am, 12:00 pm and 2:00 pm respectively and were not significantly different.

The accuracy of 1, 2 or 3 OSLER trials to estimate a (40 min) four-trial OSLER test was studied using ROC curves for the 14 different possibilities. The mean Area under the Curve (AUC) for 1, 2 or 3 trials were not statistically different compared to the four-trial OSLER test (data not shown). We also studied the difference in means between the use of 1, 2 or 3, *vs.* four-trial OSLER test by using Bland-Altman plots. We also found no statistically significant difference between deltas in means for all 14 possibilities (range 1.5 min to 1.0 min, NS). However, standard deviations for these differences were higher when only one trial was used (range 6.7 min to 10.2 min) *vs.* 3 trials (range 2.2 min to 3.4 min) with mid-results when 2 trials were used (range 4.8 min to 5.1 min). An example is shown in Figure 4 as a Bland-Altman plot. It can be seen that the data is less scarce around the identity line when using a combination of 3 trials (mean of the 8:00 am, 10:00 am and 12:00 pm trials - Figure 4, right hand panel) *vs.* a more scattered appearance around the identity line with the use of only one trial (8:00 am - Figure 4, left hand panel).

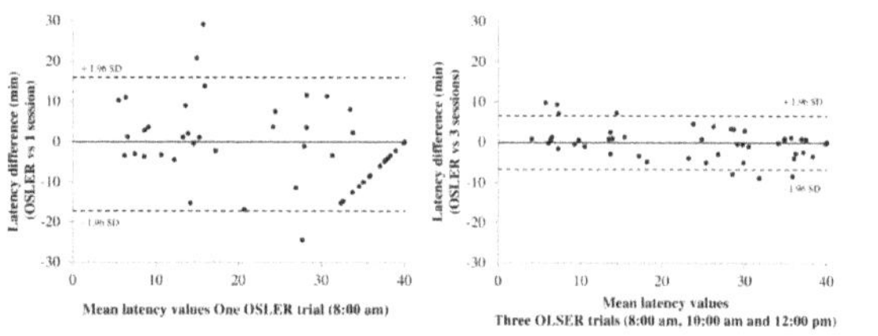

Figure 4: Assessment of the accurate number of OSLER trials to estimate the four-trial OSLER test. Bland-Altman plots showing the distribution of the differences between SOL obtained by the four-trial OSLER and the mean of 3 trials (8:00 am, 10:00 am and 12:00 pm) (left hand panel; each circle represents one patient) and one trial (8:00 am) (right hand panel; each circle represents one patient). The line of identity (OSLER and 1 or 3 OSLER trials is equal) is shown by the solid line. The broken lines represent 1.96 SD of the observed differences.

Discussion

This study assessed the accuracy of the OSLER test compared to two sets of EEG scoring using AASM criteria to score sleep in a large population mainly composed of patients with OSA on treatment referred for assessment of their daytime vigilance. Typically, patients were men, 40 years to 60 years old, with various RDI, BMI and ESS scores (Table 1).

Data	Sixty-five patients	Minimum	Maximum
Age, years	50.5 ± 10.8	23	70
Gender Men:Women	57:08:00	-	-
RDI (events/hour) (n=59)	38.9 ± 26.9	0.3	103
Body Mass Index: BMI	33.5 ± 7.9	19	58.7
ESS (n=55)	10.3 ± 6.3	1	24

Table 1: Baseline characteristics of the study patients. Baseline characteristics such as age, gender and body mass index (BMI) were collected for all patients (n=65). However, some data were not available for all the patients (respiratory disturbance index (RDI) n=59) and Epworth sleepiness scale (ESS) n=55).

The major finding of the study is that using current AASM criteria to score sleep during daytime studies, an OSLER where no sleep onset is recorded during four 40 minutes trials is reliably associated with the absence of sleep during the procedure. However, in patients with sleep onset during OSLER trials, the occurrence of EEG-determined sleep before the end of the trial occurred in about 1 out of 3 trials, which precludes the OSLER to be used as a precise surrogate to detect EEG sleep onset. Results also pointed out that at least a three-trial OSLER is necessary to estimate with good confidence the results of the four-trial OSLER.

The OSLER, either in its original [3] (or more recently modified versions [14]) is currently being used widely in the literature to assess vigilance and attention deficits in patients with sleep disorders as well as being able to reflect the presence or absence of improvement after therapy, However, it is still not clear that it can be used to detect true physiological sleep onset due to the test design itself as well as its validation in studies with small population samples and various definitions of EEG sleep onset [15,16].

On the one hand, we observed in most trials that no EEG sleep was scored although patients failed the OSLER. Since the OSLER test relies on behavior (e.g. frequency of eye blinking, fingering and fluctuation of vigilance/sustain attention system) [17], the cooperation and the motivation of the individual is essential. Therefore, false-positive results are observed (e.g. omissions without sleep).

We observed that EEG sleep onset latency is often lower than sleep onset recorded in the OSLER. The monotonous nature of the OSLER test, i.e. the constant repetitions of the diodes one second every three seconds, permits the patients to get used to the task. This could therefore explain why periods of sleep may happen with an epoch of sleep being scored according to the rule of Rechtschaffen and Kales [13]. This could also reflect the phenomenon raised by Ogilvie stating that in some patients, there is a difference in the relationship of behavioral response and EEG criteria; certain patients can remain fairly responsive in stage 1 while others do not [18].

On the other hand, we determined the optimal number of OSLER trials needed to estimate acceptable accuracy of the four-trial OSLER test. As a group, the mean values were comparable. However, we found large standard deviations around the mean (ranging from 5 min to 10 min) that, in our opinion, precludes the utilization of the test with only one or two trials. Individually, we could observe as high as a 10 min difference between the result of a single trial at 8:00 am and a four-trial OSLER test. It is not surprising that three trials are necessary given the expression of the circadian cycle, eye blinking and inter-individual differences in vigilance/attention capacities. We believe that these differences could be clinically significant. We agree with Priest who stated that at least a three-trial OSLER test was necessary [4]. The confirmation of this finding in this specific population is important since these patients were referred to objectively test their wake tendency.

This study presents some limitations. Our study was not designed to compare the OSLER test with MWT results, since no MWT was done and it is likely that the OSLER test influences waking tendency. One cannot infer from our findings that, in a given subject, the OSLER test would estimate the result of the MWT. The strength of our study is to better understand the nature of the OSLER test and its usefulness in a large sleep clinic. The EEG monitoring was used to better understand the capacities of the OSLER test to detect sleep onset utilizing a request to elicit a response. We did not take into account malingering that could have affected our results; the referring physician did not report this in any case. Our population was heterogeneous, as seen in a tertiary sleep clinic, and mostly composed of patients with sleep disordered breathing. The study did not have the statistical power to report on the reliability of the tests in sub-groups of patients (effect of stimulants, more than one diagnosis, hypersomnia not caused by sleep apnea). Finally, this study did not assess micro sleep (sleep intrusion of 3 seconds to 15 seconds in the EEG) which was almost always present when four or more consecutive LED were missed in the work of Priest [4]. The correlation of micro sleep and clinical endpoints needs more investigations since it could be useful for sleep specialists in is currently being investigated by other groups [9,10].

We conclude that, using AASM 2005 criteria to score sleep during daytime studies, patients with sleep disorders referred for assessment of their vigilance that successfully remain awake during the OSLER test (four 40 min trials) have a very low probability of EEG sleep onset during the procedure. However, patients who missed 7 consecutive stimuli and therefore have a sleep latency scored using the OSLER have a significant chance of not having EEG-recorded sleep. This precludes the OSLER to be used as a precise surrogate to detect EEG sleep onset latency. Given the large variability of the measurements, we suggest that at least three trials should be done to accurately estimate the value of the four-trial OSLER. More studies are needed to evaluate the OSLER as a tool to safely assess not only sleep onset but also attention and vigilance especially when individuals with sleep disorders are involved in tasks where this could be a concern.

Acknowledgements

The authors acknowledge the assistance of Anne-Marie Laurin, respiratory therapists and all the technicians of the Laboratoire du sommeil of Hôpital Hôtel-Dieu du Centre Hospitalier Universitaire de Montréal (CHUM). Thanks to Joseph Braidy, M.D., Mathieu Gaudet, M.D. and Zeina Kaddaha, M.D. for reviewing the manuscript. The sleep laboratory of the clinic is supported by Biron Soins du Sommeil (Québec, Canada) and Medigas (Québec, Canada).

References

1. Doghramji K, Mitler MM, Sangal RB, Shapiro C, Taylor S, et al. (1997) A normative study of the maintenance of wakefulness test (MWT). Electroencephalogr Clinical neurophysiol 103: 554-562.
2. Littner MR, Kushida C, Wise M, Davila DG, Morgenthaler T, et al. (2005) Practice parameters for clinical use of the multiple sleep latency test and the maintenance of wakefulness test. Sleep 28: 113-121.
3. Bennett LS, Stradling JR, Davies RJ (1997) A behavioural test to assess daytime sleepiness in obstructive sleep apnoea. J Sleep Res 6: 142-145.
4. Priest B, Brichard C, Aubert G, Liistro G, Rodenstein DO (2001) Microsleep during a simplified maintenance of wakefulness test. A validation study of the OSLER test. Am J Respir Crit Care Med 163: 1619-1625.
5. Bennett LS, Barbour C, Langford B, Stradling JR, Davies RJ (1999) Health status in obstructive sleep apnea: relationship with sleep fragmentation and daytine sleepiness, and effects of continuous positive airway pressure treatment. Am J Respir Crit Care Med 159: 1884-1890.
6. Chouri-Pontarollo N, Borel JC, Tamisier R, Wuyam B, Levy P, et al. (2007) Impaired objective daytime vigilance in obesity-hypoventilation syndrome: impact of noninvasive ventilation. Chest 131: 148-155.
7. Krieger AC, Ayappa I, Norman RG, Rapoport DM, Walsleben J (2004) Comparison of the maintenance of wakefulness test (MWT) to a modified behavioral test (OSLER) in the evaluation of daytime sleepiness. J Sleep Res 13: 407-411.
8. West SD, Kohler M, Nicoll DJ, Stradling JR (2009) The effect of continuous positive airway pressure treatment on physical activity in patients with obstructive sleep apnoea: A randomised controlled trial. Sleep Med 10: 1056-1058.
9. Ferreira JJ, Neutel D, Mestre TA, Galitzky M, Thalamas C, et al. (2013) Usefulness of OSLER test in Parkinson's disease. Sleep Med 14: 297-298.
10. Alakuijala A, Maasilta P, Bachour A (2014) The Oxford Sleep Resistance test (OSLER) and the Multiple Unprepared Reaction Time Test (MURT) detect vigilance modifications in sleep apnea patients. J Clin Sleep Med 10: 1075-1082.
11. Mitler MM, Gujavarty KS, Browman CP (1982) Maintenance of wakefulness test: a polysomnographic technique for evaluation treatment efficacy in patients with excessive somnolence. Electroencephalogr Clin Neurophysiol 53: 658-661.
12. American Sleep Disorders Association (1994) Practice parameters for the use of portable recording in the assessment of obstructive sleep apnea. Standards of Practice Committee of the American Sleep Disorders Association. Sleep 17: 372-377.
13. Kales A, Rechtschaffen A (1968) A manual of standardized terminology, techniques and scoring system for sleep stages of human subjects. U. S. National Institute of Neurological Diseases and Blindness, Neurological Information Network; United States.
14. Karimi M, Hedner J, Zou D, Eskandari D, Lundquist AC, et al. (2015) Attention deficits detected in cognitive tests differentiate between sleep apnea patients with or without a motor vehicle accident. Sleep Med 16: 528-533.
15. Marklund M, Carlberg B, Forsgren L, Olsson T, Stenlund H, et al. (2015) Oral Appliance Therapy in Patients With Daytime Sleepiness and Snoring or Mild to Moderate Sleep Apnea: A Randomized Clinical Trial. JAMA Intern Med 175: 1278-1285.
16. Neutel D, Peralta R, Pires J, Bentes C, Ferreira JJ (2015) End of OSLER Test Sessions in Parkinson's Disease do not Correspond to True Sleep Onset: Results from an Exploratory Study. Front Neurol 6: 200.
17. Hakkanen H, Summala H, Partinen M, Tiihonen M, Silvo J (1999) Blink duration as an indicator of driver sleepiness in professional bus drivers. Sleep 22: 798-802.
18. Ogilvie RD, Wilkinson RT, Allison S (1989) The detection of sleep onset: behavioral, physiological, and subjective convergence. Sleep 12: 458-474.

Permissions

All chapters in this book were first published in JSD&T, by OMICS International; hereby published with permission under the Creative Commons Attribution License or equivalent. Every chapter published in this book has been scrutinized by our experts. Their significance has been extensively debated. The topics covered herein carry significant findings which will fuel the growth of the discipline. They may even be implemented as practical applications or may be referred to as a beginning point for another development.

The contributors of this book come from diverse backgrounds, making this book a truly international effort. This book will bring forth new frontiers with its revolutionizing research information and detailed analysis of the nascent developments around the world.

We would like to thank all the contributing authors for lending their expertise to make the book truly unique. They have played a crucial role in the development of this book. Without their invaluable contributions this book wouldn't have been possible. They have made vital efforts to compile up to date information on the varied aspects of this subject to make this book a valuable addition to the collection of many professionals and students.

This book was conceptualized with the vision of imparting up-to-date information and advanced data in this field. To ensure the same, a matchless editorial board was set up. Every individual on the board went through rigorous rounds of assessment to prove their worth. After which they invested a large part of their time researching and compiling the most relevant data for our readers.

The editorial board has been involved in producing this book since its inception. They have spent rigorous hours researching and exploring the diverse topics which have resulted in the successful publishing of this book. They have passed on their knowledge of decades through this book. To expedite this challenging task, the publisher supported the team at every step. A small team of assistant editors was also appointed to further simplify the editing procedure and attain best results for the readers.

Apart from the editorial board, the designing team has also invested a significant amount of their time in understanding the subject and creating the most relevant covers. They scrutinized every image to scout for the most suitable representation of the subject and create an appropriate cover for the book.

The publishing team has been an ardent support to the editorial, designing and production team. Their endless efforts to recruit the best for this project, has resulted in the accomplishment of this book. They are a veteran in the field of academics and their pool of knowledge is as vast as their experience in printing. Their expertise and guidance has proved useful at every step. Their uncompromising quality standards have made this book an exceptional effort. Their encouragement from time to time has been an inspiration for everyone.

The publisher and the editorial board hope that this book will prove to be a valuable piece of knowledge for researchers, students, practitioners and scholars across the globe.

List of Contributors

Rose A Franco and Dheeraj Dhotre
Department of Medicine - Division of Pulmonary, Medical College of Wisconsin, Milwaukee, Wisconsin, USA

Jennifer C Kanady and Allison G Harvey
Department of Psychology, University of California, Berkeley, Berkeley, CA, USA

Adriane M Soehnera
Department of Psychiatry, University of Pittsburgh, School of Medicine, Pittsburgh, PA, USA

Shittu RO
Department of Family Medicine, Kwara State Specialist Hospital, Nigeria

Issa BA and Olanrewaju GT
Department of Behavioral Sciences, University of Ilorin Teaching Hospital, Nigeria

Odeigah LO
Department of Family Medicine, University of Ilorin Teaching Hospital, Nigeria

Sule AG
Department of Family Medicine, Ahmadubello University, Teaching Hospital, Nigeria

Sanni MA
Department of Hematology, Kwara State Specialist Hospital, Nigeria

Aderibigbe SA and Uthman MB
Department of Epidemiology and Community Health, University of Ilorin Teaching Hospital, Nigeria

Nyamngee AA
Department of Medical microbiology and parasitology, College of Health, Sciences, University of Ilorin, Nigeria

Mounir Chennaoui, Danielle Gomez-Merino, Pascal Van Beers, Mathias Guillard, Catherine Drogou and Clément Bougard
Institut de Recherche Biomédicale des Armées (IRBA), Département Environnements Opérationnels, 91223 Brétigny sur Orge, France
Université Paris Descartes, Hôtel Dieu, EA7330 VIFASOM (Vigilance Fatigue et Sommeil), 75004 Paris, France

Didier Lagarde
Université Paris Descartes, Hôtel Dieu, EA7330 VIFASOM (Vigilance Fatigue et Sommeil), 75004 Paris, France

G Dave Singh
BioModeling Solutions, Inc., 17933 NE Evergreen Parkway, Beaverton, USA

Tara Griffin
Emerald Coast Dental Sleep Medicine, Panama City Beach, FL 32408, USA

Samuel E Cress
Craniofacial and Dental Sleep Medicine, Sugar Land, TX 77479, USA

Diego Cohen
Admission Unit, Hospital Borda, Ramón Carrillo 375 CABA, Argentina

Ricardo Corral
Department of research and education, Hospital Borda, Ramón Carrillo 375 CABA, Argentina

Magnus Falk and Hagesund E
Division of Community Medicine, Primary Care, Department of Medicine and Health Sciences, Linköping University, Linköping, Sweden

Boniface EE
Department of Physiology, School of Basic Medical Sciences, College of Medical Sciences, University of Benin, Benin City, Edo State, Nigeria

Monika Krawietz, Carmen Garcia, Carsten Pilz, Martin Glos, Beate Diecker and Ingo Fietzeand
Charité University Medicine Berlin, Berlin, Germany

Thomas Penzel
Charité University Medicine Berlin, Berlin, Germany
International Clinical Research Center, St. Anne's University Hospital Brno, Brno, Czech Republic

Melissa Brijbassi, Takatoshi Kasai, Luigi Taranto Montemurro and T Douglas Bradley
Sleep Research Laboratory of the University Health Network Toronto Rehabilitation Institute, Toronto, Canada
Centre for sleep Medicine and Circadian Biology, University of Toronto, Toronto, Canada

Rodolfo Miralles, Isabel Celhay, Hugo Santander and Ricardo Bull
Oral Physiology Laboratory, Biomedical Sciences Institute, Faculty of Medicine, University of Chile, Santiago, Chile

Saúl Valenzuela, Aler Daniel Fuentes and Mario Felipe Gutiérrez
Oral Physiology Laboratory, Biomedical Sciences Institute, Faculty of Medicine, University of Chile, Santiago, Chile
Institute for Research in Dental Sciences, Faculty of Dentistry, University of Chile, Santiago, Chile

Rosa Cordova
Oral Physiology Laboratory, Biomedical Sciences Institute, Faculty of Medicine, University of Chile, Santiago, Chile
Institute for Research in Dental Sciences, Faculty of Dentistry, University of Chile, Santiago, Chile
Faculty of Medicine, Diego Portales University, Santiago, Chile

Valiollah Akbari
Medical Doctor, Assistant Professor of Psychiatry, Department of Psychology, University of Medical Sciences, Qom, Iran

Abbas Hajian and Mahbubeh Sadat Mirhashemi
Medical Doctor, General Practitioner, University of Medical Sciences, Qom, Iran

Gowda M, Sahoo NK and Guruprasada
Command Military Dental Centre (WC), Chandimandir, Haryana, India

Naveen KS
Army Dental Centre (R and R), Delhi, India

Verma K
Military Dental Centre (BEG), East Kirkee, Pune, India

Margaret A Madigan
Impact genomics, Inc., Lederoch, Pennsylvania, USA
Department of Clinical Neurology, Path Research Foundation, USA
Department of Personalized Genomics, IGENE LLC., USA

Marlene-Oscar-Berman
Departments of Psychiatry and Anatomy & Neurobiology, Boston University School of Medicine, and Boston VA Healthcare System, Boston, USA

Kenneth Blum
Department of Psychiatry, University of Florida, McKnight Brain Institute, USA
Impact genomics, Inc., Lederoch, Pennsylvania, USA

William Downs B
Impact genomics, Inc., Lederoch, Pennsylvania, USA

Florian Kreuk, Kristina Dushaj, Courtney Truesdell and Mona Li
Department of Clinical Neurology, Path Research Foundation, USA

Eric R Braverman
Department of Psychiatry, University of Florida, McKnight Brain Institute, USA
Department of Clinical Neurology, Path Research Foundation, USA

John Giordano and Scott Jones
Department of Holistic Medicine, National Institute for Holistic Addiction Studies, USA

Stephen Schoenthaler
Department of Holistic Medicine, National Institute for Holistic Addiction Studies, USA
Department of Sociology, California State University, USA

Joan Borsten
Department of Addiction Research & Therapy, Malibu Beach Recovery Center, USA

Thomas Simpatico
Human Integrated Services Unit University of Vermont Center for Clinical & Translational Science, College of Medicine, USA

Debmayla Barh
Institute of Integrative Omics & Applied Biotechnology, India
Department of Personalized Genomics, IGENE LLC., USA
Department of Sociology, California State University, USA

Jeffrey J Stanley
Department of Otolaryngology, Head and Neck Surgery and Neurology, University of Michigan, USA

Mohammad Ashraf Malik
Department of Psychology, Government Degree College Sopore, Jammu and Kashmir, India

Naveen Dutt, Nishant Kumar Chauhan, Ashok Kuwal, Lokesh Kumar Saini, Swetabh Purohit and Sunil Kumar
Department of Pulmonary Medicine, All India Institute of Medical Sciences, Jodhpur, India

Kirti Chaudhry
Department of Dentistry, All India Institute of Medical Sciences, Jodhpur, India

Monika Balzer-Geldsetzer and Richard Dodel
Department of Neurology, Philipps-University Marburg, Germany

Philipp Hessmann
Department of Neurology, Philipps-University Marburg, Germany
Department of Psychiatry and Psychotherapy, University Medical Center Goettingen, Germany

Jörg Heitmann
Department of Pneumology, Werra-Meissner Clinic Eschwege, Germany

Sandra Apelt
Department of Medicine, Philipps-University Marburg, Germany

Geert Mayer
Department of Neurology, Hephata Clinic Schwalmstadt-Treysa, Germany

Antonio Joaquín Gomis Devesa, Alfonso Martínez Martínez and Juan José Ortega-Albás
Clinical Neurophysiology, Sleep Disorders Unit, Hospital Universitario General de Castelló, Spain

Sameh Msaad, Nada Kotti, Sourour Abid, Mounira Hajjaji, Samia Sellami, Samy Kammoun, Ilhem Yangui and Arbi Masmoudi
Department of Pulmonology, Hedi Chaker Hospital, University of Sfax, Sfax, Tunisia

Tiina-Riitta Vuorjoki-Ranta and Antti Pihakari
Helsinki Health Centre, Unit for Specialized Oral Care in the Metropolitan Area and Kirkkonummi, Helsinki, Finland

Frank Lobbezoo
Department of Oral Kinesiology, Academic Centre for Dentistry Amsterdam (ACTA), University of Amsterdam and VU University Amsterdam, MOVE Research Institute Amsterdam, Amsterdam, The Netherlands

Henri Tuomilehto
Oivauni Sleep Clinic, Kuopio, Finland
Institute of Public Health and Clinical Nutrition, Department of Clinical Nutrition, University of Eastern Finland

Mauno Könönen
Department of Stomatognathic Physiology and Prosthetic Dentistry, Institute of Dentistry, University of Helsinki, Finland

Jari Ahlberg
Helsinki Health Centre, Unit for Specialized Oral Care in the Metropolitan Area and Kirkkonummi, Helsinki, Finland
Department of Stomatognathic Physiology and Prosthetic Dentistry, Institute of Dentistry, University of Helsinki, Finland

Irini Youssef, Haroon Kamran, Clive Goulbourne, Shweta Kumar, Jesse Kane, Haley Hoffner, Moro Salifu and Samy I McFarlane
Department of Medicine, Divisions of Endocrinology, Cardiology and Renal Medicine, State University of New York, Downstate Medical Center, Brooklyn, NY, USA

Mena Yacoub
Department of Cardiology, Northside Hospital, St. Petersburg FL, USA

Nirav Patel
Department of Cardiology, Hartford Hospital, Hartford, CT

Vadivelan M
Department of Medicine, Jawaharlal Institute of Postgraduate Medical Education and Research, Pondicherry, India

Seoyoun Kim and Hyojae Kim
Korea International High School (KIS), Jeju, Korea

Jong-Chul Yang
Department of Psychiatry, Chonbuk National University Hospital, Jeonju, Korea

Hiroyuki Nakano and Yoshihide Mori
Section of Oral and Maxillofacial Surgery, Division of Maxillofacial Diagnostic and Surgical Sciences, Faculty of Dental Science, Kyushu University, Japan

Katsuaki Mishima, Asuka Nakano, Takamitsu Mano, Shintaro Nakagawa and Mayumi Matsumura
Department of Oral and Maxillofacial Surgery, Graduate School of Medicine, Yamaguchi University, Japan

Hokuto Suga
Department of Pediatric Dentistry, Kagoshima University Graduate School of Medical and Dental Sciences, Japan

Yuichiro Miyawaki
Miyawaki Orthodontic Clinic, Japan

Yoshiya Ueyama
Department of Oral and Maxillofacial Surgery, Graduate School of Medicine, Yamaguchi University, Japan
Division of Oral and Maxillofacial Surgery, Graduate School of Dental Science, Kyushu University, Japan

Ahmed M Abdel-Khalek
Department of Psychology, University of Alexandria, Egypt

Anna Michela Gaeta, Anna Annunziata, Gianfranco Scotto Di Frega and Giuseppe Fiorentino
Division of Respiratory Physiopathology, Monaldi Hospital, Naples, Italy

Francesca Gaeta
Department of Medicine and Surgery, University of Salerno, Baronissi (Salerno), Italy

Krishna M Sundar, Mary Beth Scholand and Alika M Willis
Department of Medicine, University of Utah, Salt Lake City, Utah, USA

Subhashree Sundar
Department of Operations Management & Information Systems, David Eccles School of Business, University of Utah, USA

Nevin FW Zaki
Department of Psychiatry and Manager of Sleep Research Unit, Egypt

Rana Marzouk and Haggag A
Faculty of Medicine, Mansoura University, Mansoura, Egypt

Osman I
Faculty of Medicine, Banha University, Banha, Egypt

Alamah HY
Faculty of Medicine, Tanta University, Tanta, Egypt

Zaied WS
Faculty of Medicine, Menofia University, Egypt

Hassan A
Faculty of Medicine, Zagazig University, Zagazig, Egypt

Allam M
Faculty of Medicine, Alkasr Elainy University, Egypt

Saadeldeen O
Faculty of Medicine, Ain Shams University, Egypt

Russell Rosenberg
Atlanta School of Sleep Medicine, USA

Heidy Reiny
Fusion Sleep Atlanta Georgia, USA

Ahmed S BaHammam
The University Sleep Disorders Center, Department of Medicine, College of Medicine, King Saud University, Saudi Arabia
The Strategic Technologies Program of the National Plan for Sciences and Technology and Innovation in the Kingdom of Saudi Arabia, Riyadh, Saudi Arabia

Aida M Yousef
Department of Chest Medicine, Mansoura Faculty of Medicine, Mansoura University, Egypt

Wael Alkhiary
Department of Clinical Pathology, Mansoura Faculty of Medicine, Mansoura University, Egypt

Maryam Talebi and Kazem Rasoolzadeh Tabatabaye
Tarbiat Modares University, Tehran, Iran

Ensiye Vahedi
School of Medical Sciences, Baqiyatallah University of Medical Sciences, Tehran, Iran

Renata Pendle
Concordia University, Canada

Kathy Sexton-Radek and Fatema Marvi
Elmhurst College, USA

Priyanka Chanana and Anil Kumar
Pharmacology Division, University Institute of Pharmaceutical Sciences, UGC Centre of Advanced Study, Panjab University, Chandigarh, India

Vincent Jobin, Annie Mathieu, Geneviève Rondeau and Pierre Mayer
Department of Medicine, Centre hospitalier de l'Université de Montréal (CHUM),Canada

Pierre Rompré
Faculty of Dental Medicine, Université de Montréal, Canada

Mélanie Perraton-Brillon
Department of Pneumology, Hôpital Maisonneuve-Rosemont, Canada

Index

www.ingramcontent.com/pod-product-compliance
Lightning Source LLC
LaVergne TN
LVHW060607210926
848485LV00005B/1386